nMRCGP
Practice Papers:

Second Edition

Rob Daniels MA (Cantab)
MB BChir MRCGP

PasTest
Dedicated to your success

© 2009 PASTEST LTD
Egerton Court
Parkgate Estate
Knutsford
Cheshire
WA16 8DX

Telephone: 01565 752000

First Published 2007
Second Edition Published 2009

ISBN: 1905 635 591

978 1905 635 597

A catalogue record for this book is available from the British Library.

The information contained within this book was obtained by the author from reliable sources. However, while every effort has been made to ensure its accuracy, no responsibility for loss, damage or injury occasioned to any person acting or refraining from action as a result of information contained herein can be accepted by the publishers or author.

PasTest Revision Books and Intensive Courses

PasTest has been established in the field of postgraduate medical education since 1972, providing revision books and intensive study courses for doctors preparing for their professional examinations.

Books and courses are available for:
Medical undergraduates, MRCGP, MRCP Parts 1 and 2, MRCPCH Parts 1 and 2, MRCS, MRCOG Parts 1 and 2, DRCOG, DCH, FRCA, Dentistry.

For further details contact:

PasTest, Freepost, Knutsford, Cheshire WA16 7BR

Tel: 01565 752000 Fax: 01565 650264

www.pastest.co.uk enquiries@pastest.co.uk

Text prepared by Carnegie Book Production, Lancaster

Printed and bound in the UK by Information Press, Oxford

CONTENTS

ABOUT THE AUTHOR

Rob Daniels MA (Cantab) MB BChir MRCGP

After pre-clinical training at Selwyn College Cambridge, Rob completed his clinical training at Addenbrooke's Hospital before training as a GP in Norwich, Exeter and Western Australia. Since gaining a distinction in the MRCGP, he now works full time as a GP with special interests in ENT and diving and altitude medicine. Over the last 5 years, Rob has authored, co-authored and contributed to several PasTest titles in the GP range.

This book is dedicated to Lisa, Alex and Maddie.

This edition provides exclusive access to two papers from this book online, see www.pastest.co.uk/onlineextras.

With 'Online Extras' you can practice questions online, helping you to acquire knowledge and build confidence for the computer-based AKT exam. You can analyse your strengths and weaknesses through detailed feedback and develop your revision strategy and exam technique. 'Online Extras' also compares your performance with that of your peers, helping you to see if you are performing at the right level.

PasTest also offer an online revision subscription for the AKT, featuring over 1,500 unique questions which allow you to revise by specialty, question type, or difficulty. To maximize your study time, the subscription provides performance feedback which analyses your strengths and weaknesses so you can target your revision. It also compares your score with that of your peers so you can see whether you're performing at the right level for success. To subscribe, visit www.pastest.co.uk.

INTRODUCTION

This book is intended predominantly to help candidates prepare for the Membership examination of the Royal College of General Practitioners, which is the qualifying exam for a career in general practice. It is also hoped that this book will be useful for established GPs to identify learning needs as part of their appraisal process and perhaps prepare them for any future knowledge-based test introduced as part of revalidation.

In line with changes in other specialty exams, the MRCGP now consists of a written exam, a formal clinical skills assessment and workplace-based assessment. The written paper encompasses clinical scenarios, hot topics and critical reading, and is in the form of a 200 question MCQ exam known as the Applied Knowledge Test (AKT). The subject matter is divided between critical appraisal and evidence-based clinical practice components, which make up approximately 10% of the questions, 10% will comprise health informatics and administrative questions, with the remaining 80% clinical questions. The exam aims to test higher problem solving rather than simple fact recall. A wealth of information about the curriculum and exam format is available on the Royal College of General Practitioners' website (www.rcgp.org.uk).

The Applied Knowledge Tests take place at the end of January, May and October each year, via computer terminals at 152 Pearson Vue professional testing centres around the UK (www.pearsonvue.co.uk). Detailed feedback will be provided for candidates who are unsuccessful, allowing them to take remedial action where necessary before the next sitting. Candidates may take the exam at any point in their general practice specialty training, but it is expected that most will do so during their third year of specialty training, when they will be working in primary care. All questions will address important issues relating to general practice in the UK, and international applicants should note that the answers will relate to standard clinical practice in the UK, which may differ from their own country.

The key to successful preparation is twofold. Exam technique is vital in many medical exams and the AKT is no exception. Two hundred questions have to be completed in three hours at a rate of just over one question a minute. The questions are of the single best answer, extending matching question and algorithm completion format, and there are many examples of each type in this book. The second component of successful exam performance is an adequate knowledge base. The content of the questions in this book is based on the GP curriculum, which is available on the RCGP's website, and the questions are loosely based on my clinical experience. This GP curriculum (www.rcgp-curriculum.org.uk) is an excellent resource in planning your revision, especially in less clinical areas of the curriculum such as practice management and information technology.

The RCGP website gives the pass mark and exam feedback for each sitting. In April 2009 the pass mark was 63.3% and the pass rate was 84%. It is well worth reading the examiners reports on previous sittings as these describe areas of weak performance, which the examiners may concentrate on in future exams. Candidates usually perform well in clinical medicine, less well in critical appraisal and worst in administration questions.

The best way to prepare for clinical questions is to read up on problems that you see in general practice, ideally keeping a list of PUNs and DENs (patient's unmet needs and doctor's educational needs) encountered during each surgery. Try to do as many practice multiple choice questions as you can; the old-style MRCGP exam questions are still mostly valid and there are a number of excellent practice MCQ books still available in shops and medical libraries. PasTest also offer an online revision package specifically for the AKT, which gives instant progress feedback (www. pastest.co.uk). It should be possible to pick up on hot topics just through working in general practice and reading the *British Medical Journal* and *British Journal of General Practice*, but a 'Hot topics' course just before the exam is usually money well spent. In the previous incarnation of the MRCGP exam, editorials from the *British Journal of General Practice* had an uncanny habit of turning up as hot topic questions in the next paper. Exam questions are likely to be drawn from several well-known journals, including those listed above. The RCGP's website gives useful information on this, so keep your eyes peeled.

Information on management issues is best picked up by spending a session or two with a practice manager, attending practice meetings and doing multiple-choice questions to identify specific learning needs. It often helps to revise this area with a textbook, such as *Notes for the MRCGP*, although this is now somewhat out of date. Practising critical appraisal of journal articles with a group from your GP training scheme is a useful way of learning this skill, and a lot more enjoyable than trying to read a statistics textbook. The Bandolier website (www.jr2.ox.ac.uk/bandolier) is an excellent source of information about critical appraisal. I have included several statistics questions to illustrate various concepts, but all of the data and graphs are made up, so please do not take the results too seriously.

I have done my best to ensure that all the questions and answers are accurate and current. If you find any discrepancies or have any other comments please let me know and I will make the necessary changes.

I would like to thank the patients of Townsend House Medical Centre, whose images appear in this book, my colleagues at Townsend House for allowing me to use images from the practice collection and Mr Peter Simcock, Consultant Ophthalmologist at the Royal Devon and Exeter Hospital, for the retinal images.

Good luck!

Rob Daniels

November 2009

ABBREVIATIONS

A&E	accident and emergency
ACE	angiotensin-converting enzyme
ACL	anterior cruciate ligament
ACTH	adrenocorticotrophic hormone
ADH	antidiuretic hormone
ADHD	attention deficit hyperactivity disorder
AF	atrial fibrillation
AG	anion gap
ALP	alkaline phosphatase
ALT	alanine transaminase
ARB	angiotension receptor antagonist
ARDS	acute respiratory distress syndrome
APTT	activated partial thromboplastin time
AST	aspartate transaminase
AV	atrioventricular
BCC	basal cell carcinoma
BIPP	bismuth iodoform paraffin paste
BMI	body mass index
BP	blood pressure
CF	cystic fibrosis
CIN	cervical intraepithelial neoplasia
CK	creatine kinase
CMV	cytomegalovirus
CNS	central nervous system
COC	combined oral contraceptive
COA(P)D	chronic obstructive airway (pulmonary) disease
COX	cyclo-oxygenase
CRP	C-reactive protein
CSF	cerebrospinal fluid
CT	computed tomography
DES	direct enhanced service
DEXA	dual energy X-ray absorptiometry
DKA	diabetic ketoacidosis
DMARD	disease-modifying anti-rheumatic drug

DNA	deoxyribonucleic acid
DVT	deep vein thrombosis
EBV	Epstein–Barr virus
ECG	electrocardiogram
eGFR	estimated glomerular filtration rate
ENT	ear, nose and throat
ERCP	endoscopic retrograde cholangiopancreatography
ESR	erythrocyte sedimentation rate
FBC	full blood count
FEV_1	forced expiratory volume in 1 second
FFP	fresh frozen plasma
FRC	functional residual capacity
FVC	forced vital capacity
GFR	glomerular filtration rate
GGT	γ-glutamyl transferase
GI	gastrointestinal
GMSC	General Medical Services Contract
GPwSI	General Practitioner with a Special Interest
GUM	genitourinary medicine
hCG	human chorionic gonadotrophin
HIV	human immunodeficiency virus
HRT	hormone replacement therapy
HSP	Henoch–Schönlein purpura
ICU	intensive care unit
IOP	intraocular pressure
LES	local enhanced service
LFTs	liver function tests
LMWH	low-molecular-weight heparin
MAOI	monoamine oxidase inhibitor
MCH	mean corpuscular haemoglobin
MCV	mean corpuscular volume
MI	myocardial infarction
MMR	measles, mumps and rubella
MRI	magnetic resonance imaging
MRSA	methicillin-resistant *Staphylococcus aureus*
MSU	midstream urine
NCAA	National Clinical Assessment Authority

NICE	National Institute for Health and Clinical Excellence
NNH	number needed to harm
NNT	number needed to treat
NSAID	non-steroidal anti-inflammatory drug
NSTEMI	non-ST-elevation myocardial infarction
NYHA	New York Heart Association
OCD	obsessive–compulsive disorder
PCL	posterior cruciate ligament
PCOS	polycystic ovarian syndrome
PCT	primary care trust
PEFR	peak expiratory flow rate
PE	pulmonary embolus
PICA	posterior inferior cerebellar artery
PMR	polymyalgia rheumatica
POP	progestogen-only pill
PSA	prostate-specific antigen
PT	prothrombin time
PUVA	psoralen + UVA
RCT	randomised controlled trial
QALY	quality-adjusted life-year
QOF	Quality and Outcomes Framework
RA	rheumatoid arthritis
RICE	rest, ice, compression and elevation
RSV	respiratory syncytial virus
SCC	squamous cell carcinoma
SLE	systemic lupus erythematosus
SSRI	selective serotonin release inhibitor
STEMI	ST-elevation myocardial infarction
SVC	superior vena cava
T_3	triiodothyronine
T_4	thyroxine
TB	tuberculosis
TED	thromboembolic deterrent
TIA	transient ischaemic attack
TSH	thyroid-stimulating hormone
TFT	thyroid function test
U&Es	urea and electrolytes

UTI	urinary tract infection
UTRI	upper respiratory tract infection
VIN	vulval intraepithelial neoplasia
VRE	vancomycin-resistant enterococci
WCC	white cell count

Paper 1
Questions

Total time allowed is three hours. Indicate your answers clearly by putting a tick or cross in the box alongside each answer or by writing the appropriate letter alongside the appropriate answer.

1. **Which one of the following statements regarding frozen shoulder is correct?**

☐ A Ninety per cent of patients make a complete recovery

☑ B Frozen shoulder is more common in patients with diabetes mellitus

☐ C Frozen shoulder is usually directly attributable to injury

☐ D The mean age of onset is 20–30 years

☐ E X-rays are necessary to make a diagnosis

2. **A 22-year-old woman is going travelling around the world for 18 months and comes to see you to discuss using Implanon as a contraceptive. Which one of the following statements about this contraceptive method is true?**

☐ A Implanon causes weight gain in 50% of patients

☐ B Implanon is an intrauterine contraceptive device which releases progesterone into the lining of the womb

☐ C Implanon needs to be changed every 5 years

☑ D Irregular bleeding is the commonest side effect of Implanon

☐ E Normal fertility returns in 3–6 months in 90% of women after removal of Implanon

THEME: VOLUNTARY ORGANISATIONS

Options

A ALANON

B CLIC Sargent

C Cruse

D Gingerbread

E Marie Curie

F MIND

G Relate

H RNIB

I RNID

J Scope

K Terence Higgins Trust

L Turning Point

M None of the above

For each of the patients described below, select the organisation from the list above which would be most appropriate to offer support. Each option may be used once, more than once or not at all.

☐ **3.** Parents come to see you 2 weeks after the diagnosis of cerebral palsy in their 15-month-old son.

☐ **4.** A 78-year-old man is in the latter stages of terminal illness and wishes to die at home. His family have been sitting up with him through the night but are exhausted. They request help with night-sitters so that they can catch up on some sleep.

☐ **5.** A 47-year-old gentleman with longstanding schizophrenia is to be evicted from his rented accommodation. He is unemployed and has no family. He requests support in his search for new accommodation and employment.

☐ 6.   An unemployed 27-year-old single parent of three small children comes to see you in tears. She says she can no longer cope with looking after her children and needs a break. She has no close family or friends who can share the burden of care.

☐ 7.   The parents of a child with advanced leukaemia would like to take the family to Disney World for a final holiday together. Both parents have given up work to care for their child. They are seeking financial support and ask for help from charitable organisations.

8.   A 67-year-old man complains of pains in his legs when walking. You ask the nurses to do ankle and brachial blood pressures. These results are shown below.

Right brachial systolic pressure	150 mmHg
Left brachial systolic pressure	150 mmHg
Right dorsalis pedis systolic pressure	120 mmHg
Left dorsalis pedis systolic pressure	150 mmHg

Which one of the following statements is correct regarding this patient?

☐ A   The readings are inaccurate and should be repeated

☐ B   The readings show an ankle brachial pressure index (ABPI) of 0.8 on the left side

☐ C   The readings show an ABPI of 1.25 on the right side

☐ D   The readings suggest the presence of significant peripheral vascular disease affecting the left side only

☑ E   The readings suggest the presence of significant peripheral vascular disease affecting the right side only

PAPER 1

9. **Which one of the following statements regarding post-herpetic neuralgia is correct?**

☐ A No treatments have been shown to be effective in preventing post-herpetic neuralgia

☐ B Pregabalin has been shown to be the most effective treatment for post-herpetic neuralgia

☐ C Prodromal dermatomal pain is a risk factor for post-herpetic neuralgia

☐ D The presence of paraesthesia suggests an alternative diagnosis

☐ E The side-effect profile of amitriptyline outweighs its benefits

10. **A 15-month-old girl is brought in by her father, who has noticed that her umbilicus looks 'lumpy'. He tells you that it gets bigger when she cries or strains and is smaller when she is asleep. Her abdomen is shown below.**

What is the single most appropriate management at this stage?

☐ A Admit under the on-call surgeons

☐ B Refer urgently to surgical outpatients

☐ C Reassure the parents that it will usually resolve spontaneously in time

☐ D Reassurance that this is normal at her age

☐ E Treat with a surgical support

THEME: DRUG MANAGEMENT OF ASTHMA

Options

A   Combination of inhaled corticosteroid and long-acting β_2 agonist

B   Inhaled anticholinergic

C   Inhaled β_2 agonist

D   Inhaled long acting β_2 agonist

E   Inhaled low dose corticosteroid

F   Oral β_2 agonist

G   Oral corticosteroids

H   Oral leukotriene receptor antagonist

I   Oral theophylline

For each of the statements below regarding the drug management of asthma, select the most appropriate option from the list above. Each option may be used once, more than once or not at all.

☐ **11.** **Indicated for the maintenance of asthma and relief of seasonal allergic symptoms.**

☐ **12.** **The SMART regime allows patients to safely tailor their treatment with this drug according to their symptoms.**

☐ **13.** **This drug has a narrow therapeutic window and toxicity is increased by concurrent use of erythromycin, quinolones and cimetidine.**

☐ **14.** **Inhibits bronchoconstriction and reduces mucus secretion in the lungs.**

☐ **15.** **If used for more than 10 days consideration should be given to co-prescription of bisphosphonates.**

16. A 28-year-old man complains of knee pain after being hit below the knee by an outstretched boot in a football match. On examination there is a small effusion but no laceration and the knee is fully mobile but seems to have excessive backward movement on pushing the lower leg back. What is the single most likely diagnosis?

- ☐ A   Anterior cruciate tear
- ☐ B   Medial collateral tear
- ☐ C   Meniscal tear
- ☐ D   Patellar tendon tear
- ☑ E   Posterior cruciate tear

17. You see a 23-year-old epileptic woman for pre-conceptual advice. She is well and has had no seizures for 3 years while taking phenytoin. She would like to discuss the risks of pregnancy given her medical history. Which one of the following statements in this situation is correct?

- ☐ A   Phenytoin is not associated with congenital defects and she can be reassured
- ☐ B   She should be changed to gabapentin
- ☐ C   She should stop her anticonvulsants until after delivery
- ☐ D   She should take folic acid 5 mg once a day from pre-conception onwards
- ☐ E   Women who have previously taken anticonvulsants but are now free from medication have the same risk of congenital malformation as those who have never taken anticonvulsants

18. **Which one of the following statements is correct regarding current NICE guidelines on lipid levels?**

☐ A Ezetemibe/simvastatin combination therapy should be used first-line for patients with acute coronary syndromes

☐ B All patients at risk of ischaemic heart disease should be treated with 40 mg simvastatin and do not require follow-up cholesterol tests

☑ C Patients with acute coronary syndromes should be treated with 40 mg simvastatin

☐ D Patients with diabetes mellitus should have a total cholesterol of 5.0 mmol/l or less and an LDL level of < 3.0 mmol/l

☑ E Patients with diabetes mellitus should have a total cholesterol of 4.0 mmol/l or less and an LDL of < 2.0 mmol/l

19. **An elderly man living in a nursing home has had a catheter fitted for the last 5 weeks. One of the staff in the home has sent a routine urine specimen which has been reported as showing a pure growth of _Proteus_ sensitive to trimethoprim and ciprofloxacin. He is afebrile, with no urinary symptoms. Which one of the following would be the most appropriate management of this patient?**

☐ A Flush the catheter with citrate solution

☐ B No action required

☐ C Prescribe ciprofloxacin for 5 days

☑ D Prescribe trimethoprim for 3 days

☐ E Replace the catheter

THEME: DEATH CERTIFICATION

Options

A   Contact the police

B   Discuss the case with a doctor from a neighbouring practice

C   Discuss the case with the coroner

D   Discuss the case with the crematorium referee

E   Issue Certificate of Stillbirth

F   Issue Medical Certificate of Cause of Death

G   Issue Neonatal Death Certificate

H   None of the above

For each of the situations below select the single most appropriate action from the list of options above. Each option may be used once, more than once, or not at all.

☐ **20.** A 78-year-old woman diagnosed with untreatable metastatic bowel cancer 3 months ago is found dead in bed by her daughter. She was last seen by you 16 days ago.

☐ **21.** An 83-year-old man who has not seen a doctor for 7 years is found dead in an armchair at home. He has no medical history of note and seems to have died in his sleep.

☐ **22.** A 69-year-old former boiler-maker dies after a long illness with mesothelioma. You saw him the day before he died.

☐ **23.** A 57-year-old woman with a long history of mental illness commits suicide 2 days after a review by her consultant psychiatrist. She was last seen by you 10 days ago.

☐ **24.** A 37-year-old woman living on a remote farm who is 22 weeks pregnant goes into premature labour and rapidly delivers a baby at home. Before the paramedics can arrive. The baby did not show any sign of life and was not successfully resuscitated. You attend the woman before admission to hospital and are asked to certify the death of the baby.

☐ **25.** A 93-year-old woman dies of heart failure in a nursing home. She was seen the day before death by you but was confirmed dead by the out-of-hours service and has been taken to an undertaker 30 miles away. The family have made an appointment to register the death this afternoon and have asked you to issue a certificate.

26. A 17-year-old student requests a note for school regarding her absences from lectures. She tells you that for several months she has been finding it increasingly difficult to cope with being in public places. She admits to having been shy since childhood but is now increasingly panicky in groups and feels inadequate around others, although she copes at home. Things have escalated to the point where she has vomited on several occasions. She has no other symptoms of note. Which of the following statements regarding her management is correct?

☐ A Cognitive behavioural therapy is ineffective
☐ B Reassurance that there is no organic disease is usually sufficient
☐ C She should be treated with lithium
☐ D She should be treated with olanzapine
☐ E SSRIs should be used as first-line treatment

27. A 4-year-old girl who returned from a camping holiday at a farm in Wales 2 days ago is brought in by her parents complaining of abdominal pain, vomiting and diarrhoea. This has been going on for 3 days but the diarrhoea has now become bloody. On examination she looks listless and has a capillary refill time of 3 seconds, she has a temperature of 37.6°C, and she has generalised abdominal tenderness but no peritonism. A urine specimen shows microscopic haematuria. What is the single most appropriate management of this patient?

- [ ] A   Admit under paediatrics
- [ ] B   Advise parents regarding oral rehydration and review if no better
- [ ] C   Send urine for culture and treat if positive
- [ ] D   Send stool for culture and review with results
- [ ] E   Treat with oral trimethoprim and review in 3 days

28. Which one of the following statements regarding chronic fatigue syndrome is correct?

- [ ] A   Cognitive difficulties are unusual
- [ ] B   Exacerbations of fatigue are triggered by exertion and usually start during exertion, forcing patients to abandon the activity
- [ ] C   NICE guidelines suggest that the diagnosis should be considered in patients with unexplained fatigue of more than 6 weeks' duration
- [ ] D   The presence of chronic pain suggests an alternative diagnosis
- [ ] E   Cognitive behavioural therapy (CBT) should be offered to all patients with this condition

PAPER 1

29. A 35-year-old man complains of a tender lump on the side of his eyeball. He says that it has been there for several days and came on acutely. He has no other symptoms and his vision is normal. On examination his cornea looks clear, with a reactive pupil and no conjunctival injection. There is no foreign body and no fluorescein staining, but he has an injected nodular area close to the corneal limbus on the white of the eye. The eyeball is tender over the nodule but otherwise is soft. What is the single most likely diagnosis?

- [ ] A   Acute angle closure glaucoma
- [ ] B   Episcleritis
- [x] C   Herpes simplex keratitis
- [ ] D   Iritis
- [ ] E   Scleritis

30. A 57-year-old patient has recently been discharged from hospital after an angioplasty with stent insertion following a non-Q-wave myocardial infarction. Which one of the following statements is correct regarding antiplatelet therapy?

- [ ] A   Aspirin 150 mg once daily should be taken for life
- [ ] B   Aspirin 150 mg once daily and dipyridamole MR 200 mg twice daily should be taken for 12 months
- [ ] C   Clopidogrel 75 mg once a day should be taken for 3 months, then the patient should switch to aspirin 150 mg once a day for life
- [x] D   Clopidogrel 75 mg once daily should be taken for 12 months, then the patient should take aspirin 150 mg once a day for life
- [ ] E   Patients should be treated with warfarin to achieve an INR between 2.0 and 3.0 for life

THEME: CHILDHOOD INFECTIONS

Options

A   Group A streptococci

B   *Escherichia coli* O157

C   *Mycoplasma pneumoniae*

D   Parainfluenza virus

E   Paramyxovirus

F   Parvovirus B19

G   Poxvirus

H   Respiratory syncitial virus (RSV)

I   Rotavirus

J   Rubella

K   *Staphylococcus aureus*

L   Varicella

For each of the statements below, select the most appropriate option from the list above. Each option may be used once, more than once or not at all.

31. Causes crops of pinky-white shiny papules with a central pit.

32. Causes epidemics of respiratory illness in approximately 3-year cycles, often associated with target-like skin lesions.

33. After a prodromal fever this causes a macular rash to appear on the cheek that spreads to the trunk over several days.

34. Around 24 hours after the development of tonsillitis this causes a macular rash to appear over the whole body; 2–3 days later the skin is shed, particularly on the hands and soles.

35. After an incubation period of 14 days crops of vesicular lesions appear over the body. These heal over 2–3 days with new lesions appearing for 7–10 days.

36. A 27-year-old man complains of 3 weeks of diarrhoea and abdominal pain, with weight loss and fever. The stools are bloody on occasion. He has no recent history of travel and takes no regular medications. He reports recently being under a great deal of stress at work. On examination he is tender in the left iliac fossa with no peritonism and no perineal abnormalities. A stool sample is sent which is reported as negative for viral, bacterial and parasitic infections. What is the single most likely diagnosis?

- [ ] A   *Campylobacter*
- [ ] B   Crohn's disease
- [ ] C   Diverticulitis
- [ ] D   Irritable bowel syndrome
- [ ] E   Ulcerative colitis

37. Which one of the following statements regarding termination of pregnancy is correct?

- [ ] A   Girls under the age of 16 cannot have a termination without the consent of their parents
- [ ] B   Medical termination is only suitable in patients up to 9 weeks' gestation
- [ ] C   RU-486 (mifepristone) is safe to use in patients who are not fit for general anaesthesia
- [ ] D   Suction termination can be carried out under local anaesthesia
- [ ] E   The legal limit for abortion is 22 weeks

THEME: PERSONALITY DISORDERS

Options

A   Anankastic personality disorder

B   Antisocial personality disorder

C   Borderline personality disorder

D   Histrionic personality disorder

E   Hyperthymic personality disorder

F   Narcissistic personality disorder

G   Paranoid personality disorder

H   Schizoid personality disorder

For each of the descriptions below, select the most appropriate option from the list above. Each option may be used once, more than once or not at all.

☐ **38.** **Always happy and optimistic, but tend to make rash decisions without fully considering the consequences.**

☐ **39.** **Characterised by impulsivity, outbursts of anger and unpredictable behaviour. Often with episodes of deliberate self-harm or violence.**

☐ **40.** **A lack of adaptability to new situations, for example failing to take advantage of new opportunities, disabling perfectionism in even the most mundane tasks, and lack of imagination.**

☐ **41.** **Typified by an excessive sense of self-importance and power without warmth or empathy.**

☐ **42.** **Solitary, humourless people who tend to avoid situations where they will have to socialise.**

43. Regarding benefits and long-term sickness certification, which one of the following statements is correct?

- [ ] A Employment Support Allowance always requires a personal capability assessment
- [ ] B Med 3 certificates can be issued for an indefinite period from the outset
- [ ] C Med 5 certificates are used when a patient is awaiting a personal capability assessment
- [ ] D Patients who are registered blind are automatically entitled to incapacity benefit
- [ ] E The mobility component of Disability Living Allowance is only paid to patients with physical disability

44. A 53-year-old man had a pacemaker fitted for heart block last week. He complains that his left arm is swollen. On examination the left arm is red and swollen from the humerus down, with engorged veins that do not empty on elevating the arm. He is afebrile. What is the single most likely diagnosis?

- [ ] A Cellulitis
- [ ] B Compartment syndrome
- [ ] C Deep vein thrombosis
- [ ] D Post-operative wound infection
- [ ] E Subclavian arterial embolism

45. In a patient with symptoms of diabetes mellitus, which one of the following sets of blood tests is diagnostic of diabetes mellitus according to the WHO diagnostic criteria?

- [ ] A 4+ glucose level on urine dipstick testing
- [ ] B Capillary glucose level of 15.1 mmol/l
- [ ] C Fasting venous glucose of 8.3 mmol/l
- [ ] D Random venous glucose of 10.6 mmol/l
- [ ] E Venous glucose level of 9.8 mmol/l 2 hours after a 75-g oral glucose load

46. A 17-year-old girl with severe psoriasis has tried coal tar, dithranol, vitamin D analogues, steroids and emollients without effect and is desperate for something to be done. Which one of the following statements is true regarding further management of this condition?

- [ ] A Ciclosporin can be used in this patient
- [ ] B Oral steroids should be given at a dose of 40 mg once a day for 10 days, reducing to a maintenance dose of 10–15 mg according to response
- [ ] C Retinoids can be safely used in this patient
- [ ] D Topical potent steroids can be used long-term without side effects
- [ ] E Ultraviolet treatments are effective with no long-term complications

THEME: BIOLOGICAL THERAPIES

Options

A   Infliximab (Remicade)

B   Natalizumab (Tysabri)

C   Omalizumab (Xolair)

D   Ranibizumab (Lucentis)

E   Rituximab (Rituxan)

F   Trastuzumab (Herceptin)

For each of the diseases below, select the most appropriate treatment agent from the list above. Each option may be used once, more than once or not at all.

☐ **47.** **Allergy-mediated asthma.**

☐ **48.** **Multiple sclerosis.**

☐ **49.** **Severe psoriasis resistant to PUVA and standard systemic treatment.**

☐ **50.** **Breast cancer.**

☐ **51.** **Macular degeneration.**

52. A 39-year-old man with longstanding gastro-oesophageal reflux comes to see you about his condition. In spite of treatment with high-dose proton-pump inhibitors and alginates he is troubled by symptoms on a daily basis. He has tried lifestyle measures but feels he cannot go on. He begs you to refer him for surgery. Which one of the following statements is true regarding this treatment option?

- [ ] A Nissen fundoplication requires a laparotomy
- [ ] B Patients who have had a fundoplication have a reduced gastric capacity and have to eat regular small meals
- [ ] C Surgery is indicated in patients who do not wish to take long-term medication
- [ ] D Surgery is only suitable for patients with a sliding hiatus hernia
- [ ] E Surgery will control symptoms and eliminate the need for maintenance medication

53. A 34-year-old woman requests a blood test to see if she has a clotting tendency. Her brother has recently suffered a deep vein thrombosis after a routine arthroscopy. Which one of the following statements is true regarding thrombophillias?

- [ ] A Only patients with a family history of venous thromboembolism should be screened
- [ ] B Patients aged under 40 with one episode of unexplained venous thromboembolism should be screened
- [ ] C Patients who are negative for the factor V Leiden mutation can be reassured that they do not have a thrombophillia
- [ ] D Thrombophillia is always inherited
- [ ] E Thrombophillia screening is only indicated for recurrent venous thromboses

54. A 36-year-old woman with severe rheumatoid arthritis has been advised to start methotrexate by her rheumatologist. She comes to see you to discuss this, having read about this treatment on the internet. Which one of the following statements regarding this treatment is correct?

☐   A   If a full blood count is normal initially and 1 month after starting treatment, no further testing is required

☒   B   If LFTs increase by 10% after starting treatment the drug should be stopped

☐   C   Methotrexate can be safely used in pregnancy

☐   D   Methotrexate frequently causes menstrual disturbances

☐   E   Methotrexate should not be used in patients taking folic acid supplements

55. A 7-year-old boy is brought in to see you by his parents at the request of his schoolteachers. He has no friends in his class, is aloof, and seems to find it very difficult to interact with others. He likes to play on his own and seldom shares his experiences in the classroom. His only interest is in Thomas the Tank Engine and he plays with these toys in a repetitive manner. He also flaps his hands many times through the day. He was born at term after an uneventful delivery and showed normal speech and language development up to the age of 3 years. What is the single most likely diagnosis?

☐   A   Asperger syndrome

☐   B   Attention deficit hyperactivity disorder

☐   C   Cerebral palsy

☐   D   Normal variant

☐   E   Temporal lobe epilepsy

THEME: GENERAL PRACTICE AND GOVERNMENT POLICY

Options

A   Alternative Provider of Medical Services (APMS)

B   Carson Report

C   Darzi Review

D   Good Doctors, Safer Patients

E   Modernising Medical Careers

F   NHS Plan 2000

G   Royal College of General Practitioners Roadmap

H   Shipman Enquiry

I   Tooke Report

For each of the statements below, select the most appropriate option from the list above. Each option may be used once, more than once or not at all.

☐ **56.** Proposes that primary care be delivered in large collaborative federations of practices.

I ☐ **57.** Proposes to lengthen general practice training to 5 years.

c ☐ **58.** Proposes that GP-run health centres will be open 7 days a week from 0800 to 1800.

D ☐ **59.** Proposes a lowering in the standard of proof in medical negligence cases.

B ☐ **60.** Placed NHS Direct at the heart of the out-of-hours care model.

61. A 67-year-old lady, who is about to embark on a cruise, requests a prescription for some sea sickness tablets. Which one of the following statements is correct regarding this condition?

- [ ] A Cinnarazine is an effective treatment
- [ ] B Drug treatment has a placebo effect only
- [ ] C Hyoscine should not be used because it exacerbates motion sickness
- [ ] D Patients suffering sea sickness should be advised to avoid standing on-deck because the view of the moving sea can exacerbate symptoms
- [x] E Promethazine is effective, with minimal side effects, making it the first-line treatment for most patients

62. One of your patients has recently been diagnosed with tuberculosis. He has spent several weeks in the last 3 months in a community hospital and was a frequent visitor to the surgery. You attend a public health meeting to discuss contact tracing. Which one of the following statements regarding contact tracing is correct?

- [ ] A All contacts should be removed from patient care until they have been screened
- [ ] B Heaf testing has high sensitivity and specificity
- [ ] C Presence of a BCG scar implies immunity and these patients do not need to be screened
- [ ] D Quantiferon testing is the investigation of choice in screening contacts
- [ ] E X-ray is the most appropriate investigation in TB outbreaks

63. Which one of the following statements is correct regarding the use of hypnotics in the management of insomnia?

- [ ] A   Benzodiazepines have a short half-life and are therefore less likely to cause hangover effects than other hypnotics
- [ ] B   In the elderly, hypnotics are twice as likely to cause adverse effects as they are to improve sleep
- [ ] C   Hypnotics increase the amount of REM sleep
- [ ] D   Zopiclone is not a benzodiazepine and is therefore not associated with any risk of addiction
- [ ] E   Zopiclone is safe to use in elderly agitated patients

64. A 27-year-old man complains of pain above his right ankle after a dry ski slope session in preparation for his skiing holiday. He reports falling awkwardly and was unable to continue, but he can weight-bear. On examination he has tenderness and bruising 4 inches above his lateral malleolus, with numbness over the lateral border of the foot. What is the single most appropriate management?

- [ ] A   Advise him to return if he is still in pain when the swelling has subsided
- [ ] B   Advise rest, ice, compression and elevation (RICE)
- [ ] C   Apply a backslab cast for support
- [ ] D   Reassure him that he can weight-bear, making a fracture unlikely
- [ ] E   Refer immediately to the emergency department for X-ray

THEME: ABDOMINAL PAIN

Options

A	Abdominal aortic aneurysm	G	Diverticulitis
B	Acute appendicitis	H	Gastric carcinoma
C	Acute cholecystitis	I	Irritable bowel syndrome
D	Acute pancreatitis	J	Peptic ulcer
E	Crohn's disease	K	Renal colic
F	Colonic carcinoma	L	Ruptured ectopic pregnancy

For each of the clinical scenarios described below, select the most appropriate diagnosis from the list of options above. Each option may be used once, more than once or not at all.

65. A 76-year-old man complains of recurrent attacks of colicky left iliac fossa pain. On examination he has left iliac fossa tenderness but no peritonism.

66. A 39-year-old man complains of acute colicky pains radiating from his back to his groin and coming in waves.

67. A 33-year-old woman complains of 3 months of diarrhoea, weight loss and abdominal pain. On examination she has a right iliac fossa swelling and fleshy skin tags around her anus.

68. A 44-year-old woman complains of fever, vomiting and pain in her shoulder. On examination she is tender in the right upper quadrant.

69. A 67-year-old man complains of several weeks of dysphagia, weight loss and, more recently, epigastric pain. On examination he is cachectic with generalised abdominal tenderness.

70. A 56-year-old diabetic lady who takes simvastatin has come to see you after reading an article in her daily newspaper about the dangers of taking statins. She would like your advice on whether to continue. Which one of the following statements about the side effects of cholesterol-lowering treatment is true?

- [ ] A Ezetimibe has been reported to be associated with an increased risk of cancer
- [ ] B Patients with familial hypercholesterolaemia should all be treated with 40 mg simvastatin
- [ ] C Patients with mixed hyperlipidaemias should be treated with a statin and a fibrate
- [ ] D Simvastatin is the only statin which interacts significantly with other drugs
- [ ] E Sleep disturbance is rare

71. A 33-year-old woman complains of several months of bilateral breast pain, starting in her mid-cycle and associated with an increase in breast size. Her symptoms resolve with the onset of her period. She has no discharge, skin changes or lymphadenopathy. Examination is unremarkable. Which one of the following statements regarding her management is correct?

- [ ] A The breast pain is likely to improve during pregnancy
- [ ] B Combined oral contraceptive pills inhibit ovulation and therefore improve menstrual breast pain
- [x] C Evening primrose oil is the most effective treatment
- [ ] D She should be warned that her symptoms will worsen after the menopause
- [ ] E Topical NSAIDs are effective in relieving pain

72. **The figures below show changes in the incidence of prostate cancer and death rates over the last 10 years.**

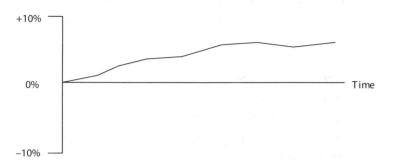

Figure (a) Percentage change in new cases of prostate cancer diagnosed per year.

Figure (b) Percentage change in deaths from prostate cancer per year.

Which one of the following is the most likely explanation for this data?

- ☑ A   Advances in treatment have led to improved survival rates
- ☐ B   Changes in lifestyle have increased the risk of developing cancer
- ☐ C   Clinically asymptomatic cancers are being diagnosed earlier
- ☐ D   New cases are being diagnosed at the same rate as survival is increasing
- ☐ E   Newer treatments do not improve life expectancy

PAPER 1

73. Which one of the following statements regarding the ASCOT study (Anglo-Scandinavian Cardiac Outcomes Trial) is correct?

- [ ] A   It demonstrated significant benefits in treating hypertensive patients with calcium antagonists and ACE inhibitors compared with β blockers and thiazides

- [ ] B   There was found to be an increased risk of diabetes in the calcium antagonist arm compared with the thiazide arm

- [ ] C   It showed no difference in cardiac disease between the three treatment arms of thiazides, calcium antagonists or ACE inhibitors

- [ ] D   The trial compared aggressive treatment of hypertension with watchful waiting

- [ ] E   This was a secondary prevention study

74. A 47-year-old man complains of recurrent episodes of fleeting pain radiating from his tonsils to his right ear. He describes the pain as like an electric shock typically lasting a few seconds. The only obvious trigger he can identify is eating certain foods. Examination of the head and neck is unremarkable, with no skin lesions or lymphadenopathy. He has no associated vertigo, deafness or tinnitus. What is the single most likely diagnosis?

- [ ] A   Glossopharyngeal neuralgia
- [ ] B   Ménière's syndrome
- [ ] C   Ramsay Hunt syndrome
- [ ] D   Tonsillar carcinoma
- [ ] E   Trigeminal neuralgia

75. A 73-year-old man comes to see you to discuss medication recommended by the local neurologist following a transient ischaemic attack. He has been advised to take aspirin and dipyridamole but is allergic to aspirin. Which one of the following would be an appropriate alternative regime?

- [ ] A   Clopidogrel
- [ ] B   Dipyridamole alone
- [ ] C   Dipyridamole and clopidogrel
- [ ] D   Low-molecular-weight heparin
- [ ] E   Warfarin

76. Comparing retrospective with prospective studies, which one of the following statements is true?

- [ ] A   Retrospective studies are less prone to bias than prospective studies
- [ ] B   Retrospective studies are more expensive to conduct than prospective studies
- [ ] C   Retrospective studies are quicker to conduct than prospective studies
- [ ] D   Results from retrospective studies carry more statistical significance than prospective studies
- [ ] E   Prospective studies are designed to detect differences in populations and therefore always produce statistically significant data

THEME: DERMATOLOGICAL TREATMENTS

Options

A	Azathioprine	F	Prednisolone
B	Betnovate	G	PUVA
C	Ciclosporin	H	Roaccutane
D	Dermovate	I	Tacrolimus
E	Diclofenac gel		

For each of the situations below, select the most appropriate treatment from the list above. Each option may be used once, more than once or not at all.

77. A 76-year-old man with an area of solar keratosis on his scalp declines treatment with cryotherapy because he has experienced severe blistering in the past.

78. A 6-year-old girl has severe eczema which she can only control using daily Betnovate. Her parents are concerned about the risks of long-term steroid use.

79. A 36-year-old woman with acne on her face and back has tried Dianette and oral antibiotics without success. Her acne is ruining her life and she demands treatment.

80. A 45-year-old lifelong psoriasis sufferer who has had no benefit from coal tar, emollients, topical steroids or vitamin D analogues now has severe psoriasis which causes him a great deal of distress.

81. A 35-year-old businessman has been treated unsuccessfully for a flare of his eczema with emollients and Betnovate. He has avoided all soaps and cannot identify any other obvious triggers.

82. A 33-year-old woman who is 33 weeks into her second pregnancy presents with reduced fetal movements. She has no abdominal pain or bleeding but has not felt the baby move since the previous evening. On examination her abdomen is soft, with fundal height consistent with dates. Which one of the following is the single most appropriate management of this situation?

☒ A Admit under on-call obstetric team

☐ B Ask her to contact the midwife if she has not felt ten movements by 1700 the following day

☐ C Do cervical examination to assess for pre-term labour

☐ D Reassure her that this is normal in the last trimester

☐ E Refer directly to the antenatal unit for biophysical profile

83. Which one of the following statements regarding the management of tension-type headache is correct?

☐ A First-line treatment for tension-type headaches should be codeine 30–60 mg up to four times daily as required

☐ B Preventative treatment should be used only where rescue treatment is required more than three times a week

☐ C Propranolol is the most effective prophylactic treatment

☐ D Tricyclic antidepressants are associated with increased risk of tension-type headache

☐ E Use of opioid or combination analgesics is associated with an increased risk of medication-overuse headache compared with use of non-opioid analgesics

84. A 27-year-old marketing executive asks for advice about her nails. She has recently been through a stressful relationship break-up and is applying for new jobs. She is self-conscious about the appearance of her thumbnails, shown below.

Which one of the following would be the most appropriate management of this condition?

- [ ] A   Amorolfine nail lacquer
- [ ] B   Avoidance of nail rubbing
- [ ] C   Calcium supplementation
- [ ] D   Reassurance
- [ ] E   Terbinafine tablets

85. A 56-year-old woman who had a wide local excision of a breast cancer and axillary clearance 5 years ago presents with a 3-month history of an increasingly swollen arm on the side of her previous surgery. On examination the oedema is non-pitting, with no erythema and minimal tenderness. Which one of the following is the single most likely diagnosis?

- [ ] A   Cellulitis
- [ ] B   Deep vein thrombosis
- [ ] C   Lymphoma
- [ ] D   Lymphoedema
- [ ] E   Recurrent breast cancer

86. A 56-year-old man attends for routine blood tests in the surgery. He has a history of chronic obstructive pulmonary disease (COPD), with an FEV_1 of 75% of predicted, and also suffers from essential hypertension. Unfortunately he continues to smoke 10–20 cigarettes a day. A full blood count is taken and the results are shown below.

Haemoglobin	19.6 g/dl (NR 13.5–18.0 mg/dl)
WCC	$6.7 \times 10^9/l$ ($4.0–11.0 \times 10^9/l$)
Platelets	$276 \times 10^9/l$ ($150–400 \times 10^9/l$)

What would be the single most appropriate initial management step in this case?

- [ ] A Prescribe aspirin 300 mg once daily
- [ ] B Reassure him that these results are normal
- [ ] C Refer under 2-week rule to haematology
- [ ] D Start a smoking cessation programme and repeat the blood tests in 4 weeks
- [ ] E Venesect until the haemoglobin is in the normal range

87. While visiting your parents your mother asks you if you can have a look at a mole she is worried about. She tells you that she doesn't particularly like her own GP due to his rudeness and is too busy to see one of the other doctors at the surgery. Which one of the following would be the most appropriate response in this situation, according to General Medical Council guidelines?

- [ ] A Encourage her to complain to the practice manager about the doctor's rudeness
- [ ] B Examine the mole and advise her on management accordingly
- [ ] C Suggest she sees another doctor at the practice
- [ ] D Refer her to a local dermatologist
- [ ] E Telephone her GP and explain the situation

THEME: UPPER GASTROINTESTINAL DISORDERS

Options

A   Achalasia

B   Barrett's oesophagus

C   Coeliac disease

D   Hiatus hernia

E   Maltoma

F   Oesophageal cancer

G   Oesophageal dysmotility

H   Oesophageal stricture

I   Plummer–Vinson syndrome

J   Reflux oesophagitis

For each of the statements below, select the option from the list above that is most appropriate. Each option may be used once, more than once or not at all.

88. Associated with *Helicobacter pylori* infection.

89. Causes a slowly progressive, intermittent dysphagia, often causing chest infections.

90. Associated with a 1% annual risk of developing oesophageal cancer.

91. Usually presents with bolus obstruction.

92. Causes dysphagia in association with glossitis, koilonychia and angular stomatitis.

93. Which one of the following statements about NICE guidance on the management of menorrhagia is correct?

☐ A Sixty per cent of women presenting in primary care will ultimately have a hysterectomy

☐ B Endometrial ablation is an effective treatment that avoids hysterectomy, thus preserving fertility

☐ C Menorrhagia is a clinical diagnosis and does not require any investigations

☐ D Mirena coils are the most effective medical treatment for menorrhagia

☐ E Oral progestogens given in the luteal phase are effective in those unfit for surgery

94. A 43-year-old man has recently discovered that his father has Huntington's disease. He has been tested and does not have the disease. He has two small children and would like to know their risk of developing the disease. There is no family history of Huntington's disease in the mother's pedigree. Which one of the following statements is true regarding this situation?

☐ A Each child has a 25% chance of being affected

☐ B Each child has a 25% chance of being a carrier

☐ C Each child has a 0% chance of being affected

☐ D He has a 25% chance of being a carrier

☐ E He has a 50% chance of being a carrier

95. A 29-year-old woman comes to see you for advice. She is due to get married in 3 weeks and is concerned that she will have a flare of her cold sores, which always seems to occur when she is stressed. She asks if anything can be done to prevent this. Which one of the following statements is correct regarding this scenario?

- [ ] A   Cold sores are caused by infection with *Staphylococcus aureus* and using flucloxacillin will usually prevent an exacerbation
- [ ] B   Cold sores are caused by primary infection with herpes simplex virus and can be prevented by taking oral aciclovir
- [ ] C   Exacerbations are more common in the winter
- [x] D   Topical aciclovir is an effective prophylactic treatment
- [ ] E   Ultraviolet light used at the onset of symptoms will abort the attack

96. A 45-year-old woman complains of pain on the radial side of her wrist which came on after a weekend spring trimming flowers for a wedding display. On examination she has tenderness and swelling along the radial border of the thumb with maximal tenderness over the head of the radius. Resisted abduction exacerbates the pain. What is the single most likely diagnosis?

- [ ] A   Carpal tunnel syndrome
- [ ] B   De Quervain's tenosynovitis
- [ ] C   Lateral epicondylitis
- [ ] D   Medial epicondylitis
- [ ] E   Osteoarthritis of the first metacarpophalangeal joint

97. A 34-year-old man has a renal ultrasound carried out to investigate renal colic. He is shocked to be told he that has a duplex ureter on the right and comes to see you to discuss the significance of this. Which one of the following statements about this condition is true?

- [ ] A   Duplex ureters are of no clinical significance
- [ ] B   Pelvi-ureteric junction (PUJ) obstruction is more common in patients with duplex ureters
- [ ] C   Surgery is indicated in all cases
- [ ] D   This condition is extremely rare
- [ ] E   Treatment with an ACE inhibitor is indicated to prevent nephropathy

98. A 2-year-old boy is brought to see you by his mother, who is concerned that he is developing a squint. On examination he appears to have a right-sided squint and also when you look at his eyes with an ophthalmoscope you see that he has a white pupillary reflex on that side. He was adopted at birth and his parents have no knowledge of his family or antenatal history. Which one of the following would be the most appropriate management for this child?

- [ ] A   Reassure the mother and arrange to review him in 4 weeks
- [ ] B   Refer to ophthalmology for assessment of vision
- [ ] C   Refer to optician for glasses
- [ ] D   Refer to the orthoptic department for patching
- [ ] E   Refer under the 2-week rule

99. A 53-year-old woman complains of increasing difficulties with her figure. She tells you that she has always had a slim figure but that over the last 6 months she has noticed her waist is getting bigger in spite of regular exercise and dieting. She also reports new onset of urinary frequency and constipation. On examination she has some dullness in her flanks but no other obvious abnormalities on abdominal palpation. Which one of the following would be the most appropriate next step in her assessment?

- [ ] A   Bimanual examination
- [ ] B   Check thyroid function
- [ ] C   Refer for colonoscopy in view of change in bowel habit
- [ ] D   Refer for ultrasound scan
- [ ] E   Trial of anticholinergic

100. A 9-year-old boy is brought into the surgery by his mother after an episode of frank haematuria. This seems to have started after a viral infection and he has complained of loin pain over the last 24 hours. On examination he appears well with no fever or oedema and no masses in his abdomen. Urinalysis is positive for blood but negative for nitrites and leukocytes, with protein 1+. Reviewing his notes you discover he was treated last year for a suspected urinary tract infection by a locum after presenting with macroscopic haematuria. What is the single most likely diagnosis?

- [ ] A   Beetroot consumption
- [ ] B   IgA nephropathy
- [ ] C   Polycystic kidneys
- [ ] D   Urinary tract infection
- [ ] E   Wilms' tumour

PAPER 1

101. A 44-year-old man attends for a routine insurance medical. While taking his blood pressure you notice an unusual area of skin on his elbow. He does not have any patches elsewhere apart from his other elbow, and is otherwise well. He has mild hypertension treated with ramipril and suffered from eczema when he was younger, but takes no other medication. A photograph of his arm is shown below.

What is the most likely cause of this appearance?

- [ ] A   Drug reaction
- [ ] B   Lichenification
- [ ] C   Tinea
- [ ] D   Traumatic depigmentation
- [ ] E   Vitiligo

102. Which one of the following should be part of a routine 8-week check for newborn infants?

- [ ] A   Coordination
- [ ] B   Cover test for squint
- [ ] C   Guthrie test
- [ ] D   Hearing
- [ ] E   Presence of cataracts

103. A 41-year-old woman complains of sudden onset of visual loss in her right eye which she noticed on waking. She also complains of discomfort in the eye which is worse when looking upwards. On examination she has a central defect on field testing and a relative afferent pupillary defect, although her fundus looks normal. The contralateral eye is normal. What is the single most likely diagnosis?

- [ ] A Acute glaucoma
- [ ] B Amaurosis fugax
- [ ] C Central retinal vein occlusion (CRVO)
- [ ] D Optic neuritis
- [ ] E Papilloedema

104. You meet a new patient for the first time at his new patient check. He had a thyroidectomy for thyroid cancer 25 years ago and has been taking thyroxine ever since. He tells you that he has not had his thyroid function tested for some time so you send him for a blood test. Which one of the following statements is correct regarding this situation?

- [ ] A He should stay on his current dose and does not need thyroid function tests
- [ ] B He should have a TSH level within the normal range
- [ ] C His T_4 level should be within the normal range
- [ ] D His T_3 level should be within the normal range
- [ ] E His TSH should be < 0.01 µU/l

THEME: STATISTICAL TERMS

Options

A   False positive

B   False negative

C   Incidence

D   Odds ratio

E p value

F   Prevalence

G   Sensitivity

H   Specificity

I   Standard deviation

J   Standard error of the mean

K   Standardised mortality rate

L   True positive

M   True negative

For each of the statements below, select the most appropriate term from the list above. Each option may be used once, more than once or not at all.

☐ **105.** Quantifies the spread of the distribution of data within a series; is equal to the square root of the variance.

☐ **106.** An estimate of risk used in case–control studies.

☐ **107.** An estimate of statistical significance.

☐ **108.** The proportion of new cases of a disease diagnosed within a specified time period.

☐ **109.** The proportion of people without a condition diagnosed as being disease-free with a particular screening test.

110. One of your patients has recently had an upper gastrointestinal endoscopy which has shown Barrett's oesophagus. He is concerned that this means that he will get cancer and comes to see you to discuss this diagnosis. Which one of the following statements regarding this condition is true?

- [ ] A Barrett's oesophagus is a benign condition with no long-term complications
- [ ] B Barrett's oesophagus will often resolve if *Helicobacter pylori* infection is treated
- [ ] C Patients with Barrett's oesophagus should be referred for oesophagectomy
- [ ] D There is a 1% annual risk of developing malignancy in patients with Barrett's oesophagus
- [ ] E There is no treatment for Barrett's oesophagus other than surveillance

111. One of your patients complains of persistent pain and crunching in his knees. He had a meniscectomy in his thirties and on examination he has clinical signs of osteoarthritis. Which one of the following statements regarding evidence-based management of this condition is correct?

- [ ] A Acupuncture can be effective in relieving pain
- [ ] B Glucosamine use is not supported by the evidence and it cannot be prescribed on an FP10
- [ ] C Patients should be advised to avoid exercise as this will exacerbate symptoms
- [ ] D Steroid injections into affected joints have no beneficial effect but expose patients to risks of infection and avascular necrosis
- [ ] E Topical NSAIDs have a placebo effect only

112. A 47-year-old lady with a history of focal migraine comes to you with 3-hour history of severe headache centred around her right eye, with loss of vision in that eye and nausea and vomiting. On examination her conjunctiva is injected and her pupil does not constrict to light. What is the single most likely diagnosis?

- [ ] A   Acute angle closure glaucoma
- [ ] B   Cluster headache
- [ ] C   Giant-cell arteritis
- [ ] D   Focal migraine
- [ ] E   Subarachnoid haemorrhage

113. A 56-year-old man with no previous history of note complains of a hot, red and swollen left calf. He cannot recall any obvious triggers. On examination he has an erythematous, swollen calf with generalised tenderness. Bloods are sent which provide the following results:

Haemoglobin	13.6 g/dl
WCC	$10.8 \times 10^9/l$ (NR 3.6–11.0/l)
Platelets	$375 \times 10^9/l$ (150–400 $\times 10^9/l$)
Neutrophils	$7.7 \times 10^9/l$ (1.8–7.5 $\times 10^9/l$)
Lymphocytes	$2.2 \times 10^9/l$ (1.1–3.5 $\times 10^9/l$)
Monocytes	$0.50 \times 10^9/l$ (0.2–0.8 $\times 10^9/l$)
Eosinophils	$0.30 \times 10^9/l$ (0.04–0.4 $\times 10^9/l$)
D-Dimer	390 ng/ml (0–230 ng/ml)
CRP	17 mg/l (0–5 mg/l)

What is the single most likely diagnosis?

- [ ] A   Cellulitis
- [ ] B   Deep vein thrombosis
- [ ] C   Fungal infection
- [ ] D   Ruptured Baker's cyst
- [ ] E   Varicose eczema

114. **Which one of the following statements regarding the management of migraine is true?**

☐ A Ergotamine can be used in an acute attack in patients who have taken a triptan without effect

☐ B Lifestyle measures are important in the management of recurrent migraine

☐ C NSAIDs are ineffective in migraine

☐ D Triptans are licensed for children over the age of 6 years

☑ E Where patients are needing triptans more than twice a month they should be treated with valproate as a prophylactic

115. **A 33-year-old farm labourer complains that he has developed a cough, chest tightness and breathlessness, with myalgia. He has had this in the past and has been treated with a salbutamol inhaler with slight benefit. He is well most of the year but reports getting these symptoms at certain times of the year when he is working indoors. On examination he is afebrile and has a respiratory rate of 30/minute with fine crepitations in both lung fields. He has no wheeze or finger clubbing. Which one of the following is the most likely diagnosis?**

☐ A Asthma

☐ B Atypical pneumonia

☐ C Bronchiectasis

☐ D Extrinsic allergic alveolitis

☐ E Pulmonary fibrosis

116. Which one of the following statements regarding evidence-based management of dysmenorrhoea is correct?

☐ A Aspirin is the most effective NSAID in the management of primary dysmenorrhoea

☐ B The combined oral contraceptive has a number needed to treat of 5 for management of primary dysmenorrhoea

☐ C COX-2 inhibitors have been shown to have no additional efficacy compared with placebo

☐ D Paracetamol is as effective as ibuprofen, with fewer side effects

☐ E Spinal manipulation has been proved to be of benefit in primary dysmenorrhoea

117. Which one of the following statements regarding partnership agreements is correct?

☐ A A partnership agreement does not need to be updated to reflect partnership changes, as long as new partners agree to the terms of the old agreement

☐ B A partnership without a formal partnership agreement is not considered to be a legal partnership

☐ C Only qualified general practitioners can legally be partners in a medical practice

☐ D Under the Partnership Act 1890 all financial decisions made by a partnership must be unanimous

☐ E Where a partnership agreement does not exist, the partnership can be terminated at any time by one of the partners

THEME: LEARNING AND TEACHING METHODS

Options

A   Cathartic

B   Counselling

C   Didactic

D   Heuristic

E   Reflective

F   Socratic

For each of the descriptions of teaching methods below, select the most appropriate option from the list above. Each option may be used once, more than once or not at all.

☐   **118.   Facilitates learning through awareness-raising questions.**

☐   **119.   Explores feelings and assumptions.**

☐   **120.   Promotes learner autonomy and self-directed learning.**

☐   **121.   A formal lecture style.**

122. Your practice is updating its protocols for the management of type 2 diabetes and you wish to make this process evidence-based. Which one of the following statements regarding the drug management of type 2 diabetes is true?

☐ A   All diabetics, regardless of age and the presence of risk factors, should be treated with a statin

☐ B   Glitazones should be used as first-line treatment in the overweight

☐ C   Metformin should not be used in patients on glitazones due to the risk of heart failure

☐ D   The ADVANCE trial showed that addition of perindopril and indapamide to the treatment of patients with diabetes, regardless of the presence of hypertension, reduces the risk of cardiovascular events

☐ E   The ACCORD (Action to Control Cardiovascular Risk in Diabetes) trial confirmed the benefits of aggressive control of blood sugar levels

123. A 23-year-old woman comes to see you for her 6-week check after delivering a boy by caesarian section. She is breastfeeding and has not had a period yet, but would like to discuss contraception. Which one of the following statements is true?

☐ A   A negative pregnancy test is required before starting the contraceptive pill if periods have not yet returned

☐ B   A combined oral contraceptive pill (COCP) can be started at any time from 1 week after the birth onwards

☐ C   The earliest possible fertile ovulation is around 28 days post-partum

☐ D   Ovulation does not occur until after the return of periods

☐ E   Progesterone-only pills interfere with breastfeeding and should be avoided in lactating mothers

THEME: MANAGEMENT OF BACK PAIN

Options

A   Discharge

B   GP management

C   NSAIDs

D   Physiotherapy

E   Red flag symptoms

F   Refer to back school

G   Refer to secondary care

H   Review in 2 weeks

I   Review in 4 weeks

J   Strong opioids

The local physiotherapy department have developed a new spinal triage system to simplify the management of mechanical back pain. They wish to simplify this with a flowchart. Complete the figure below from the list of options above. Each option may be used once, more than once or not at all.

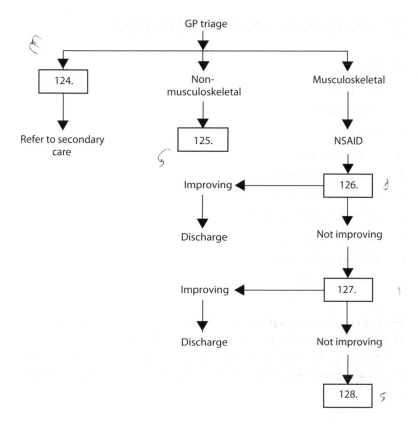

129. You receive a telephone call from a concerned mother. Her 17-month-old son had his MMR vaccination at 14 months. There have been six confirmed cases of measles at her son's crèche and she asks your advice as to what precautions she should take. Which one of the following is the most appropriate advice in this case?

- ☐ A He should have a MMR booster at 4½ years of age
- ☐ B He should have a measles booster vaccine
- ☐ C He should have an MMR booster immediately
- ☐ D He should have blood sent to assess if he is immune
- ☐ E She should be reassured that no further vaccinations are required

130. A 35-year-old woman is diagnosed with a heart murmur at a routine employment medical. A subsequent echocardiogram shows mitral valve prolapse. She comes to see you to discuss the implications of this. Which one of the following statements is correct regarding this condition?

- [ ] A   All patients should be referred for valve replacement
- [ ] B   It commonly causes congestive cardiac failure
- [ ] C   It is usually caused by streptococcal infection
- [ ] D   It can be associated with palpitations
- [ ] E   Patients should be anticoagulated with warfarin

131. A 48-year-old man complains of 6 months of loss of smell and reduced taste. He reports that his symptoms are constant and seemed to have started for no obvious reason. He is a lifelong hay fever sufferer but says he can breathe through his nose. You do not have a Thudichum's nasal speculum in the surgery but limited examination of the nose with an otoscope does not show any obvious pathology. Which one of the following is the most likely diagnosis?

- [ ] A   Deviated nasal septum
- [ ] B   Frontal lobe tumour
- [ ] C   Head injury
- [ ] D   Nasal polyps
- [ ] E   Overuse of decongestant

THEME: CAUSES OF PNEUMONIA

Options

A   Aspergillosis

B   Actinomycosis

C   *Coxiella burnetii* pneumonia

D   Cytomelagovirus

E   Legionnaire's disease

F   Measles

G   *Mycoplasma* pneumonia

H   *Pneumocystis carinii* pneumonia

I   Psittacosis

J   Q fever

K   Tuberculosis

L   Varicella

For each of the descriptions below, select the most appropriate option from the list above. Each option may be used once, more than once or not at all.

☐ **132.** **Epidemics occur in 3–4-year cycles, predominantly affecting children.**

☐ **133.** **Causes a prodromal illness with fever, coryza, conjunctivitis and cough, followed by the development of a rash starting on the neck.**

☐ **134.** **Affects the immunocompromised, causing a suppurative pneumonia; has a poor prognosis.**

☐ **135.** **Causes a primary viral pneumonia in adults.**

☐ **136.** **Causes a prodromal illness with fever, diarrhoea, headache and myalgia, followed by the development of respiratory symptoms; hyponatraemia is often found.**

137. A 65-year-old woman develops a painful rash on her back. On examination she has numerous circular target lesions over her back and torso. These have a central blister. Which one of the following statements is correct regarding this scenario?

- [ ] A These lesions are never seen in the mouth
- [ ] B This condition is iatrogenic and a full drug history should be taken
- [ ] C This condition often has an infectious cause
- [ ] D This condition usually resolves spontaneously in 3–5 days
- [ ] E This patient has erythema nodosum and should have a chest X-ray to exclude sarcoidosis

138. A 48-year-old woman complains of a sore throat. While talking to her you notice that she has a swollen neck and on examination she has a smooth swelling, more pronounced on the right side, which moves with swallowing. She thinks this has been present for a number of years. There are no palpable lymph nodes. She is otherwise well. Blood tests reveal a normal full blood count, normal renal and liver function, and normal thyroid function. Which one of the following statements regarding her management is correct?

- [ ] A She should have a blood sent for thyroid autoantibodies and if these are normal she should be reassured
- [ ] B She should be prescribed levothyroxine 100 micrograms once a day initially
- [ ] C She should be reassured
- [ ] D She should be referred for an ultrasound examination
- [ ] E She should be referred under the 2-week rule

139. A 78-year-old man is thought to have an irregular heartbeat at a blood pressure check. The nurse who sees him takes an electrocardiogram which is shown below.

Which one of the following is the correct diagnosis of this ECG trace?

- A Atrio-ventricular dissociation
- B Paroxysmal atrial fibrillation
- C Ventricular bigeminy
- D Wenckebach phenomenon
- E 2:1 heart block

140. A 79-year-old man complains of deafness. On examining his ears you find wax impaction on both sides but also note the following lesion on his pinna. He reports that this has been present for a number of years and bleeds occasionally

What is the single most likely diagnosis?

☐ A Actinic keratosis

☐ B Basal cell carcinoma (BCC)

☐ C Chondrodermatitis nodularis helicis

☐ D Keratoacanthoma

☐ E Squamous cell carcinoma (SCC)

THEME: DIFFICULT PATIENTS

Options

A   Dependent clingers
B   Entitled demanders
C   Frequent attenders
D   Heartsink patient
E   Manipulative help rejector
F   Self-destructive denier
G   None of the above

For each of the descriptions below, select the most appropriate option from the list above. Each option may be used once, more than once or not at all.

141.   Often try to take control of the doctor–patient relationship.

142.   More commonly identified by male rather than by female GPs.

143.   Unconsciously engages in behaviour that is likely to be detrimental to the patient's own health.

144.   Seem to derive satisfaction from the physician's inability to treat their symptoms.

145.   An objective description that is medicolegally appropriate.

146. A 39-year-old schoolteacher complains that her right eye seems to be protruding more than the left. She has no visual symptoms or pain. Previous history is unremarkable other than chronic rhino-sinusitis for which she takes nasal steroids. On examination she does appear to have some asymmetry and proptosis. She saw her optician prior to this visit and has normal visual acuity, colour vision, fundoscopy and visual fields. She has no headache or any symptoms of hypothyroidism or hyperthyroidism. Blood tests, including thyroid function, are normal. What is the single most appropriate next step in her management?

- [ ] A   Check thyroid autoantibodies
- [ ] B   Check for anti-acetylcholine receptor antibodies
- [ ] C   Reassure her that this is normal
- [ ] D   Refer under the 2-week rule for suspected brain tumour
- [ ] E   Treat with broad-spectrum antibiotics

147. Your local water supply has been temporarily suspended due to the discovery of *Cryptosporidium* in a reservoir. A number of your patients have come to see you, concerned that they might have been exposed prior to the shutdown. Which one of the following statements is true regarding this situation?

- [ ] A   *Cryptosporidium* affects all age groups, causing severe diarrhoea and vomiting
- [ ] B   *Cryptosporidium* can be resistant to chlorination of water
- [ ] C   *Cryptosporidium* in children causes a mild diarrhoea that lasts less than 48 hours
- [ ] D   *Cryptosporidium* can cause haemoytic uraemic syndrome
- [ ] E   Humans are a secondary host and do not transmit the infection to others

THEME: TRAVEL MEDICINE

Options

A   Cholera

B   Dengue

C   Diphtheria

D   Hepatitis A

E   Hepatitis B

F   Hepatitis C

G   Japanese B encephalitis

H   Leishmaniasis

I   Meningitis A and C

J   Rabies

K   Schistosomiasis

L   Tetanus

M   Tuberculosis

N   Typhoid

O   Yellow fever

Regarding travel advice and immunisations, for each of the statements below select the single most appropriate option from the list above. Each option may be used once, more than once or not at all.

☐ **148.** Recommended for travellers staying in rural areas of India, Nepal and South-East Asia for more than 4 weeks during the rainy season.

☐ **149.** Recommended particularly for Hajj pilgrims.

☐ **150.** Evidence of vaccination is required for entry into many countries in Africa.

☐ **151.** Recommended particularly for travel to Russia.

☐ **152.** Requires pre- and post-exposure inoculations to be effective.

153. Which one of the following statements regarding hypertrophic obstructive cardiomyopathy (HOCM) is true?

A   The cause is usually viral
B   It is a cause of sudden death in young athletes
C   It is a benign condition
D   Treatment with β blockers will increase life expectancy
E   It usually presents with signs of congestive cardiac failure

154. Which of the following statements about the side effects of painkillers is true?

A   Buprenorphine cannot be taken with other opioids
B   Co-proxamol is toxic and is no longer available
C   Tramadol is not an opioid and is not associated with nausea or constipation
D   Transdermal fentanyl patches are not associated with constipation
E   Transdermal opioid patches do not reach steady-state analgesic levels for 24 hours

PAPER 1

155. A 25-year-old nulliparous woman complains of breakthrough bleeding most months on her 30-microgram COCP. She has been taking this for 12 months now, takes no other medications and does not miss pills. Examination is unremarkable and she recently had a cervical smear which was reported as negative. She does not get any post-coital bleeding and high vaginal swabs and chlamydial swabs were recently negative. Which one of the following is the most appropriate management?

- [ ] A Advise her to take two pills a day
- [ ] B Change to a triphasic pill
- [ ] C Change to the mini-pill for better cycle control
- [ ] D Suggest a Mirena intrauterine device (IUD)
- [ ] E Reassure her that this is normal and that no action is needed

156. Which one of the following statements about the management of problem drinking is true?

- [ ] A Acamprosate reduces the desire to drink
- [ ] B Antabuse (disulfiram) is safe to use in the community
- [ ] C Non-specialist interventions do not lead to statistically significant reductions in alcohol use
- [ ] D Only 10% of problem drinkers are abstinent at 1 year
- [ ] E The aim in managing problem drinking should always be abstinence

THEME: TREATMENT OF PROSTATE CANCER

Options

A   Brachytherapy

B   Cryotherapy

C   Cyproterone acetate

D   Docetaxel

E   External-beam radiotherapy

F   LHRH analogue

G   Orchidectomy

H   Radical prostatectomy

I   Watchful waiting

For each of the statements below regarding the management of prostate cancer, select the most appropriate option from the list above. Each option may be used once, more than once or not at all.

157.   Associated with a 10% risk of proctitis.

158.   Shown in the Scandinavian Prostate Cancer Group Study to be as effective as radical prostatectomy in terms of its effect on overall mortality.

159.   Indicated for non-hormone-sensitive recurrent disease in patients who have previously been treated with radiotherapy.

160.   Useful in patients with metastatic disease who cannot tolerate LHRH agonist treatment.

161.   Causes an initial increase in testosterone production.

162. **Which one of the following statements about gout is true?**

- [ ] A   Colchicine should be prescribed as 1 tablet every hour until the pain resolves or diarrhoea develops
- [ ] B   Dietary factors are the commonest triggers for an acute attack of gout
- [ ] C   Joint aspiration typically reveals cloudy fluid and this is diagnostic in larger joints
- [ ] D   Normal serum uric acid during an acute attack of arthritis excludes gout
- [ ] E   Patients who are intolerant of colchicine or NSAIDs should be treated with prednisolone

163. **A 27-year-old nulliparous woman has had a lump in her breast for several months. She has had no discharge or skin changes. On examination she has a firm, mobile, non-tender lump in the outer quadrant of her left breast, with no lumps in her axilla or supraclavicular area. What is the single most likely diagnosis?**

- [ ] A   Breast carcinoma
- [ ] B   Ductal carcinoma *in situ* (DCIS)
- [ ] C   Fibroadenoma
- [ ] D   Galactocele
- [ ] E   Paget's disease of the breast

164. **Regarding vaginal infections, which one of the following statements is true?**

- [ ] A   A fishy smell suggests candidal infection
- [ ] B   Bacterial vaginosis is always symptomatic
- [ ] C   Candidal infection is more common in pregnancy
- [ ] D   *Trichomonas* does not cause disease in men
- [ ] E   Where bacterial vaginosis is confirmed, the partner must also be treated to prevent re-infection

165. A pilot weight-loss clinic has been running for 12 months and the PCT would like to extend the service based on its results. The results are shown below (BMI, body mass index; CI, confidence interval; N/A, not applicable).

Time since start (months)	Number of patients	Mean weight change (kg)	95% CI	Mean BMI (kg/m²)
0	1500	N/A	N/A	32
1	1200	−2.6	−4.1 to +1.3	31
2	1000	−3.1	−3.9 to +0.5	29
3	900	−3.3	−3.4 to −1.8	28
6	600	−3.4	−3.6 to −2.5	28
12	300	−2.9	−3.2 to −2.6	29

Which one of the following statements about these data is correct?

- [ ] A On an intention-to-treat basis the data show a mean weight loss of −2.9 kg at 12 months

- [ ] B The data show a statistically significant weight loss at 3 months

- [ ] C The data show high levels of concordance

- [ ] D The majority of patients who complete 12 months' treatment achieve a normal BMI

- [ ] E Weight loss is maintained at 12 months in the majority of patients

THEME: ANTIHYPERTENSIVE MEDICATIONS

Options

A   Aliskiren

B   α Blocker

C   Angiotensin-converting enzyme inhibitor

D   Angiotensin II-receptor antagonist

E   β Blocker

F   Calcium-channel blocker

G   Methyldopa

H   Moxonidine

I   Thiazide diuretic

J   Verapamil

For each of the statements below regarding antihypertensive medication, select the most appropriate drug from the list of options above. Each option may be used once, more than once or not at all.

- ☐ **166. Associated with erectile dysfunction.**
- ☐ **167. Associated with stress incontinence.**
- ☐ **168. Can precipitate gout.**
- ☐ **169. Indicated for pregnancy-induced hypertension.**
- ☐ **170. First line treatment for African–Caribbean patients with essential hypertension.**

171. A 6-year-old girl comes to see you with her mother. She has been complaining of 6 months of intermittent pain in the right side of her groin and she has a persistent limp. She is otherwise well but seems to be limping most of the time. On examination she has a full range of movement on the left side of her hip but movements on the right side are limited in all directions. Examination of the groin reveals no hernia and no lymphadenopathy. Blood tests are taken which are normal. What is the single most likely diagnosis?

- [ ] A Congenital dislocation of the hip
- [ ] B Irritable hip
- [ ] C Perthe's disease
- [ ] D Septic arthritis
- [ ] E Slipped upper femoral epiphysis

172. Which one of the following statements regarding the management of osteopenia and osteoporosis is correct?

- [ ] A Bisphosphonates are only available in oral formulation
- [ ] B Bisphosphonates have been shown to increase bone density but not to reduce fractures
- [ ] C Patients diagnosed with osteoporosis should be investigated for coeliac disease
- [ ] D Patients diagnosed with post-menopausal osteoporosis should be treated with bisphosphonates for life
- [ ] E A T score < 1.5 is diagnostic of osteoporosis

173. Which one of the following statements regarding the management of Parkinson's disease is true?

☐ A Early treatment improves the long-term prognosis

☐ B Parkinson's disease is a purely motor disorder

☐ C Postural hypotension is a common symptom of Parkinson's disease

☐ D Ropinirole should be used as first-line treatment

☐ E The presence of hallucinations suggests concurrent mental illness

174. Which one of the following statements regarding evidence-based medicine is true?

☐ A Application of evidence-based practice results in cost savings

☐ B Evidence-based medicine involves statistical analysis of data

☐ C The advantage of evidence-based practice is that it requires no formal training or resources

☐ D The practice of evidence-based medicine is applicable to quantitative research as well as to qualitative research

☐ E Where there is a lack of robust evidence for a particular treatment it should not be pursued

THEME: MANAGEMENT OF ABNORMAL SMEARS

Options

A   Refer for colposcopy

B   Refer under 2-week rule

C   Repeat in 1 month

D   Repeat in 6 months

E   Repeat in 1 year

F   Repeat in 3 years

G   Repeat in 5 years

H   Smear no longer necessary

Regarding the management of cervical smear results, for each of the situations described below select the most appropriate management option from the list above. Each option may be used once, more than once or not at all.

- [ ] **175.** **A 34-year-old woman has had a smear reported as 'borderline, with endocervical changes'. She has not previously had abnormal smears.**

- [ ] **176.** **A 27-year-old woman with a history of previous chlamydial infection has had two consecutive inadequate smears.**

- [ ] **177.** **A 63-year-old woman who has not had any previous abnormal smears has a normal smear. She enquires about follow-up smears.**

- [ ] **178.** **A 36-year-old woman with no history of abnormal smears has a smear reported as showing mild dyskariosis.**

- [ ] **179.** **A 31-year-old woman has a smear which shows suspected carcinoma *in situ*.**

180. A 24-year-old girl attends for a new-patient check. She asks if there is anything else she can use for the rash on her arms. She has had this for most of her life and uses regular moisturisers; otherwise the skin becomes dry. She also reports that the rash improves when she is away from the stress of the office on holiday. The rash is shown below.

What would the single most appropriate management be in this instance?

- [ ] A   Prescribe topical steroids
- [ ] B   Prescribe topical tacrolimus
- [ ] C   Prescribe vitamin D analogues
- [ ] D   Refer for PUVA therapy
- [ ] E   Treat with antifungal treatment

181. A 17-year-old girl has a lump in her lower eyelid that has been present for 9 months and which is slowly enlarging. She reports that this started after she developed a stye, but she is becoming increasingly self-conscious and would like your advice on management. Which one of the following is the single most appropriate action?

- [ ] A   She should be offered incision and curettage
- [ ] B   She should be told that it is unlikely to resolve spontaneously
- [ ] C   She should be referred immediately to ophthalmology outpatients for excision
- [ ] D   She should be treated with antibiotic ointment
- [ ] E   She should be treated with cryotherapy

182. A 34-year-old unemployed man comes to you with a 3-month history of back pain. He reports that he has tried numerous drugs and a course of physiotherapy to no avail and would like to apply for incapacity benefit. Which one of the following statements is true regarding this situation?

- [ ] A   Absence from work for more than 4 weeks is associated with only a 20% chance of returning to work within 12 months
- [ ] B   Chiropractic is superior to physiotherapy in the management of chronic back pain
- [ ] C   Incapacity benefit rules require the patient to have been seen by a spinal specialist
- [ ] D   The presence of yellow flag symptoms should prompt referral
- [ ] E   There is no evidence for the benefit of 'back schools' in this situation

183. A 36-year-old woman with no previous history of note complains of nausea and vomiting with fever, followed by watery diarrhoea and abdominal pain, which started 12 hours after attending a wedding with a buffet reception. Which one of the following is the most likely organism responsible?

- ☐ A *Campylobacter*
- ☐ B *Cryptosporidium*
- ☐ C *Salmonella*
- ☐ D *Shigella*
- ☐ E Typhoid

184. With regard to cardiopulmonary resuscitation, which one of the following statements regarding the current guidelines (2005) is correct?

- ☐ A Automated external defbrillators (AEDs) should not be used on patients with pacemakers
- ☐ B Compression to ventilation ratio should be 10 to 1
- ☐ C Compression to ventilation ration should be 15 to 2
- ☐ D Compression to ventilation ratio should be 30 to 2
- ☐ E In cases of anaphylaxis, adrenaline (epinephrine) should be given down an endotracheal tube

185. A 78-year-old man complains of mid-thoracic backache for the last 3 months. He looks pale and has lost weight. On examination he has some tenderness over his 8th thoracic vertebra, but there are no other obvious signs. You arrange for some blood tests, which show raised plasma viscosity, a normochromic normocytic anaemia with normal WCC and platelets, a raised calcium, and an eGFR of 42 ml/minute. What is the single most likely diagnosis?

- [ ] A   Chronic lymphocytic leukaemia (CLL)
- [ ] B   Lung cancer
- [ ] C   Multiple myeloma
- [ ] D   Prostate cancer
- [ ] E   Sarcoma

186. A 32-year-old woman has recently been discharged from hospital after having a molar pregnancy. She comes to see you to discuss the implications of this diagnosis. Which one of the following statements is true?

- [ ] A   Ninety per cent of patients with a molar pregnancy will go on to develop neoplastic disease within 2 years
- [ ] B   Prognosis is poor In patients who develop neoplastic disease
- [ ] C   Patients should be monitored with regular β-hCG levels for 2 years
- [ ] D   Recurrence risk is high and patients should be advised to have sterilisation
- [ ] E   The COCP is suitable contraception in the β-hCG monitoring phase

THEME: THE MENTAL HEALTH ACT

Options

A   Section 2
B   Section 3
C   Section 4
D   Section 7
E   Section 12

F   Section 17
G   Section 135
H   Section 136
I   None of the above

For each of the situations described below, select the single most appropriate option from the list above. Each option may be used once, more than once or not at all.

187. A 23-year-old man who has been living with his mother has developed an addiction to heroin. He refuses treatment but his mother asks you to have him sectioned so that he can be treated.

188. A 77-year-old man is found confused and wearing only his pyjamas in the street in the middle of the night in early February. He is unable to give his name to the police or explain why he is there, but refuses to go with them. They feel he is at risk and would like to take him to a safe place.

189. A 31-year-old paranoid schizophrenic has stopped taking his medication and is refusing to leave the house where he lives with his mother. He has started to self-harm and will not see his doctor, who he believes is the devil.

190. A 52-year-old man with severe learning disabilities due to Down syndrome can no longer be looked after by his elderly mother, but refuses to go into a residential home. Social services have requested that he be admitted to one under the provisions of the Mental Health Act.

191. The 31-year-old paranoid schizophrenic has been assessed and treated in hospital and it is felt that he needs a further period of supervised patient treatment, but that this can be given in the community. He has a history of non-compliance and subsequent relapse.

THEME: MANAGEMENT OF HEAVY MENSTRUAL BLEEDING

Options

A   Contraceptive pill

B   Danazol

C   Fibroids present on ultrasound

D   Luteal phase progestogens

E   Mirena

F   Normal ultrasound

G   Refer routinely

H   Refer under the 2-week rule

I   Tranexamic acid

The algorithm below describes the management of women with heavy menstrual bleeding. From the list of options above, select the most appropriate management for each missing step. Each option may be used once, more than once or not at all.

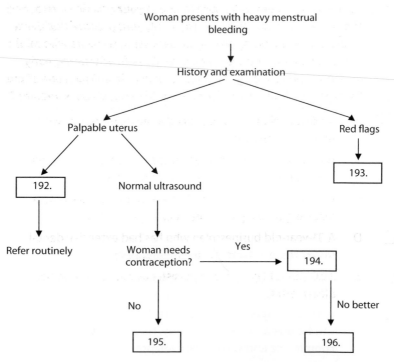

197. A 37-year-old man comes to see you with his new wife. They have only been married for 3 months but already she has had to resort to sleeping in the spare room because of his snoring. He has no symptoms or signs of sleep apnoea, and is otherwise well. On examination he has a collar size of 15 inches, a BMI of 27 kg/m² and examination of his nose and throat are normal. Which one of the following is the most appropriate action in this situation?

- [ ] A   Advise the patient that his snoring is harmless and no treatment is needed
- [ ] B   Check thyroid function
- [ ] C   Prescribe sedatives for his wife
- [ ] D   Refer for continuous positive airway pressure (CPAP) treatment
- [ ] E   Refer for uvulopalatoplasty (UVPP)

198. Following a needlestick injury to one of your practice nurses and the subsequent significant-event audit, your practice decides to undertake an active approach to identifying patients who might have hepatitis C. This would have the benefit of treating early infection and reducing the risk of transmission. Which one of the following patients are at risk and would benefit from screening?

- [ ] A   A 56-year-old man who worked as an oil worker in West Africa for many years
- [ ] B   A 23-year-old man who has recently returned from a year travelling in South-East Asia with a new tattoo
- [ ] C   A 38-year-old woman who had a 4-unit blood transfusion following a post-partum haemorrhage in 1988
- [ ] D   A 31-year-old businessman who has had extensive dental treatment in a dental facility in Singapore
- [ ] E   A 56-year-old man with a persistently raised GGT on his blood results

199. Which one of the following statements regarding the use of opioids in non-malignant chronic pain is correct?

- [ ] A Fentanyl patches should be considered when patients on codeine have adequate pain control but are experiencing significant side effects

- [ ] B Combination analgesics, eg co-codamol, do not offer additional benefits in terms of pain control but are associated with increased side effects

- [ ] C The use of strong opioids for chronic pain is frequently associated with withdrawal symptoms on reducing the dose

- [ ] D When titrating the dose of a strong opioid, eg morphine, a quantity of 5 mg MST tablets should be supplied to take on an as-required basis between morning and evening doses; a record should be kept of consumption and this can then be used to adjust the twice-daily dosage

- [ ] E Where a weak opioid (eg codeine) is ineffective an alternative weak opioid (eg dihydrocodeine) should be tried before a strong opioid

200. You are asked to give a talk to the local school about the hazards of recreational drug use. Which one of the following statements is true?

- [ ] A Cannabis use in the short term (less than 6 months) does not lead to psychological problems

- [ ] B Cocaine use is associated with cardiovascular and rhinological side effects but not psychological

- [ ] C Heroin use can cause heart failure

- [ ] D Ketamine use is associated with respiratory depression

- [ ] E Side effects from ecstasy use are due to water intoxication and can be avoided through limiting consumption

Paper 1
Answers

1.   B: Frozen shoulder is more common in patients with diabetes mellitus

Long-term studies suggest that only 39% of patients make a full recovery, although another 54% have no functional limitation despite a small reduction in mobility. Secondary frozen shoulder is rare, while diabetes increases the risk by up to 36%. Mean age of onset is 40–60 years. The diagnosis is essentially a clinical one, although X-rays or blood tests might be necessary to exclude other pathology if clinically suspected.

2.   D: Irregular bleeding is the commonest side effect of Implanon

Implanon capsules are inserted in the skin above the elbow and consist of a single capsule changed every 3 years, unlike Norplant, which consisted of five rods that were changed every 5 years. Irregular bleeding is common in Implanon users, and can be treated with the combined contraceptive pill or tranexamic acid in the first 6 months, after which it usually settles down. Acne is common, but there is no evidence of an effect on mood, weight or libido. Around 50% of women become amenorrhoeic on Implanon. After removal, blood levels of etonogestrel are undetectable within 1 week and ovulation occurs in 90% of women within 3 weeks. The implants are changed after 3 years and the pregnancy rate in users is less than 0.1 in 100 women over 3 years.

3.   J: Scope

Scope was formerly known as The Spastics Society and provides support on all levels to patients and their families who are suffering from the effects of cerebral palsy.

4.   E: Marie Curie

Marie Curie will often provide night-sitters for people close to the end of life, as well as providing emotional support.

5.   F: MIND

MIND will often act as the advocate for patients with mental illness and provide practical support during difficult times, as well as providing a mentoring role.

6.   D: Gingerbread

The Gingerbread charity provides support for one-parent families and might be able to help with respite in cases such as these.

7.   B: CLIC Sargent

CLIC Sargent provides support to patients with cancer under the age of 21 and their families. This support can be financial or in the form of respite.

8.   E: The readings suggest the presence of significant peripheral vascular disease affecting the right side only

The ABPI is 0.8 on the right side and 1.0 on the left. An ABPI of < 0.9 suggests the presence of significant peripheral vascular disease, while an ABPI < 0.8 suggests a risk of ulceration. Once the ABPI is < 0.5 this indicates critical ischaemia. ABPI readings > 1.0 can be seen where the patient is not supine or where there is reduced arterial compliance, as in atherosclerosis.

9.   C: Prodromal dermatomal pain is a risk factor for post-herpetic neuralgia

Risk factors for post-herpetic neuralgia include age > 50, prodromal pain, and severe pain and rash during the attack. Prompt use of antivirals reduces the incidence of post-herpetic neuralgia by up to 50%. Systematic review suggests the best evidence is for tricyclic antidepressants, while there is also evidence for anticonvulsants, 5% lidocaine plasters, opiates and capsaicin. Severe intractable pain might be helped by ketamine injections.

10. C: Reassure the parents that it will usually resolve spontaneously in time

This is a para-umbilical hernia. Spontaneous closure is the norm and surgery is only indicated if closure fails to occur. These are more common in African-Caribbean children and occur twice as commonly in boys as girls. Incarceration is uncommon below the age of 3 years, so there is usually no indication for surgical treatment below this age and 93% close without any intervention. Some surgeons advocate taping the skin over the hernia to bring the edges of the hernia together in an attempt to hasten closure, but this is not usually necessary.

11. H: Oral leukotriene receptor antagonist

Leukotriene receptor antagonists are of no value in acute asthma but have a role in the maintenance treatment of asthma. They also have some benefits in allergic rhinitis. They are licensed in children and can be useful as a steroid-sparing agent.

12. A: Combination of inhaled corticosteroid and long-acting β_2 agonist

The SMART (Symbicort as maintenance and reliever therapy) approach allows patients to self-manage their asthma according to their symptoms. It has been shown to reduce the use of oral steroids and the number of doctor consultations.

13. I: Oral theophylline

Theophylline is rarely used due to the risk of adverse effects, including arrythmias, nausea and diarrhoea. Particular care should be taken to ensure patients are not using inhaled theophylline before starting oral treatment due to the risk of toxicity.

14. **B:** **Inhaled anticholinergic**

Inhaled anticholinergics reduce vagal tone and have the benefit of reducing mucus secretion, which makes them useful in patients with chronic obstructive pulmonary disease.

15. **G:** **Oral corticosteroids**

Long-term (> 3 months) oral steroids at a dose greater than 5 mg a day should prompt the use of bisphosphonates to prevent osteoporosis. The Royal College of Physicians further recommends that three separate short courses over a 12-month period should be considered to be equivalent to 3 months' prescribing.

16. **E:** **Posterior cruciate tear**

The positive drawer test indicates a posterior cruciate tear. This injury is typically seen in patients who have received a blow to the proximal tibia with the knee flexed, for example in a road traffic accident or by falling onto a flexed knee. Management involves a splint initially, followed by physiotherapy. Anterior cruciate tears are associated with a positive anterior drawer test. In younger patients surgery is usually necessary, particularly in sportsmen. Patellar tendon tears result in an inability to extend the knee. Medial and lateral collateral tears are associated with laxity when the knee is stressed laterally or medially.

17. **D:** **She should take folic acid 5 mg once a day from pre-conception onwards**

Women who have taken anticonvulsants in the past remain at increased risk of fetal abnormalities, especially neural tube defects, and should be counselled accordingly. All epileptic women should take folic acid 5 mg a day rather than 400 micrograms a day. Phenytoin is associated with cleft lip and heart defects. There is no evidence that newer anticonvulsants are safer. Expert advice should be sought in epileptic women who are planning pregnancy so that they can be changed onto a regime with the lowest risk while minimising the risk of seizures in the changeover period.

18.   E: Patients with diabetes mellitus should have a total cholesterol of 4.0 mmol/l or less and an LDL of < 2.0 mmol/l

Recent NICE guidance suggested that patients with diabetes mellitus should be treated to a target of 4/2. The current (2008/9) QOF targets are a total cholesterol of 5.0 mmol/l, but this might be revised in future years. In the Heart Protection Study all patients were treated with 40 mg simvastatin with no further testing but the NICE guidance recommends treating to target. Patients with acute coronary syndromes should be treated with a high-intensity statin such as atorvastatin. Inegy, a combination of simvastatin and ezetimibe has been associated with increased risk of cancer in some studies. It is recommended for patients who cannot tolerate a sufficient dose of simvastatin to reach target levels.

19.   B: No action required

The presence of asymptomatic bacteriuria is common in catheterised patients and no action is necessary unless they are unwell. *Proteus* is often associated with urinary stones or foreign bodies. Replacing the catheter would increase the risks of infection by causing local trauma, and irrigation would simply flush bacteria into the bladder.

20.   C: Discuss the case with the coroner

Where a patient has not been seen in the last 14 days you cannot issue a death certificate without discussing the case with the coroner. In a situation such as this the coroner will usually allow a death certificate to be issued.

21.   A: Contact the police

Sudden deaths should be referred to the police who will arrange appropriate investigation and a post-mortem examination. You cannot issue a death certificate in this situation.

22.   C   Discuss the case with the coroner

Where industrial disease is implicated the employment box should be ticked on the death certificate and the coroner informed.

23.   C: Discuss the case with the coroner

Unnatural deaths should always be referred to the coroner.

24.   H: None of the above

A stillborn baby can only be certified on a Certificate of Stillbirth after 24 weeks of pregnancy. If the baby does breathe after birth, no matter what gestation, a neonatal death form should be used. This case should be referred to the obstetrics and gynaecology department to arrange investigation and appropriate counselling, and to liaise with the coroner.

25.   F: Issue Medical Certificate of Cause of Death

Death certificates do not require the doctor to have seen the body after death, as long as another medical practitioner has seen the body and confirmed death.

26.   E: SSRIs should be used as first-line treatment

Social phobia has a lifetime risk of 13% and is particularly common in women from lower social classes. Affected people experience feelings of panic in public situations and nausea and vomiting are common. Management comprises CBT where available and SSRIs in the short term. Benzodiazepines or β blockers can also help with crises.

27.   A: Admit under paediatrics

This patient has haemolytic uraemic syndrome, which may follow Escherichia coli O157 infection. Risk factors include extremes of age. Clinical suspicion should be raised in children with bloody diarrohea. Oliguria and dehydration are common and thrombocytopenic purpura can be seen. Treatment is supportive, although some patients need short-term dialysis.

28.   E: CBT should be offered to all patients with chronic fatigue syndrome

The diagnosis of chronic fatigue syndrome should be considered in patients with unexplained fatigue lasting more than 3 months in a child or 4 months in an adult. Chronic pain, sleep disturbance and cognitive difficulties are common. Exacerbations usually start 24–48 hours after exertion. The treatment of this condition involves graded exercise and CBT. The prognosis is extremely variable, with some patients making a quick recovery and others developing chronic disease. The disease has been reported to follow infection with a number of viruses, and it is estimated that 10% of patients with clinical Epstein–Barr virus infection will develop chronic fatigue syndrome.

29.   B: Episcleritis

Episcleritis is a localised, self-limiting condition affecting the sclera. Iritis can be excluded on examination and scleritis is usually a severe boring pain rather than a dull ache. Scleritis is usually bilateral and associated with connective tissue disease. The inflammation in episcleritis is usually limited to a small sector and typically settles over 7–10 days. Topical non-steroidal drops might accelerate this process and steroid drops are also helpful, but should only be given after expert assessment to exlude keratitis. Keratitis is usually obvious on fluorescein staining but a slit lamp should be used. Acute angle closure glaucoma usually causes stony-hard eyes and vomiting with severe pain.

30.   D: Clopidogrel 75 mg once daily should be taken for 12 months, then the patient should take aspirin 150 mg once a day for life

Following stent insertion patients should take clopidogrel for 12 months and then switch to aspirin.

31.   G: Poxvirus

Molluscum contagiosum causes crops to appear and spread through auto-inoculation. They are typically seen in the pre-school age-group and individual lesions can last from 2–3 weeks to several months. No specific treatment is needed and they regress spontaneously.

32.   C: *Mycoplasma pneumoniae*

Mycoplasma causes respiratory symptoms in young children and can be associated with erythema multiforme. These patients usually respond to oral macrolides, eg erythromycin.

33.   F: Parvovirus B19

Parvovirus B19 (also called erythrovirus B19) causes a mild, self-limiting disease in children but unexposed pregnant women can develop fetal hydrops as a result of this infection.

34.   A: Group A streptococci

Scarlet fever follows infection with β-haemolytic streptococci and can cause rheumatic fever or glomerulonephritis. Children should be treated with at least 10 days of penicillin V and excluded from school until the antibiotics are started.

35.   L: Varicella

Varicella need only be treated in adults, neonates or the immunocompromised.

36.   E: Ulcerative colitis

Ulcerative colitis often presents as an isolated proctitis and attacks can start after periods of stress. The diagnosis is usually made at proctoscopy, where a typical granular and ulcerated appearance is seen. Crohn's disease is the major differential in this age group but is often associated with piles or fistulas and tends to cause more systemic features. Management usually consists of rectal steroids or aminosalicylates; loperamide should not be used as it does not work and can increase the risk of toxic megacolon. Long-term management is usually with aminosalicylates. Patients with ulcerative colitis are at increased risk of colorectal cancer and should be screened regularly.

37.   D: Suction termination can be carried out under local anaesthesia

Mifepristone can be used for late abortions (> 15 weeks) with prostaglandin pessaries and is an alternative to surgical termination. It cannot be used in women with a history of cardiac or respiratory disease. Two doctors must sign the certificate before a termination can take place and if they feel that a patient is Gillick-competent the parents need not be informed. The legal limit for termination is 24 weeks but there is some debate about lowering this to 22 weeks. At present fewer than 1% of abortions take place after 20 weeks.

38.   E: Hyperthymic personality disorder

Hyperthymic personality is characterised by persistent enthusiasm and optimism that is associated with rash judgements (eg poor financial investments).

39.   C: Borderline personality disorder

Borderline personality disorders are typified by young men who frequently get drunk and are involved in fights or acts of vandalism. They are often lonely and crave company, but are unable to develop rewarding relationships.

40.   A: Anankastic personality disorder

Anankastic personality disorders show considerable overlap with obsessional neurosis and these people are often ill at ease in company and are very sensitive to criticism.

41.   F: Narcissistic personality disorder

Narcissistic personality types also are very sensitive to criticism, but are easily bored and have difficulty forming emotional attachments to others.

42.   H: Schizoid personality disorder

Schizoid personality types are typically seen as aloof or boring and are happiest in their own company.

43.   A: Employment Support Allowance always requires a personal capability assessment

Patients who are registered blind are usually entitled to Disability Living Allowance but do not automatically have a right to incapacity benefit. Individual cases are assessed on their merits, and the mobility component is based on mobility difficulties rather than on physical disability. A Med 5 certificate is used for patients who have been seen by the treating physician but where he has not given a sick certificate, for example a patient presenting to her GP for a sick note after being discharged from hospital after a hysterectomy where the gynaecologist didn't give a sick note. Med 4 certificates are used to certify people awaiting a personal capability assessment. During the first 6 months a Med 3 can only be issued up to 6 months, after which they can be indefinite. An ESA 113 form can be used by GPs for patients who are too severely incapacitated to attend an assessment.

44.   C: Deep vein thrombosis

DVT is a complication of pacemaker placement and should be treated with tinzaparin and warfarinisation, as for other thromboembolic disease. Cellulitis or wound infection should be considered in the differential but would be unusual in the absence of fever. Arterial embolism would normally cause pain, pulselessness and pallor.

45.   C: Fasting venous glucose of 8.3 mmol/l

The WHO criteria require a positive history and a fasting glucose > 7.0 mmol/l or a random venous glucose level > 11.1 mmol/l. After an oral glucose tolerance test, a 2-hour level of > 11.1 mmol/l is diagnostic. The diagnosis cannot be made on capillary or urinary testing.

46.   A: Ciclosporin can be used in this patient

Oral steroids and prolonged use of topical potent steroids have unacceptable side effect profiles. Retinoids are teratogenic and this effect can persist for up to 2 years, making them unsuitable for young women or for those wishing to start a family. UV treatments are effective but can cause cataracts and skin cancers.

47.   C: Omalizumab (Xolair)

Omalizumab is useful in allergy-mediated asthma. Patients need to have elevated IgE levels, and it is not suitable for other forms of asthma. It is given by regular injection.

48.   B: Natalizumab (Tysabri)

Natalizumab acts on T cells to reduce severity of symptoms in multiple sclerosis. It is licensed as monotherapy for relapsing MS and is given by injection. It can reduce the frequency of attacks and slow down the accumulation of disability. It might also be helpful in Crohn's disease.

49. **A: Infliximab (Remicade)**

NICE guidance recommends the use of infliximab for severe psoriasis (a Psoriasis Area Severity Index > 20) in patients not responding to or not suitable for PUVA or ciclosporin and other systemic treatments. It also has a role in acute Crohn's disease and in rheumatoid arthritis.

50. **F: Trastuzumab (Herceptin)**

Trastuzumab acts on the HER2 receptors on malignant cells, and is accordingly licensed for HER2-positive patients. It reduces the risk of early recurrence by 50%. NICE recommends its use following surgery, chemotherapy and radiotherapy if appropriate. It can cause congestive cardiac failure and cardiac work-up is required.

51. **D: Ranibizumab (Lucentis)**

Ranibizumab is licensed for wet macular degeneration and is given as an injection into the eye. It has been shown to stabilise eyesight in the majority of patients and 30–40% of patients experience an improvement in their visual acuity.

52. **C: Surgery is indicated in patients who do not wish to take long-term medication**

Indications for surgery include severe oesophagitis, long-term complications, and inability or unwillingness to take long-term medication. Surgical options include laparoscopic fundoplication, laparoscopic placement of a silastic prosthesis or use of the falciform ligament to reduce the hernia and maintain it, and open fundoplication. Long-term follow-up studies suggest that about a third of patients need proton-pump inhibitors after surgery, compared to two-thirds of patients managed medically. Surgery is useful in sliding and rolling hernias; rolling hernias are more likely to obstruct. Patients should be able to eat normally after surgery.

53. **B:** **Patients aged under 40 with one episode of unexplained venous thromboembolism should be screened**

Thrombophillia can be due to factor V Leiden, protein C or protein S deficiency or lupus anticoagulant. Patients should be screened if they have an unexplained venous thrombosis below the age of 40, below the age of 60 with an affected first-degree relative, below the age of 60 with an unusual site (eg mesenteric vein), or in recurrent miscarriage. Patients aged under 40 with arterial thromboses (eg stroke) should also be tested for thrombophillia. Lupus anticoagulant and anti-cardiolipin are acquired disorders.

54. **D:** **Methotrexate frequently causes menstrual disturbances**

Full blood count and LFTs should be done pre-treatment, after the initial dose and after dose changes. Once stable they can be done every 2–3 months. Falls in WCC and platelets, or increase in LFTs by a threefold factor or more should prompt cessation. A mild increase in LFTs is common but a fall in albumin of > 5 g/l is an early sign of liver toxicity. Folic acid is given on the 6 days a week when methotrexate is not taken. Methotrexate is teratogenic.

55. **A:** **Asperger syndrome**

This child has typical features of Asperger's. Children with this condition have a specific impairment in social functioning but have a normal IQ and often excel in certain areas. Patients can have a normal vocabulary but struggle with abstract language and metaphors, and have significant difficulties interpreting and using non-verbal communication.

56. **G:** **Royal College of General Practitioners Roadmap**

The RCGP Roadmap acknowledges the challenges that are faced by general practice but suggests that, rather than following the Darzi model of polyclinics, individual practices come together in federations to share services along the lines of GP cooperatives which formerly delivered out-of-hours care.

57.   I: Tooke Report

The Tooke Report was commissioned after problems with applications for speciality training. One of the key recommendations for primary care was that after the F1 year trainees would apply for 3 years of hospital specialty training and then 2 years in general practice, with training overseen by NHS: Medical Education England, who are responsible to the Chief Medical Officer.

58.   C: Darzi Review

The key aspirations of the Darzi Review were to increase access both in terms of opening hours and provision of health centres in deprived areas, and to increase access to specialists in the community.

59.   D: Good Doctors, Safer Patients

The CMO's report proposes that there will be two tiers of regulation, a local one administered by PCTs, who will be responsible for maintaining registers of approved GPs and dealing with complaints, and the GMC who will deal with more serious issues. Where necessary, referrals to the GMC will now be handled by an independent investigative panel before being judged by the GMC, thus separating the roles of investigator and adjudicator. There will be a simultaneous reduction in the standard of proof from 'beyond reasonable doubt' to 'the balance of probability'.

60.   B: Carson Report

The Carson Report into out-of-hours care attempted to redefine out-of-hours care from the patient's perspective. It proposed a model in which NHS Direct would handle all telephone calls and triage them appropriately to a number of different out-of-hours providers, including mental health, dental and medical organisations. It also instigated rigorous care standards for out-of-hours providers.

61. A: Cinnarazine is an effective treatment

Hyoscine is the most effective treatment, especially when used as a patch. Cinnarazine and promethazine are helpful but promethazine causes sedation and for most patients this limits its use, although it may be useful in children. Patients should be advised to stay on-deck where possible, with a view of the horizon, and to try and stay in the middle of the boat where motion is minimal. Alcohol, heavy meals and pungent odours can exacerbate symptoms. Homeopathic treatments might be effective but trials have not shown any benefit from acupressure bands.

62. D: Quantiferon testing is the investigation of choice in screening contacts

Quantiferon is a highly sensitive and specific test for TB-sensitised T cells and patients with a positive test should be given chemoprophylaxis. Heaf testing is suitable for mass screening of populations while Mantoux testing is more specific and is a better choice for screening healthcare workers where quantiferon is not available, although false positives can occur. Chest X-rays will only pick up pulmonary TB. Heaf testing might be positive in patients who have had avian TB or previous BCG vaccination.

63. B: In the elderly, hypnotics are twice as likely to cause adverse effects as they are to improve sleep

A meta-analysis in the *BMJ* (Glass et al., Sedative hypnotics in older people with insomnia: meta-analysis of risks and benefits. *BMJ* 2005; 331: 1169.) concluded that adverse effects were particularly likely in the elderly. Z-drugs have a rapid onset of action and shorter half-lives than benzodiazepines and so are less likely to cause hangover, but this symptom, together with tolerance and addiction are risks of all hypnotics. Hypnotics and alcohol produce sedation but not restful sleep.

64.   E: Refer immediately to the emergency department for X-ray

This patient has symptoms of a fractured fibula, commonly seen after a fall wearing ski boots or inline skates. The common peroneal nerve might be damaged, causing numbness over the lateral border of the foot and weak dorsiflexion. Surgery might be necessary to keep the fibula reduced. Undisplaced fractures of the mid-shaft might not need a cast but where there are signs of damage to the common peroneal nerve this should be treated actively to avoid lasting disability.

65.   G: Diverticulitis

This pattern of recurring attacks of left iliac fossa pain is usually due to diverticulitis. Colonic cancer would be the main differential in this age group and can be differentiated on barium enema or colonoscopy. In younger patients, irritable bowel syndrome can cause similar symptoms.

66.   K: Renal colic

Renal colic tends to radiate to the scrotum or labia and typically comes in waves. Dipstick testing usually shows haematuria.

67.   E: Crohn's disease

Crohn's usually starts in the terminal ileum or proximal colon and a mass can form in this part of the bowel. Diarrhoea, weight loss and fever are common. Diagnosis is usually made on endoscopy.

68.   C: Acute cholecystitis

Referred pain to the shoulder is usually a sign of diaphragmatic irritation, in this case due to inflammation of the gallbladder. Ectopic pregnancy or chlamydial perihepatitis should also be considered as possible causes in women. In cholecystitis there is right upper quadrant tenderness that is worse on inspiration.

69. H: Gastric carcinoma

Progressive dysphagia with weight loss suggests a diagnosis of gastric or oesophageal cancer. An epigastric mass might be palpable and hepatomegaly is common.

70. A: Ezetimibe has been reported to be associated with an increased risk of cancer

The SEAS (Simvastatin and Ezetimibe in Aortic Stenosis) trial looked at use of ezetimibe in combination with simvastatin in patients with mild aortic stenosis. It found no significant reduction in cardiovascular endpoints but did find increased incidence of all cancers. Ezetimibe is a cholesterol absorption inhibitor that has been shown in trial data to reduce low-density lipoproteins (LDL) but it did not reduce clinical endpoints. Patients with a mixed hyperlipidaemia should be treated with a statin initially. Macrolides and antifungals interact with simvastatin and atorvastatin and should be used with caution in all patients on statins. Sleep problems are common, and there are increasing reports of impotence with statins. Patients with familial hyperlipidaemias should be treated to target.

71. E: Topical NSAIDs are effective in relieving pain

Most women require only reassurance that they do not have breast cancer. Where symptoms have started after initiation of the pill or HRT, this should be reviewed. The condition is unaffected by pregnancy. Suppression of the ovarian hormonal axis with LHRH analogues will cure symptoms but the side effects do not justify treatment. Symptoms usually cease at the menopause. Soft support bras, worn at night, and topical NSAIDs are the most effective treatments, and some women find increased dietary soya to be helpful. There is no evidence of benefit from evening primrose oil.

PAPER 1

72.   C: Clinically asymptomatic cancers are being diagnosed earlier

The most likely explanation for the increase in cancer diagnoses over a short period is improved case-finding. The time-course is too short for a change in true prevalence and prostate cancer has a long lead-time before symptoms appear. The lack of change in the death rate suggests that these cancers are not associated with reduced life expectancy, ie they are being diagnosed earlier but treatment and individual life expectancy is the same. Changes in life expectancy with new treatments can only be compared on a case-control basis. Advances in treatment might have led to improved life expectancy for individual patients, but many patients are treated with watchful waiting and die of other causes.

73.   A: The trial demonstrated significant benefits in treating hypertensive patients with calcium antagonists and ACE inhibitors compared with β blockers and thiazides

The ALLHAT study showed that thiazides were as effective as calcium antagonists and ACE inhibitors in preventing coronary heart disease. The ASCOT study showed that aggressive treatment with calcium antagonist followed by ACE inhibitor was significantly superior to β blockade followed by thiazide for overall mortality, stroke and diabetes. The study was a primary prevention study involving hypertensive patients with at least one other risk factor.

74.   A: Glossopharyngeal neuralgia

Glossopharyngeal neuralgia is less common than trigeminal neuralgia but causes similar symptoms in the distribution of the glossopharyngeal nerve. Initial assessment should aim to exclude facial nerve involvement, tonsillar tumour and herpes zoster. Treatment usually aims to provide reassurance and avoidance of trigger factors where possible. Anticonvulsants can be helpful in some cases.

75.   A: Clopidogrel

Clopidogrel should be used when aspirin is genuinely contraindicated. Warfarin is only indicated if patients are found to be in atrial fibrillation or have other risk factors which require anticoagulation. There is no evidence that the combination of dipyridamole and clopidogrel is more effective than clopidogrel alone. Where patients are experiencing dyspepsia with aspirin, co-prescription of a proton-pump inhibitor should be tried.

76.   C: Retrospective studies are quicker to conduct than prospective studies

Retrospective studies are more prone to bias but are cheaper and quicker to conduct. They have the advantage that the two groups are known to have different rates of a disease, whereas prospective studies do not have this advantage. It is not uncommon for an intervention group and a control group to have a statistically insignificant difference in event rates at the end of a long and expensive trial.

77.   E: Diclofenac gel

Solar keratosis can be treated with 5-fluorouracil, cryotherapy or diclofenac gel. Imiquod can be useful in refractory lesions.

78.   I: Tacrolimus

Topical tacrolimus is licensed as a steroid-sparing agent in the treatment of eczema.

79.   H: Roaccutane

Roaccutane is particularly useful in older women whose acne is often unresponsive to antibacterials. It should not be given to women who could be pregnant as it is teratogenic, and adequate contraception is necessary.

80.   G: PUVA

PUVA (psoralen plus UVA) is effective for all forms of psoriasis. It can cause erythema and irritation. Combination with other treatments such as calcipotriol reduces the amount of radiation required.

81.   D   Dermovate

Dermovate is a high-potency steroid that is suitable for short-term treatment of psoriasis and eczema that is not responding to treatment with milder steroids. It should be applied for a maximum of 4 weeks and a maximum of 50 g should be applied per week.

82.   E: Refer directly to the antenatal unit for biophysical profile

Reduced fetal movements are a common concern in the third trimester. Mothers should be asked to choose a set time every day and record how long it takes to feel ten movements. If these are not felt she should be referred to the antenatal unit for a biophysical profile, comprising cardiotocography (CTG), ultrasound examination of liquor volume, fetal tone, movements and breathing movements, giving a numerical score with 10 the maximum. If the score is between 0 and 2 immediate delivery is indicated, while a score of 8 or more is normal.

83.   E: Use of opioid or combination analgesics is associated with an increased risk of medication-overuse headache compared with use of non-opioid analgesics

First-line treatment for tension-type headache should be a non-steroidal. Where analgesics are taken on more than 15 days a month there is a risk of overuse headache, which is more common with opioid or combination treatments. Amitriptyline should be the first-line prophylactic but patients should be warned about sedation and the dose should be titrated slowly.

84.   B: Avoidance of nail rubbing

This condition is seen in people under stress who rub their thumbnails, causing typical central nail damage. Where this condition is unilateral, trauma to the nail bed should be considered. In fungal nail infections the infection normally starts distally, with discoloration of the nail, while a low calcium level causes brittle nails. Reassurance alone will not improve the condition and sometimes CBT might be appropriate to break up the stress response.

85.   D: Lymphoedema

Lymphoedema is a common incurable complicaton of breast cancer surgery, particularly where this involves axillary clearance. The arm is typically oedematous with no erythema and with non-pitting oedema. Infection can develop and fibrosis is common. Management involves elevation and massage, and four-layer bandaging followed by compression hosiery can be effective. Lymphoma would not normally affect a whole arm, while cellulitis and DVT are usually associated with erythema and tenderness.

86.   D: Start a smoking cessation programme and repeat the blood tests in 4 weeks

This pattern of blood results usually reflects secondary polycythaemia due to chronic hypoxia from COPD and smoking. Smoking cessation might be sufficient to bring his haemoglobin back to normal limits. If this fails to occur he should be investigated to confirm whether this is primary or secondary polycythaemia. Primary polycythaemia is associated with the *JAK2* mutation and can be tested in most laboratories. The mainstay of management is venesection once secondary causes have been addressed.

87.   C: Suggest she sees another doctor at the practice

GMC guidelines state that you should avoid treating people you are close to. Obviously, in life-or-death situations this can be waived but convenience is not a reason to enter into a clinical situation where one's judgement might be impaired. If one has serious concerns about patient safety it would be appropriate to raise these but clash of personalities is not an appropriate reason to instigate a complaint. GMC guidance further recommends that you should only provide treatment where you have adequate knowledge of the patient's health, and in the scenario described here there could be issues in your mother's medical history of which you are unaware.

88.   E   Maltoma

Non-Hodgkin's lymphoma affecting the mucosal associated lymphoid tissue (MALT) of the stomach is the commonest non-epithelial malignancy of the stomach and accounts for 3% of stomach tumours. These tumours are associated with _H. pylori_ infection and in low-grade tumours regression can occur after eradication of the infection.

89.   A: Achalasia

Achalasia is due to failure of relaxation of the gastro-oesophageal junction, resulting in progressive dilatation of the oesophagus. Regurgitation is common and many patients develop aspiration pneumonia. The symptoms progress more slowly than oesophageal cancer but often cause chronic malnourishment. In South America this condition is often seen in association with cardiomegaly in Chagas' disease, a trypanosomal infection.

90.   B: Barrett's oesophagus

Barrett's oesophagus is associated with a small risk of developing cancer and many authorities advocate routine endoscopic surveillance. The presence of dysplasia in biopsies is suspicious but at repeat endoscopy 75% of these will have resolved. Where this has not occurred surgery should be considered.

91.   H: Oesophageal stricture

Oesophageal stricture is usually caused by acid reflux and often presents as bolus obstruction, but upper gastrointestinal endoscopy and biopsy are manadatory to exclude an underlying malignancy. Dilation can be carried out at the time of endoscopy.

92.   I: Plummer–Vinson syndrome

Plummer–Vinson syndrome (also know as Patterson–Brown–Kelly syndrome) causes an oesophageal web and therefore dysphagia, together with iron-deficiency anaemia. It is associated with a significant increase in risk of oesophageal cancer.

93.   D: Mirena coils are the most effective medical treatment for menorrhagia

In the 1990s the hysterectomy rate was around 60%, but the introduction of Mirena coils and endometrial ablation has revolutionised the management of menorrhagia. Current NICE guidance recommends Mirena as the first-line medical treatment, although many patients prefer to try oral medication first. Tranexamic acid, the combined oral contraceptive and norethisterone all have a place, but danazol and luteal-phase progestogens do not. LHRH analogues are effective in the short term (eg pre-hysterectomy) but are not suitable in the long term. Endometrial ablation is effective but causes infertility. Examination to exclude fibroids might require imaging.

94.   C: Each child has a 0% chance of being affected

Huntington's disease is an autosomal dominant trait which presents in middle age. Children of affected parents therefore have a 50% risk of inheriting the gene (assuming the named parent is indeed the biological parent) and in time of becoming affected. If they are affected they will therefore have a 50% chance of passing the disease to each of their children, but if they are unaffected they will not have any risk of being a carrier or of developing the disease.

95.   E: Ultraviolet light used at the onset of symptoms will abort the attack

Cold sores are caused by reactivation of latent herpes simplex in the trigeminal ganglion, rather than primary infection. Attacks are often triggered by ultraviolet. There is no evidence that topical aciclovir is effective but there is some evidence of efficacy for oral aciclovir. However oral aciclovir is expensive and is not considered cost-effective. Where attacks are triggered by UV light, sunscreens might be effective. Small hand-held ultraviolet light emitters are available on FP10 to be used at the onset of tingling and have been shown to abort or shorten the duration of an attack.

96.   B   De Quervain's tenosynovitis

De Quervain's tenosynovitis is inflammation of the extensor pollicis brevis and abductor pollicis longus tendons. Finkelstein's test is positive if resisted abduction is painful. Treatment is usually steroid injection and a splint, but surgical decompression might be required in chronic cases. Carpal tunnel syndrome causes pain on pressure over the carpal tunnel (Tinel's test) or through forced flexion of the wrist (Phalen's test). Medial and lateral epicondylitis cause tenderness over the medial and lateral epicondyles respectively.

97.   B: Pelvi-ureteric junction obstruction is more common in patients with duplex ureters

Duplex ureter is seen in 0.2% of live births, and is more common in patients with a positive family history. It is usually picked up on antenatal ultrasound but in older patients might be discovered on routine ultrasound scanning. PUJ obstruction and urinary tract infection are more common in patients with this condition and this might require active management. Surgery is seldom necessary.

98.   **E:**   **Refer under the 2-week rule**

This child has symptoms of retinoblastoma and should be referred under the 2-week rule. Early treatment carries a good prognosis because these tumours tend to metastasise late. Any child with new-onset squint, leukocoria or uveitis needs urgent assessment. The condition is familial and often there will be an affected first-degree relative.

99.   **A:**   **Bimanual examination**

This lady has symptoms of an ovarian tumour and abdominal examination alone will miss pelvic tumours. Vaginal examination is mandatory in these cases and where a mass is found referral under the 2-week rule is indicated. Ovarian tumours are often clinically silent in their early stages, only becoming apparent when they reach sufficient size to cause pressure effects or ascites and a high index of suspicion should be maintained in patients with new symptoms, particularly those affecting the bladder or bowel, or those who have clinical evidence of ascites.

100.   **B:**   **IgA nephropathy**

IgA nephropathy is the underlying pathology in 50% of cases of recurrent frank haematuria. It is usually seen in children and young adults and is more common in boys. Episodes are usually triggered by viral infections and usually resolve over days or weeks. Oral steroids are often used. Most patients have a good prognosis, but 15–20% of patients go on to develop chronic renal failure. Poor prognosis is associated with heavy proteinuria and hypertension. Bladder cancer would be very unusual in this age group. Wilms' tumours usually present in infancy and are palpable on examination as a flank mass, with microscopic haematuria. Polycystic kidneys are usually evident from birth in children, or develop in adulthood in the case of adult polycystic kidney disease.

101.   D: Traumatic depigmentation

Long-term eczema can result in lichenification (thickening of the skin), thinning due to long-term steroid use or loss of pigment due to scratching. Vitiligo can produce a similar appearance but is usually evident elsewhere. Tinea causes colour changes but there is usually scaling. Drug reactions usually cause darker macules.

102.   E: Presence of cataracts

The Guthrie test is done shortly after birth and involves taking a heel-prick test for congenital hypothyroidism. Coordination and patch-testing are done at a later date when these skills have started to develop, usually by health visitors at the 8-month and 18-month checks and by an orthoptist around the age of 3 years. Newborn babies all have oto-acoustic emission testing shortly after birth. Congenital cataracts must be picked up early to avoid amblyopia.

103.   D: Optic neuritis

This patient is suffering from retrobulbar neuritis, usually caused by multiple sclerosis. Papilloedema typically causes a peripheral visual field loss with normal acuity. CRVO usually causes engorgement of the retinal veins and a sunset appearance of the retina. Acute glaucoma causes severe pain in the eye, while amaurosis fugax causes retinal pallor and loss of vision in the whole eye and lasts for seconds or minutes.

104.   E: His TSH should be < 0.01 µU/l

Patients with a previous history of thyroid cancer should be treated until they have a TSH < 0.01 µU/l to prevent stimulation of any residual thyroid tissue. Often this requires high doses of levothyroxine than are normally used but there is no set dose and the dose should be given at the lowest level that suppresses TSH, to avoid excess symptoms of hyperthyroidism. T_4 and T_3 levels do not need to be measured because the goal of treatment is suppression of TSH rather than biochemical euthyroidism.

105. **I:** **Standard deviation**

Standard deviation.

106. **D:** **Odds ratio**

The odds ratio is the ratio of the risk for a condition in one group compared with another.

107. **E:** *p* value

A *p* value of < 0.05 is generally accepted as the threshold of statistical significance, ie the risk of the finding occurring by chance is 1:20.

108. **C:** **Incidence**

The incidence is the rate of new diagnoses; the prevalence is the number of people suffering from a condition at a given time.

109. **H:** **Specificity**

Specificity is the number of true negatives; sensitivity is the number of true positives.

110. **D:** **There is a 1% annual risk of developing malignancy in patients with Barrett's oesophagus**

Barrett's oesophagus is metaplastic change in the distal oesophagus caused by longstanding acid reflux. There is a 1% annual risk of malignant transformation and many centres carry out routine surveillance. Treatment is of the underlying reflux, with medication and lifestyle measures. Photodynamic therapy is available in some centres. There is no association between *H. pylori* and Barrett's oesophagus.

111.   A: Acupuncture can be effective in relieving pain

Acupuncture has been shown to benefit pain and function. All patients should be advised to take regular aerobic exercise and a referral to physiotherapy is often helpful in developing specific exercises. Topical NSAIDs have been shown to be effective. There is some evidence for glucosamine and it can be prescribed on an FP10. Steroid injections can be beneficial in the short term, for example for acute flares, but repeated injections should be avoided due to the risk of cartilage damage.

112.   A: Acute angle closure glaucoma

This is a typical history of acute angle closure glaucoma. On examination the pupil is often fixed in a semi-dilated position and is oval. The eye feels stony-hard and the pain is extreme. Cluster headache can cause pain localised around the eye but is not usually associated with fixation of the pupil. Anyone with a temporal headache should be examined to exclude temporal arteritis. Migraine would not normally cause pupillary changes and subarachnoid haemorrhage causes a more generalised headache with no loss of vision, although cranial nerve lesions can be seen.

113.   A: Cellulitis

D-Dimer is an acute phase protein and a low-level increase in combination with a raised CRP and neutrophil count suggests infection rather than clot. Where CRP and white cell count are normal, an ultrasound or venogram is often necessary to rule out clot. A ruptured Baker's cyst should be considered in the differential for a DVT but can only be diagnosed on ultrasound at the time of imaging the veins. Varicose eczema is unlikely in the absence of history or signs of venous hypertension.

114.   B: Lifestyle measures are important in the management of recurrent migraine

Triggers (eg menses, food, stress, lack of sleep) should always be explored in patients with recurrent migraine and avoidance of any obvious triggers explored. Triptans are effective but should not be used in those with cardiovascular risk factors or in the under-12s. First-line prophylactic treatment is with β blockers, while valproate and topiramate can be used if these are ineffective. Ergotamine cannot be used with triptans, although NSAIDs can, and many patients find diclofenac suppositories helpful.

115.   D: Extrinsic allergic alveolitis

This patient has symptoms of farmer's lung, an acute extrinsic allergic alveolitis. Symptoms typically come on 4–8 hours after exposure to fungal spores and in time the condition can progress to pulmonary fibrosis. Similar symptoms are seen with bird fanciers, maltworkers and mushroom farmers. An occupational history is vital in diagnosing these patients. Management is with avoidance and with steroids if severe. Bronchiectasis would tend to present with recurrent chest infections from childhood, while pulmonary fibrosis would usually be associated with chronic rather than relapsing and remitting symptoms, and clubbing.

116.   B: The combined oral contraceptive has a number needed to treat of 5 for management of primary dysmenorrhoea

A Bandolier review found that, in general, NSAIDs are the most effective treatment, with ibuprofen having the best risk to benefit ratio. Aspirin was the least effective. COX-2 inhibitors are effective, with good tolerability. There is no evidence to support the use of spinal manipulation and paracetamol has very weak efficacy in pain relief in this condition.

117.   E: Where a partnership agreement does not exist, the partnership can be terminated at any time by one of the partners

Where no formal partnership agreement exists, the partnership is considered a 'partnership at will' and can be terminated at any time without prior discussion. A partnership agreement should include all names and profit shares and therefore should be updated with all partnership changes. All decisions are by a majority, unless specified in the partnership agreement. Non-GP partners are legal, but might require complex calculations regarding remuneration.

118.   F: Socratic

119.   B: Counselling

120.   D: Heuristic

121.   C: Didactic

Didactic teaching is the traditional form of medical school teaching typified by lectures. The Socratic approach encourages the learner to become more self-aware and the role of the teacher is to raise this self-awareness, while the heuristic approach aims to empower the learner to practice lifelong self-directed learning. The counselling style is particularly useful for mentoring roles. A detailed discussion on this subject can be found in Roger Neighbour's book, *The Inner Apprentice*.

122. **D:** The ADVANCE trial showed that addition of perindopril and indapamide to the treatment of patients with diabetes, regardless of the presence of hypertension, reduces the risk of cardiovascular events

Metformin can be used with glitazones or sulphonyureas, but should be used with caution in those with renal impairment or heart failure. Glitazones should not be used in people with heart failure. They have been shown to reduce HbA1c but not reduce clinical endpoints. The ACCORD study looked at intensive treatment to an HbA1c of < 6.0% compared with usual care and found an increase in adverse events, including death.

123. **C:** The earliest possible fertile ovulation is around 28 days post-partum

Ovulation precedes the onset of a period so patients should be advised not to have unprotected sex before their first period after childbirth. The pill should not be used in the early post-partum phase due to the risk of thromboembolism. In the absence of breastfeeding, the earliest the pill should be considered is 21 days, but patients who have suffered from HELLP syndrome or pregnancy-induced hypertension are at increased risk of thrombosis and should not start the COCP until biochemically normal and normotensive. The COCP interferes with breastfeeding, so the mini-pill is a better choice in lactating mothers. Mothers should be warned that breastfeeding has poor efficacy as a contraceptive.

124. **E:** Red flag symptoms

125. **B:** GP management

126. **H:** Review in 2 weeks

127. **D:** Physiotherapy

128.   G: Refer to secondary care

129.   C: He should have an MMR booster immediately

A single dose of MMR confers immunity in 70–85% of patients. In the case of an outbreak, a booster dose is recommended which will boost coverage to 95%, and can be given from 4 weeks after the previous dose. Single measles vaccines are not licensed or available in the UK. Failure to vaccinate with the booster at this time makes him prone to infection and carriage of the vaccine. Where children have received a booster before the age of 18 months, the usual pre-school booster should also be given because response below the age of 18 months can be suboptimal.

130.   D: It can be associated with palpitations

The typical patient with mitral valve prolapse is a young slim woman. It is frequently asymptomatic and is often picked up on routine examination as a diastolic murmur or systolic click. It is associated with atypical chest pain and palpitations, and rarely causes congestive cardiac failure or embolic phenomena. Beta blockers or antiplatelet therapy might be indicated. Patients with no other abnormalities on echocardiography and no other cardiac risk factors have a long-term survival rate similar to that of the general population.

131.   D: Nasal polyps

Nasal polyps are by far the commonest cause of reduced smell and taste. Tumours of the frontal lobe, meningiomas or ethmoid tumours are all very rare and are usually associated with other symptoms. Overuse of decongestants causes rhinitis rather than loss of smell. Nasal polyps can cause reduced sense of smell without complete nasal obstruction and are often not visible without a Thudichum speculum. A trial of steroids, either nose drops or orally, will produce a dramatic improvement if nasal polyps are the cause. They can be removed surgically, but 50% recur within 2 years.

132.   G: *Mycoplasma* pneumonia

Mycoplasma pneumonia causes a flu-like respiratory illness that affects children. It can be associated with erythema multiforme, myalgia and diarrohea. Treatment is with a macrolide or tetracycline for 10–14 days.

133.   F: Measles

Measles starts with a prodromal illness with respiratory symptoms and can go on to develop into pneumonia in around 1 in 6 patients, with bronchiectasis as a late complication.

134.   A: Aspergillosis

Aspergillosis tends to affect people with HIV or on immunosupressants or the chronically ill. It is usually diagnosed in patients who fail to respond to antibiotic therapy. It has been noted at post-mortem in 4% of patients dying in hospital.

135.   L: Varicella

Varicella frequently causes a primary viral pneumonia in adults but less commonly in children. X-rays show multiple small pulmonary lesions. Treatment is with aciclovir.

136.   E: Legionnaire's disease

Legionella has an incubation period up to 10 days and is often associated with altered mental status. Respiratory symptoms and signs are often mild initially, and renal failure can develop. Treatment is with a macrolide and supportive care.

137.   C: This condition often has an infectious cause

There are many causes of erythema multiforme. *Mycoplasma* and herpesvirus infections are common causes and should be excluded, particularly if oral steroids are contemplated. Itch often responds to antihistamine or topical steroids. This condition can be associated with mouth and genital ulcers in Stevens–Johnson syndrome or with toxic epidermal necrolysis. Erythema nodosum causes tender nodules on the legs that fade to look like bruises.

138.   D: She should be referred for an ultrasound examination

Multinodular goitres are common but where there is a dominant nodule the patient should be referred for excision in order to prevent malignant change. This occurs in about 5% of multinodular goitres. Indications of malignancy that should prompt 2-week referral include rapid growth, tracheal compression, laryngeal nerve involvement, irregular nodules, lymphadenopathy and a history of neck irradiation.

139.   C: Ventricular bigeminy

This ECG shows ventricular bigeminy, where a normal sinus beat is followed by a premature ventricular contraction. There is often a compensatory pause after the ectopic beat. In the absence of other cardiovascular disease it is seldom of consequence. A history should be taken, aimed at identifying any factors that might increase ectopic activity, such as thyroid disease, caffeine or alcohol, but usually no treatment is needed. Paroxysmal atrial fibrillation consists of runs of atrial fibrillation interspersed with normal sinus rhythm while Wenkebach phenomenom is characterised by an increasing PR interval until a ventricular beat is missed. AV dissociation shows atrial activity and ventricular activity that are not coordinated, while 2:1 heart block shows 2 P waves for each QRS complex.

140.   E: Squamous cell carcinoma

The appearance of an ulcerated lesion on the ear suggests either an SCC or a BCC. In this case there is no pearly rolled edge and there is a crust with underlying ulceration, suggestive of an SCC. Keratoacanthomas usually develop over a fairly rapid time-course but are similar histologically and clinically, often making excision necessary for diagnosis. Chondrodermatitis is usually seen higher up on the pinna and is a painful nodule. Actinic keratosis does not usually ulcerate.

141.   B: Entitled demanders

Entitled demanders seek medical attention and try to control the direction through intimidation and inducing guilt. They might also attempt to use litigation or the threat of this to get their own way.

142.   D: Heartsink patient

'Heartsinks' are a function of the doctor–patient relationship rather than purely a character trait of the patient. Female GPs identify fewer heartsinks than their male colleagues and doctors who are stressed and showing signs of burnout typically report higher numbers of heartsinks.

143.   F: Self-destructive denier

The possibility of underlying depression should be considered in these patients, but often these patients seem to derive satisfaction from their plight, in an extension of the sick role. An example would be the poorly controlled diabetic who is rapidly going blind but who continues to ignore advice on diet and medication.

144. E: Manipulative help rejector

Manipulative help rejectors are usually pleasant in a consultation but believe that they are beyond help and seem to enjoy the physician's inability to cure them of their symptoms, which are usually mild and not life-threatening. Where a symptom is cured they will often present with a new, equally difficult symptom.

145. C: Frequent attenders

One should always avoid subjective terms that imply a character judgement such as 'dependent clinger' or 'heartsink' when writing in medical notes.

146. A: Check thyroid autoantibodies

The most likely cause in this patient is thyroid eye disease, usually seen in Graves' disease, but it can precede the development of hyperthyroidism. Myasthenia gravis causes ptosis rather than proptosis and can be tested for with anti-acetylcholine receptor antibodies. A brain tumour would not usually cause proptosis and tumours in the orbit would usually cause visual signs and pain. Orbital cellulitis can cause proptosis but is usually clinically obvious, with erythema, pain and fever, together with ophthalmoplegia and, later, loss of colour vision. Following blood tests for Graves' disease, she should be referred to ophthalmology.

147. B: *Cryptosporidium* can be resistant to chlorination of water

Some strains are resistant to chlorination, although all strains of these organisms should be killed by chlorine dioxide ozone if used correctly. Transmission is faeco-oral, with humans or animals passing spores in the faeces. Affected children should remain off school until 48 hours after symptoms have settled. Most cases are mild but children and the immunocompromised can develop a chronic illness. Transmission is usually through drinking, but can also be through swimming in lakes and rivers, drinking from streams (eg when hiking) or through sexual intercourse.

148. G: Japanese B encephalitis

Japanese B encephalitis is a viral disease spread by mosquitoes. It is commonly seen in areas where pigs and humans cohabit, ie rural areas. Students on gap-year projects in rural communities and aid workers should be vaccinated if they will be in these areas in July–December (India/Nepal) or May–September (SE Asia). Patients with clinical infection have a 25% mortality and long-term neurological effects are seen in 30–70% of survivors.

149. I: Meningitis A and C

Over recent years there have been a number of outbreaks of meningitis amongst Hajj pilgrims, who often travel and sleep in crowded conditions.

150. O: Yellow fever

Yellow fever is a viral disease spread by mosquitoes that is endemic in Africa and South America. A single dose of vaccine gives protection for 10 years and can only be given in designated centres. A certificate of vaccination is required for entry into several countries.

151. C: Diphtheria

Diphtheria is endemic in Russia because of the low vaccination rates among children there, and between 1990 and 1998 there were 157 000 cases and 5000 deaths. The relatively high standard of living in much of Russia might mean that travellers underestimate the risks of this infection. Diphtheria vaccination is highly effective but booster doses are needed.

152.   J: Rabies

Rabies vaccination should be given to those who are at high risk, for example bat-handlers or those working with animals in an endemic area, or those who are travelling to a remote endemic area where they would struggle to obtain prompt medical assistance in the event of an animal bite. Where a significant risk of infection occurs (eg a dog bite) two post-exposure doses are required. Patients who have not been vaccinated require five doses post-exposure.

153.   B: It is a cause of sudden death in young athletes

HOCM is the commonest genetic cardiac disease and is inherited as an autosomal dominant trait, although many cases are the result of spontaneous mutation. It frequently presents with sudden death in young athletes, and in some countries high-school athletes are required to have echocardiography as a screening test. Less frequently it can present with chronic heart failure or arrhythmia, but treatment usually controls symptoms only without affecting outcome. It can also be detected as an asymptomatic finding in older patients.

154.   E: Transdermal opioid patches do not reach steady-state analgesic levels for 24 hours

Transdermal patches require 24 hours to reach a steady state and additional breakthrough analgesia might be required during this time. Co-proxamol is toxic in overdose but is available on a named-patient basis. Buprenorphine is a partial agonist but can be taken with other opioids, although it makes more sense to use additional buprenorphine tablets for breakthrough pain.

155. B: Change to a triphasic pill

Breakthrough bleeding is common in the first 6 months on the combined pill. If it persists and no other cause can be found, the patient should be changed to a higher oestrogen dose pill or a triphasic pill. There is little justification for taking two combined pills a day as the dose of oestrogen would pose a significant risk of side effects. The mini-pill is a common cause of spotting and would not be an appropriate alternative in this instance. A Mirena IUD would be technically difficult to fit in a nulliparous woman but might be appropriate if symptoms could not be controlled with medication or if oestrogen was contraindicated.

156. A: Acamprosate reduces the desire to drink

Acamprosate works on CNS GABA receptors to reduce the desire for alcohol and is licensed for use in prevention of relapse. Antabuse produces an unpredictable reaction and can cause severe illness. It should only be used under consultant supervision for new patients, although it might be an effective longer-term treatment once abstinence is established. Brief interventions, with assessment, education and advice on drinking have been shown to reduce alcohol consumption by 20%. Many patients with no long-term damage can safely reduce their drinking to normal levels without the need for abstinence, which in many cases is socially difficult, for example in remote communities. Long-term follow-up of survivors shows that at 4 years 28% of patients have been abstinent for 6 months and 18% are drinking asymptomatically (Rand report).

157. E: External-beam radiotherapy

Approximately 12% of patients receiving external-beam radiotherapy suffer proctitis and haemorrhage. This is significantly less common with brachytherapy.

158.   I: Watchful waiting

Radical prostatectomy was shown to reduce deaths from prostate cancer but not overall mortality when compared with watchful waiting.

159.   D: Docetaxel

Docetaxel chemotherapy can be effective in non-hormone-responsive recurrences. Bisphosphonates might be useful in managing bone pain as an adjunct to radiotherapy or NSAIDs.

160.   G: Orchidectomy

NICE recommend offering bilateral orchidectomy to all patients with hormone-sensitive tumours as an alternative to LHRH agonists.

161.   F: LHRH analogue

LHRH analogues cause an initial flare in testosterone production followed by suppression to the equivalent of castration. Initial treatment should be covered with an anti-androgen to prevent tumour flare, especially where there are spinal metastases. Cord compression has been reported in some patients in whom LHRH analogues are used alone.

162.   E: Patients who are intolerant of colchicine or NSAIDs should be treated with prednisolone

Most cases of gout are due to an inherited metabolic defect or are iatrogenic, common triggers including thiazides, furosemide and low-dose salicylates. The traditional purine-rich duet is rarely seen as a cause. Uric acid often drops during an acute attack. Joint aspiration reveals clear fluid, with crystals seen on microscopy. Colchicine should be given as 500 micrograms three times a day. Prophylaxis should be considered if patients are having more than two attacks a year but should not be started during an acute attack, and patients should be warned that prophylaxis can trigger an acute attack.

163.   C: Fibroadenoma

Fibroadenomas are often described as 'breast mice' because they often seem to run away on examination. They are benign and can be removed for reassurance in the young after definitive diagnosis with cytology and ultrasound. In the over-40s all breast lumps should be removed. If left, one in four will regress spontaneously. They can cause diagnostic confusion on mammograms, particularly in the elderly, because of calcification. Paget's disease is a localised cancer causing skin changes. DCIS is usually diagnosed on mammography but occasionally is seen as a firm (non-mobile) mass. A galactocoele is seen in women after finishing lactating and is cystic. Suspicious features in any breast lump are fixation, associated skin changes or discharge, lymphadenopathy and growth.

164.   C: Candidal infection is more common in pregnancy

A fishy smell suggests bacterial vaginosis or *Trichomonas*. These are both treated with metronidazole orally or clindamycin pessaries. There is no need for condoms or partner treatment with bacterial vaginosis. Bacterial vaginosis is often discovered incidentally on swabs or smears. Thrush is more common in the sexually active, pregnant and immunocompromised. Trichomoniasis is a sexually transmitted disease that causes a urethritis in men and a foul-smelling mucopurulent discharge in women. Diagnosis is on microscopy.

165.   B: The data show a statistically significant weight loss at 3 months

The data show an 80% drop-out rate by 12 months. The data are not presented on an intention-to-treat basis. Assuming that the patients who drop out regain their weight loss, the average weight loss is likely to be less than 1 kg. The high drop-out rates imply poor concordance with treatment. Weight loss is maintained in the 20% of patients who are still in the programme at 12 months.

166. E: β Blocker

Beta blockers are commonly associated with erectile dysfunction, poor exercise tolerance and nightmares. They can also precipitate wheeze in asthmatics.

167. B: α Blocker

Alpha blockers are useful in men with prostate problems but can cause incontinence in women.

168. I: Thiazide diuretic

Thiazides, furosemide and aspirin are common causes of gout.

169. G: Methyldopa

Methyldopa is seldom used outside pregnancy due to sedation but very few antihypertensives are safe for use in pregnancy, hence its continued use.

170. I: Thiazide diuretic

African-Caribbean patients tend to have low-renin hypertension that is salt-sensitive, so drugs acting on the angiotensin system are less effective. Thiazides or calcium-channel blockers are the most appropriate first-line treatment.

171. C: Perthe's disease

Perthe's disease, avascular necrosis of the femoral head, is usually seen in children between the ages of 5 and 10 years, and 80% of cases are seen in boys. Initially it presents as an irritable hip but later the joint becomes fixed and movements improve, albeit with a positive Trendelenburg gait. Congenital dislocation of the hip usually presents earlier as asymmetrical creases, or is picked up at child health surveillance. Slipped upper femoral epiphysis is typically seen in boys between the ages of 10 and 15 years and presents with a shortened and rotated leg. Septic arthritis is usually associated with a raised CRP and WCC. The main differential is irritable hip but this does not usually persist as long and can be excluded on X-ray.

172.   C: Patients diagnosed with osteoporosis should be investigated for coeliac disease

Bisphosphonates are available in oral and intravenous formulations. They have been proved to increase bone density and reduce fractures. In patients who are intolerant, strontium can be used as a second-line treatment, or HRT can be used in younger, post-menopausal patients. A T score < 2.5 is diagnostic, and all patients should be assessed to exclude secondary osteoporosis, for example due to coeliac disease or hypogonadism. Bisphosphonates should usually be prescribed for 5 years. Where patients have refractory osteoporosis, PTH or teriparatide can be used under specialist supervision.

173.   C: Postural hypotension is a common symptom of Parkinson's disease

Parkinson's disease is associated with a number of non-motor symptoms, ranging from pain, postural hypotension and bladder problems to hallucinations, particularly in patients being treated with levodopa. These can be difficult to treat and many antipsychotics make motor symptoms worse. There is no evidence favouring any treatment early on, and treatment should be started once symptoms interfere with daily life. There is some evidence that ropinirole is associated with a lower frequency of nausea but overall drop-out rates are the same as for levodopa.

174.   D: The practice of evidence-based medicine is applicable to quantitative research as well as to qualitative research

Evidence-based practice requires both skills in searching and critical appraisal and the equipment to access them, such as computers with internet connections. Qualitative outcomes are as important if not more important than quantitative ones; it is patient outcomes that should drive the search for evidence. Lack of evidence of effect is not evidence of lack of effect; it should prompt the search for more evidence rather than discourage the use of a certain treatment. As seen by the effect of NICE guidance in many areas, application of evidence-based practice often increases healthcare costs.

175.   A: Refer for colposcopy

Patients with 'borderline change with endocervical changes' should be referred for colposcopy after one abnormal smear. Patients with 'borderline smear with squamous changes' should be referred after three abnormal smears.

176.   D: Repeat in 6 months

Three inadequate smears should prompt referral for colposcopy.

177.   H: Smear no longer necessary

Local protocols vary but most areas invite women for their first smear at 25, then 3-yearly to 49, and 5-yearly to 64. Patients aged over 65 need only have a smear if they have had a previous abnormal result.

178.   D: Repeat in 6 months

Again, local protocols vary but it is considered acceptable after one smear showing mild dyskariosis to repeat this and refer for colposcopy if the follow-up smear is abnormal.

179. B: Refer under 2-week rule

Smears which are suspicious of cancer should be referred under the 2-week rule. Note that cervical smears are a screening test rather than a diagnostic test and cannot rule out cancer. Where a cervix looks abnormal or there is a suspicious history, a clinical diagnosis should prompt a 2-week referral.

180. C Prescribe vitamin D analogues

This patient has psoriasis. The use of emollients will often improve the dry scaly appearance, leaving red papules. The improvement in symptoms with ultraviolet light is characteristic. Steroids will often produce a dramatic improvement, which relapses however on cessation of the steroid. Vitamin D analogues are the first-line treatment for most patients. Patients with new-onset psoriasis should have a thorough drug history to exclude causative agents such as β blockers.

181. A: She should be offered incision and curettage

Chalazions are cysts that develop in the meibomian glands. They often enlarge slowly but a third resolve within 3 months and almost all resolve within 2 years. If they become infected they should be treated with a short course of antibiotic ointment. Definitive treatment is incision and curettage which can be done in general practice if the right equipment is available. If large they can compress the eyeball, causing astigmatism. Lesions around the eye should always be examined for evidence of malignancy (eg basal cell carcinoma, squamous cell carcinoma), although this would be unusual in this age group. Cryotherapy is not appropriate in this area due to the risk of cicatrising scars.

182. **A:** **Absence from work for more than 4 weeks is associated with only a 20% chance of returning to work within 12 months**

Yellow flag symptoms predicting increased risk of chronic pain include poor social situation, affective disorder, poor engagement with therapy, and chronic symptoms. Patients off work for more than 3 months will often never return to work. There is no consistent evidence of increased benefit from chiropractic, osteopathy or physiotherapy – they all seem to work. Back schools encourage rehabilitation and often include elements of cognitive behavioural therapy, which have been shown to be helpful in chronic cases. Perineal numbness and continence problems are red flag symptoms, and these should prompt urgent referral.

183. **C:** *Salmonella*

Salmonellosis has an incubation period of 12–48 hours and typically causes vomiting followed by diarrhoea, which usually settles over 72 hours. In some cases it can cause a reactive arthritis and approximately 1% of patients go on to become carriers. Treatment is supportive, and antibiotics are not recommended for most patients. *Campylobacter* causes diarrhoea and malaise but vomiting is rare; prolonged excretion can occur and this might be relevant for care-home or nursing staff. *Shigella* is unusual in the UK but should be suspected in travellers who return with bloody diarrohea. *Cryptosporidium* usually affects children, while typhoid has a much longer incubation period and a more protracted clinical course.

184. **D:** **Compression to ventilation ratio should be 30 to 2**

The most recent guidelines (2005) suggest a ratio of 30 to 2 although there is some evidence that ventilation is not of any additional benefit in patients with ventricular fibrillation. Adrenaline (epinephrine) should be given by the intramuscular route if intravenous access is not available. AEDs can be used on patients with pacemakers but the electrodes should not be placed over the pacemaker.

185.   C: Multiple myeloma

This pattern of symptoms and blood results is suggestive of myeloma. Urine should be sent for Bence Jones protein and he should be referred under the 2-week rule. CLL would usually cause a raised white cell count and symptoms are unusual, while lung cancer would usually cause respiratory symptoms. Metastatic prostate cancer can cause bony pain but would be unusual in patients without urinary symptoms. Persistent backache in young patients with systemic signs should prompt investigation to exclude sarcoma or infection.

186.   C: Patients should be monitored with regular β-hCG levels for 2 years

Around 10% of molar pregnancies go on to develop neoplastic disease, but if treated early there is a very good prognosis. Recurrence risk for molar pregnancy is approximately 1 in 80 and most women go on to have a normal pregnancy afterwards. The COCP should not be used until β-hCG levels are undetectable because it can delay tumour regression. All patients should be referred to specialist centres for follow-up.

187.   I: None of the above

Detention is specifically excluded in patients without mental illness but who are sexually deviant, suffer from drug and alcohol addiction, who commit disorderly acts or on the grounds of religious or cultural beliefs.

188.   H: Section 136

Section 136 allows the police to take a patient to a place of safety for up to 72 hours. They cannot enter a private residence without consent to do so, however.

189.   C: Section 4

Section 4 of the Mental Health Act allows admission for 72 hours for assessment and allows for emergency detention and assessment. It requires one doctor and the application can be made by the nearest relative or an Approved Mental Health Professional. It should be used only where delay would pose a significant risk of harm to the patient or others.

190.   I: None of the above

Severe learning disabilities in the absence of other mental health problems are specifically excluded under the 2007 amendments to the Mental Health Act. This situation would best be resolved through the courts.

191.   F: Section 17

Section 17 is an amendment introduced in 2007 to allow supervised community treatment orders and includes provision for failure to comply and the conditions under which re-admission would be needed.

192.   C: Fibroids present on ultrasound

193.   H: Refer under 2-week rule

194.   A: Contraceptive pill

195.   I: Tranexamic acid

196.   E: Mirena

197.   B: Check thyroid function

Simple snoring can have a significant impact on quality of life of spouses and many snorers only present because of spousal pressure. Sleep apnoea should be excluded on the history and significant causes of obstruction such as large tonsils, a large tongue base or nasal obstruction identified. Simple measures that can help include weight loss, avoidance of sedatives and alcohol, and positional measures if the snoring is postural. Thyroid function should always be checked. Where simple measures fail, UVPP might be considered but it is very painful and is associated with a significant risk of nasal escape.

198.   B: A 23-year-old man who has recently returned from a year travelling in South-East Asia with a new tattoo

At-risk groups include those who have had blood transfusions before 1987, those who have had dental treatment, invasive medical procedures or body piercing in the developing world, those with a history of intravenous drug use, people with a raised ALT level and people who have had contact with these groups. Singapore is a developed country and not high-risk; patients who live abroad as expats but who do not use local facilities for health care are not at risk.

199. **C:** **The use of strong opioids for chronic pain is frequently associated with withdrawal symptoms on reducing the dose**

Strong opioids used for chronic pain are often associated with physiological withdrawal symptoms and many patients need to go onto Oramorph to allow slow weaning off morphine. Fentanyl patches should be used when patients have inadequate pain control and do not wish to take, or are unable to take, oral opioids. Where pain control is adequate but associated with side effects an alternative to weak opioids is low-strength buprenorphine patches. Oramorph should be used to titrate MST dose. If a weak opioid is ineffective at maximal dose, a stronger opioid should be used. Where combination analgesics are used, the higher strength (eg co-codamol 30/500) should be used. Weaker strengths have opioid side effects but without the efficacy of the stronger formulations.

200. **C:** **Heroin use can cause heart failure**

Ecstasy causes malignant hyperthermia and this can progress to rhabdomyolysis. It is also associated with low mood and reduced intellectual performance. Intravenous drug use can cause infective endocarditis, particularly right-sided, and deep vein thrombosis. Cocaine can cause anxiety, depression and psychosis, as well as its better known side effects of rhinitis, myocardial infarction and septal perforation. Cannabis strength is increasing and psychosis is becoming increasingly common, even with short-term use. Ketamine is an anaesthetic agent that is sometimes used recreationally as 'Special K'. It is associated with hypertension but does not usually suppress respiration.

Paper 2
Questions

*Total time allowed is three hours. Indicate your answers clearly by putting a
tick or cross in the box alongside each answer or by writing the appropriate
letter alongside the appropriate answer.*

1. A 65-year-old man with no previous medical history of note has
    just been discharged from hospital after a pulmonary embolus.
    There was no obvious precipitating factor and he has never had
    one before. He was intensively investigated in hospital and no
    cause was found. Which of the following statements about the
    duration of his anticoagulation is true? Select one option only.

☐ A   He should take warfarin for 6 weeks after discharge
☐ B   He should take warfarin for 6 months after discharge
☐ C   He should be on warfarin for life
☐ D   He should take warfarin for 12 months after discharge
☐ E   He should be tested for thrombophilia now, and if this is
      negative may stop after 3 months

2. A 7-year-old boy is seen with his mother complaining of a 6-
    week history of joint pain, lethargy and headache. He has been
    getting recurrent episodes of sore throat and has persistently
    enlarged lymph nodes. On examination he is pale and has
    some petechiae on his back. Which of the following is the most
    appropriate next step in this patient? Select one option only.

☐ A   Prescribe a 10-day course of phenoxymethylpenicillin
      (penicillin V)
☐ B   Reassure the mother that he probably has post-viral fatigue
      and review in 6 weeks if no better
☐ C   Check his full blood count (FBC)
☐ D   Prescribe a non-steroidal drug for his arthralgia
☐ E   Reassure the mother that the probable diagnosis is Henoch–
      Schönlein purpura, which should resolve without any
      complications

THEME: TREATMENT OF SYMPTOMS IN CANCER

Options

A   Baclofen

B   Cholestyramine

C   Chlorpromazine

D   Dexamethasone

E   Gabapentin

F   Haloperidol

G   Hyoscine hydrobromide

H   Morphine

I   Pamidronate

J   Phenytoin

For each of the symptoms described below, select the most appropriate treatment from the list of options. Each option may be used once, more than once or not at all.

☐   **3.   Hypercalcaemia.**

☐   **4.   Anorexia.**

☐   **5.   Pruritus.**

☐   **6.   Muscle spasm.**

☐   **7.   Hiccoughs.**

8. **Which one of the following statements about recent developments in the management of rheumatoid arthritis is true?**

☐ A Mortality is decreased in patients with rheumatoid arthritis taking long-term, low-dose steroids

☐ B According to the FIN-RACo study, aggressive treatment of rheumatoid arthritis should be reserved for patients with advanced disease

☐ C Etanercept does not offer any significant benefit in patients who have failed to tolerate methotrexate

☐ D Intensive (monthly) follow-up does not show any benefits compared with regular care

☐ E Patient-initiated outpatient follow-up reduces outpatient visits by 38%

9. **Which of the following statements about screening for congenital dislocation of the hip is true? Select one option only.**

☐ A The Ortolani test is used to detect a dislocatable hip

☐ B The Barlow test is used to detect a dislocated hip

☐ C Ultrasonography is much more sensitive and specific than clinical testing

☐ D Most children who are discovered to have the condition will require surgery

☐ E Breech presentation is a risk factor

PAPER 2

10. A 37-year-old man complains of pain every time that he passes a stool. He has noticed fresh blood on the toilet paper. He has tried Anusol with no effect. Which of the following is the most appropriate management in this case? Select one option only.

☐ A   Topical glyceryl trinitrate

☐ B   Anal stretch

☐ C   Instillagel

☐ D   Ciprofloxacin

☐ E   Haemorrhoidectomy

11. A 67-year-old man has been suffering from metastatic lung cancer for the last 18 months. He has been using fentanyl patches at home for the last few weeks but is now getting very distressed. You decide to start a syringe driver. Which of the following statements is correct about the use of syringe drivers in palliative care? Select one option only.

☐ A   Morphine may suppress respiration and therefore should not be used in patients with a lung primary

☐ B   When converting a patient to a morphine syringe driver from fentanyl, it is best to start at a low dose and titrate upwards to achieve pain control

☐ C   Levomepromazine (Nozinan) will help with agitation and nausea

☐ D   Morphine is effective only for visceral pain

☐ E   Midazolam and morphine cannot be mixed in the same syringe driver because of precipitation

12. A 74-year-old former boilermaker complains of progressive dyspnoea and weight loss over the last 18 months. He is an ex-smoker but has no other previous medical history of note. On examination he has bilateral inspiratory crackles and is clubbed. You arrange a chest radiograph, which shows diffuse shadowing and pleural plaques. What is the most likely diagnosis? Select one option only.

☐ A   Asbestosis

☐ B   Bronchogenic carcinoma

☐ C   Extrinsic allergic alveolitis

☐ D   Left ventricular failure

☐ E   Chronic obstructive airway disease

13. An 8-month-old boy is brought in by his parents who think that he has a lazy eye. Which of the following statements is true about this condition? Select one answer only.

☐ A   The affected eye relaxes fixation on an object when the contralateral eye is covered with a hand or mask

☐ B   The aim of treatment in patching is to cover the bad eye, thus allowing the good eye to send unambiguous messages to the brain

☐ C   Lazy eye may be caused by retinoblastoma

☐ D   It does not run in families

☐ E   It is always obvious from infancy

THEME: CONTRACTUAL STATUS OF GENERAL PRACTICE

Options

A APMS

B GMS

C LIFT

D PMS

E PMS plus

F Private contractor status

For each description below, select the most appropriate contractual status from the list of options. Each option may be used once, more than once or not at all.

- [ ] **14.** This is a nationally negotiated contract.

- [ ] **15.** A practice takes over the running of local district nursing services.

- [ ] **16.** It supports the redevelopment of primary care premises.

- [ ] **17.** It covers a GP doing GPwSI sessions in dermatology.

- [ ] **18.** It is subject to a reduction in Quality and Outcomes Framework (QOF) points.

19. A 67-year-old woman presents with dizziness and fatigue. Her electrocardiogram (ECG) is shown below (heart rate 32/minute, QT interval 604 ms).

Heart Rate: 32 bpm

QT Interval: 604 ms

Which one of the following statements is true with regard to this case?

- [ ] A The diagnosis is Mobitz type 2 heart block
- [ ] B She should be treated with a cardioselective β blocker
- [ ] C This condition is usually iatrogenic
- [ ] D If the patient is well in herself she can be referred to the outpatients department
- [ ] E She should be treated with a permanent pacemaker

20. One of your patients comes to see you to request a vasectomy. He has four children already and feels that he cannot afford to have anymore. You counsel him about the pros and cons of vasectomy. Which of the following statements about vasectomy is true? Select one option only.

- [ ] A   It is usually carried out under general anaesthetic
- [ ] B   Sterility is immediate after the procedure
- [ ] C   Bruising is uncommon and should be investigated
- [ ] D   The lifetime failure rate is approximately 1%
- [ ] E   Vasectomy is reversible in only 50% of cases

21. With regard to the management of epistaxis in a 76-year-old man, which of the following statements is correct? Select one option only.

- [ ] A   Most bleeds are posterior
- [ ] B   Bleeding comes from branches of the internal jugular vein
- [ ] C   The majority of cases are caused by high blood pressure
- [ ] D   Anterior bleeds are never fatal
- [ ] E   Silver nitrate cautery may cause septal perforation
- [ ] F   BIPP packing should be used if bleeding fails to settle with pressure

22. A 56-year-old man presents with a painful red eye of 3 days' duration. He has had a small amount of mucopus but has not responded to chloramphenicol. Examination reveals reduced corneal sensation and fluorescein staining reveals the appearance below.

Which of the following is the most likely diagnosis?

- A   Dendritic ulcer
- B   Iritis
- C   Acute conjunctivitis
- D   Corneal foreign body
- E   Recurrent corneal erosion

23. **Which one of the following statements about assisted suicide is true?**

☐ A Assisted suicide is legal in the UK as long as certain legal criteria are met

☐ B Rates of physician-assisted suicide have risen consistently since legalisation in the Netherlands

☐ C Physician-assisted suicide accounts for 17% of deaths in the Netherlands

☐ D Neuromuscular relaxants are the drug of choice in the Netherlands

☐ E The 'doctrine of double effect' refers to the use of a drug primarily to bring about death in assisted suicide

24. **A 76-year-old man is brought into the surgery by his wife. He claims not to know why he is there but she tells you that she is worried that he may be starting to develop dementia. Which of the following statements is NOT true about dementia? Select one option only.**

☐ A Dementia is usually associated with altered cognition and consciousness

☐ B It is usually seen in many spheres of intellectual function

☐ C All patients should have baseline biochemical and haematological investigations before referral

☐ D Gingko biloba is of some benefit in slowing memory impairment

☐ E HIV testing is appropriate in young patients

THEME: LIVER FUNCTION TESTS

Options

A   Gallstones

B   Gilbert's syndrome

C   Haemochromatosis

D   Haemolysis

E   Hepatitis

F   Iatrogenic

G   Malnutrition

H   Physiological

For each of the descriptions below, select the most appropriate diagnosis from the list of options. Each option may be used once, more than once or not at all.

☐ **25.** A 34-year-old man has recently suffered flu-like symptoms. His bloods show a raised bilirubin only and a normal FBC.

☐ **26.** A 56-year-old man attends for liver function tests (LFTs) as part of an insurance medical. He has a raised GGT, normal bilirubin, ALT (alanine transferase) and alkaline phosphatase (ALP).

☐ **27.** A 12-year-old girl has blood tests as part of investigations for recurrent urinary tract infections. Her ALP level is raised, although bilirubin and ALT are normal.

☐ **28.** A 34-year-old man has recently returned from a holiday where he had a brief romance. He has now developed jaundice. His blood tests show an ALT five times normal levels, bilirubin elevated and a normal ALP.

☐ **29.** A 47-year-old woman presents with acute abdominal pain. Her urine has darkened and her stools are pale. Bloods show raised ALT, raised bilirubin and raised ALP. GGT (γ-glutamyltransferase) is normal.

30. A 76-year-old woman who has been treated for a recurrence of breast cancer has a fungating wound. She is particularly concerned about the odour. She has been told that she is incurable. Which of the following palliative treatments may help? Select one option only.

- ☐ A An absorbent dressing will remove exudates and minimise odour
- ☐ B Admission for a short course of intravenous antibiotics will reduce bacterial load and thus the odour
- ☐ C Topical metronidazole is effective
- ☐ D Skin grafting will close the wound and reduce the odour
- ☐ E Treatment should be directed at helping her cope psychologically

31. A 45-year-old man presents with acute onset of severe pain in his loin that is radiating to the flank and groin. On examination he is slightly tender in the renal angle but has no fever. His urine is positive to blood on dipstick testing. Which one of the following statements about this situation is true?

- ☐ A He should be given fluids and a broad-spectrum antibiotic
- ☐ B This condition is usually the result of raised urate levels
- ☐ C A non-steroidal anti-inflammatory drug (NSAID) is contraindicated due to the risk of renal failure
- ☐ D Plain radiographs will usually show a stone if one is present
- ☐ E This could be a presentation of a renal tumour

THEME: ERECTILE DYSFUNCTION

Options

A   All of them

B   Caverject

C   MUSE (Medicated Uretheral System for Erection)

D   None of them

E   Sildenafil

F   Tadalafil

G   Vacuum pump

For each statement relating to treatments for erectile dysfunction, select the most appropriate treatment from the list of options. Each option may be used once, more than once or not at all.

☐ **32.** **The treatment may cause disturbance of colour vision.**

☐ **33.** **It is contraindicated in sickle cell disease.**

☐ **34.** **It is contraindicated in urethral stricture.**

☐ **35.** **Its efficacy may persist for 36 hours after use.**

☐ **36.** **It may be prescribed on the NHS to men with Parkinson's disease.**

37.   A local reflexologist writes to your practice asking if you would like to set up a reflexology service under practice-based commissioning. She cites a recent paper which showed significant benefits for patients with depression. You look the paper up on the internet and find the following abstract:

Qualitative study of the efficacy of reflexology in patients with mild depression

A retrospective postal survey was sent to 18 patients who had received reflexology for mild depression in the 6 months before the survey. The survey dealt with efficacy and satisfaction measures using a 10-point scale. The results showed that 16/18 (89%) of patients reported improvement in their depression after treatment, while no patients reported adverse effects; 13/18 described themselves as very satisfied with the service and 5/18 were quite satisfied. The mean number of sessions was 11, with each session lasting 45 minutes. These data suggest that reflexology is a cost-effective and efficacious alternative to drugs in the management of depression.

Which one of the following statements is true with regard to this research?

- [ ] A   The data support the suggestion that reflexology is a cost-effective alternative to drug therapy
- [ ] B   The study follows a valid protocol
- [ ] C   Qualitative studies are less prone to bias than quantitative studies
- [ ] D   The results should be treated with caution because of inclusion bias
- [ ] E   The improvement rates are significantly better than those seen with antidepressants

38. A 53-year-old woman presents with mild right iliac fossa pain of 2 months' duration. Examination shows no abnormality but blood tests show a mild iron-deficiency anaemia. Which of the following statements regarding investigation is correct? Select one option only.

☐ A Refer for barium enema

☐ B Refer for sigmoidoscopy

☐ C If a barium enema is normal she may be reassured

☐ D Refer for ultrasonography

☐ E A raised ESR suggests that infection is a probable cause

39. Which one of the following statements about suicide is true?

☐ A Approximately 4000 people a year commit suicide in England and Wales

☐ B Young women are a high-risk group

☐ C It is more likely in those living in rural communities

☐ D Cutting the wrists is the most common mode of attempted suicide

☐ E There is a 20% risk of a patient who has had an episode of deliberate self-harm committing suicide within the next 12 months

THEME: PAEDIATRIC SYNDROMES

Options

A   Charcot–Marie–Tooth syndrome

B   Down syndrome

C   Edwards syndrome

D   Fragile X syndrome

E   Klinefelter syndrome

F   Noonan syndrome

G   Patau syndrome

H   Turner syndrome

I   Williams syndrome

For each description below, select the most appropriate diagnosis from the list of options. Each option may be used once, more than once or not at all.

☐   **40.**   A chromosome 18 trisomy with a ventricular septal defect and pulmonary stenosis.

☐   **41.**   A child with upslanting eyes, prominent epicanthic folds, reduced muscle tone and spots on the iris.

☐   **42.**   It accounts for 5–10% of severe learning difficulties in boys; often skips a generation.

☐   **43.**   It affects boys only, with delayed puberty, crypto-orchidism and learning difficulties.

☐   **44.**   It is characterised by elfin facies, aortic stenosis and hypercalcaemia.

45. Your practice manager has been reviewing the private fees charged in your practice and has suggested that these are increased. Which one of the following statements is true with regard to private services?

☐ A Private fees can be set at whatever level the practice wishes

☐ B The British Medical Association publishes recommended levels for each service annually

☐ C Private fees cannot increase by more than the level of inflation

☐ D Private fees are covered by the GMS Contract

☐ E Private fees can be charged only if the practice is registered for VAT

46. A 61-year-old woman comes to see you for advice about whether she should have her hip replaced (as recommended by her orthopaedic surgeon). Which one of the following statements about hip replacements is true?

☐ A Ninety per cent of hip replacements last for more than 10 years

☐ B There is a 10% infection risk for hip replacement surgery

☐ C Once pain free, there are no restrictions on movement

☐ D The incidence of DVT is 10% after total hip replacement

☐ E Hip resurfacing is superior to conventional arthroplasty in advanced osteoarthritis

THEME: BENEFITS

Options

A   Bereavement payment
B   Carers' Allowance
C   Child benefit
D   Crisis loan
E   DS1500
F   Disability Living Allowance
G   Incapacity Benefit
H   Income Support
I   None of them
J   Working families' tax credit

For each situation described below, select the most appropriate benefit from the list of options. Each option may be used once, more than once or not at all.

☐ **47.** A 53-year-old woman whose husband dies after a long illness has been left with large bills to pay.

☐ **48.** A new mother whose partner is a barrister.

☐ **49.** A 13-year-old girl with cystic fibrosis who has severe illness and is unable to attend school.

☐ **50.** A 76-year-old man who has just been discharged from hospital with a diagnosis of inoperable pancreatic cancer. He has been told his life expectancy is 2–3 months.

☐ **51.** The mother of the 13-year-old girl with cystic fibrosis is a full-time carer.

52. A 3-year-old boy is brought in by his mother with a 6-day history of fever, conjunctivitis, cracked lips and a red tongue, with red swollen hands and feet. She reports that in the first few days of the illness he had a rash on his abdomen but this has now faded. On examination of his heart sounds he has a gallop rhythm and the heart sounds appear muffled. Which of the following is the likely diagnosis? Select one option only.

- [ ] A   Kawasaki's disease
- [ ] B   Takayasu's disease
- [ ] C   Measles
- [ ] D   Rubella
- [ ] E   Scarlet fever

53. A 73-year-old man with a history of hypertension and diabetes presents with 4 weeks of increasing breathlessness on exertion. Over the last 10 days he has had trouble sleeping and cannot get his shoes on as a result of swollen legs. On examination he is afebrile with a regular pulse, which you measure as 100 at rest. Which of the following diagnoses is probable in this case? Select one option only.

- [ ] A   New-onset atrial fibrillation (AF)
- [ ] B   Pulmonary fibrosis
- [ ] C   Right ventricular failure
- [ ] D   Cor pulmonale
- [ ] E   Biventricular failure

PAPER 2

54. A 5-year-old boy is brought in by his father because he says that it hurts to pass urine. On examination he has balanitis. Which of the following statements is true with regard to management of this condition? Select one option only.

- [ ] A *Staphylococcus aureus* is the most common organism
- [ ] B Topical treatment is rarely helpful
- [ ] C All patients should be referred for circumcision
- [ ] D It may cause phimosis
- [ ] E Ninety per cent of 6 year olds should be able to retract the foreskin

55. A 19-year-old medical student complains of hair loss during the build-up to his first year exams. This has caused great distress because it has forced him to cut off his ponytail. On examination he has a discrete patch of hair loss on the back of his head, there is no inflammation or scarring, and he is otherwise well. Which of the following statements about this condition is NOT true? Select one option only.

- [ ] A The condition usually resolves over 3–6 months
- [ ] B It may be associated with thyroid disorders
- [ ] C Corticosteroids are a useful first-line therapy if used early
- [ ] D Spontaneous regrowth occurs in 75% of patients
- [ ] E It may be associated with nail changes

56. Which one of the following statements about the success of NHS reforms is true?

A The proportion of patients receiving thrombolysis within 30 minutes of arrival in hospital has risen from 39% to 50% since 2000

B The number of teenage pregnancies has been cut by 50% since 1997

C Of 2-week referrals, 99% are seen within 2 weeks

D Cancer mortality has fallen by 35% since 1995

E The higher performance in the QOF is associated with higher hospital admission rates

57. A 13-year-old girl attends with her mother. She is becoming increasingly concerned about the appearance of her back and has stopped going swimming because of this. On examination she has a prominent scoliosis. Which of the following statements about scoliosis is true? Select one option only.

A Spontaneous resolution never occurs

B Scoliosis is always evident from infancy

C Scoliosis in adolescence is more common in boys

D Scoliosis usually affects the lumbar spine

E Scoliosis may be associated with deformity of the skull and ribcage

F All of the above

PAPER 2

THEME: BLEEDING IN EARLY PREGNANCY

Options

A   Blighted ovum

B   Cervical incompetence

C   Complete abortion

D   Ectopic pregnancy

E   Missed abortion

F   Septic abortion

G   Threatened abortion

For each of the descriptions below, select the most appropriate diagnosis from the list of options. Each option may be used once, more than once or not at all.

☐ **58.** A woman with heavy bleeding in week 7 of pregnancy which initially settled. She now feels unwell and has an offensive vaginal discharge.

☐ **59.** A woman with a positive pregnancy test has bleeding and abdominal pain in the sixth week of her pregnancy. Ultrasonography shows an empty uterus. Her quantitative β-hCG (β-human chorionic gonadotrophin) level is maintained over 72 hours.

☐ **60.** A woman with a previous history of dilatation and curettage presents with bleeding and mild cramps in week 14 of pregnancy.

☐ **61.** A woman with painless bleeding in week 7 of pregnancy. On examination her external os is closed.

☐ **62.** This is usually accompanied by light bleeding only and severe abdominal pain.

63. A 3-month-old baby is brought to the out-of-hours treatment centre by his parents with a cough and failure to feed. He had previously been well and was born after an uneventful pregnancy. He has had coryzal symptoms for the last 3 days. On examination he is tachypnoeic, cyanosed and has a temperature of 40°C. Examination of his chest reveals widespread wheeze and crepitations. What is the most likely diagnosis? Select one option only.

- [ ] A   Pneumonia
- [ ] B   Inhaled foreign body
- [ ] C   Asthma
- [ ] D   Bronchiolitis
- [ ] E   Pertussis

64. One of your receptionists decides to retire and and you advertise for a replacement. Several of the applicants are aged over 60 years. The practice retirement age is set at 60. Which one of the following statements is true about this situation?

- [ ] A   Age discrimination laws are designed specifically to protect elderly people
- [ ] B   Mandatory retirement is 60 years for women and 65 years for men
- [ ] C   Employers must write to employees in advance of their retirement date and advise them of their rights to apply to work beyond this date
- [ ] D   Employment benefits with length of service are legal as long as the length of service to qualify is no more than 10 years
- [ ] E   Dismissal on the basis of age is unlawful regardless of age

65. You are updating your practice protocols for the management of stroke and ischaemic heart disease and would like to make these evidence-based. Which one of the following statements about the use of blood-thinning agents in cardiovascular disease is true?

☐ A British Hypertension Society guidelines recommend aspirin as primary prevention in those with a 10-year cardiovascular risk > 15%

☐ B The MATCH trial (Management of ATherothrombosis with Clopidogrel in High-risk patients) showed that addition of aspirin to clopidogrel is more effective than aspirin alone in preventing recurrent stroke

☐ C The ESPRIT trial (European/Australasian Stroke Prevention in Reversible Ischaemia Trial) showed that an aspirin and dipyridamole combination is effective in secondary prevention of ischaemic stroke and transient ischaemic attacks (TIAs)

☐ D The CAPRIE trial (Clopidogrel versus Aspirin in Patients at Risk of Ischaemic Events) showed clopidogrel to be no more effective than aspirin for secondary prevention

☐ E Self-monitoring of warfarin causes an increase in bleeding rates

66. A 76-year-old man with controlled hypertension is diagnosed with pneumonia. Which of the following statements about management is correct? Select one option only.

☐ A He should receive a broad-spectrum cephalosporin

☐ B He should be treated with a macrolide

☐ C First-line treatment should be amoxicillin 250 mg three times daily

☐ D If he fails to respond to a first-line antibiotic the dose should be increased

☐ E If *Staphylococcus sp.* is suspected flucloxacillin should be added

67. A 28-year-old man and his partner are seen together. Since being together he has been plagued by premature ejaculation and this is starting to cause problems in their relationship. Which of the following statements about management of this condition is true? Select one option only.

☐ A The problem affects 5% of men questioned in surveys

☐ B Clomipramine taken before intercourse is no more effective than placebo

☐ C Paroxetine can increase the period before ejaculation up to eight times longer than placebo

☐ D Fluoxetine is very effective when taken once a day

☐ E Chlorpromazine is the treatment of choice for resistant patients

THEME: HEPATITIS

Options

A   Epstein–Barr virus

B   Hepatitis A

C   Hepatitis B

D   Hepatitis C

E   Hepatitis D

F   Hepatitis E

For each of the following descriptions, select the most appropriate diagnosis from the list of options. Each option may be used once, more than once or not at all.

☐ **68.** It is spread predominantly by intravenous drug use; there are mild symptoms in most patients with a 20% risk of cirrhosis.

☐ **69.** It is seen only in association with hepatitis B virus, enhancing the severity of this infection.

☐ **70.** It is spread by the faeco-oral route, and affects all age groups.

☐ **71.** It may be endemic in residential institutions.

☐ **72.** It may be spread parenterally or through unprotected sex. More than 90% of patients make a full recovery.

73. A 31-year-old woman presents with her 32-year-old husband about their inability to have children. They are concerned that it might be a result of her age and would like referral. You take a full history and examine them both. Which one of the following is NOT a cause of infertility?

☐ A   Endometriosis

☐ B   Alcohol consumption

☐ C   Smoking

☐ D   High body mass index (BMI)

☐ E   Tight underwear

74. A 67-year-old hypertensive woman is started on aspirin and ramipril after suffering a transient ischaemic attack. One week after starting the ramipril she attends for renal function testing and her creatinine has increased from 83 to 133 μmol/l. Which of the following statements about her management is true? Select one option only.

☐ A   The dose of ramipril should not be increased further and she should have a repeat blood test in 1 week

☐ B   As long as she is not hypotensive and her creatinine < 150 μmol/l she can be reassured

☐ C   The ramipril should be stopped and specialist advice sought

☐ D   The ramipril should be changed to an angiotensin II receptor blocker

☐ E   She should have her aspirin stopped

75. After morning surgery one of the practice nurses comes to see you with concerns about the competence of one of your colleagues. She reports that she has noticed several occasions recently where he has given inappropriate medical treatment and feels duty-bound to report her concerns. When you attempt to bring this up with the doctor concerned he becomes aggressive and irritable. Which one of the following would be the appropriate step to take at this stage?

- [ ] A Report him to the General Medical Council
- [ ] B Discuss his performance with other members of the practice team to see if there are other concerns
- [ ] C Contact his appraiser to express your concerns
- [ ] D Refer him to the National Clinical Assessment Authority (NCAA)
- [ ] E Refer him to the Local Medical Committee

76. A 54-year-old woman presents with vertigo. Which of the following symptoms would be consistent with a diagnosis of benign paroxysmal positional vertigo? Select one option only.

- [ ] A Hallpike testing provokes instantaneous onset of symptoms
- [ ] B It worsens with repeat Hallpike testing
- [ ] C It is typically triggered by particular head movements
- [ ] D It is associated with unilateral tinnitus
- [ ] E It requires MRI to confirm the diagnosis
- [ ] F It may be treated with stemetil

77. A 32-year-old woman attends for a mole check after reading a newspaper article about skin cancer. The lesion shown below is particularly worrying her, because it has recently grown significantly.

What is the likely diagnosis? Select one option only.

☐ A   Seborrhoeic keratosis

☐ B   Intradermal naevus

☐ C   Histiocytoma

☐ D   Malignant melanoma

☐ E   Squamous cell carcinoma (SCC)

78. Which one of the following statements is true with regard to anorexia nervosa?

☐ A   Patients can be screened for this condition using the SCOFF questionnaire

☐ B   The prevalence in the UK is estimated to be 10%

☐ C   It is seen exclusively in females

☐ D   It is characterised by obsession with exercise

☐ F   It can be diagnosed in those with a BMI < 20 kg/m² and food avoidance

THEME: CARDIOVASCULAR DRUGS

Options

A	Amiodarone	I	Metoprolol
B	Atorvastatin	J	Ramipril
C	Clopidogrel	K	Simvastatin
D	Dipyridamole	L	Sotalol
E	Flecainide	M	Spironolactone
F	Furosemide	N	Valsartan
G	Indapamide	O	Verapamil
H	Isosorbide mononitrate	P	Warfarin

For each clinical scenario above, select the most appropriate therapy from the list of options. Each option may be used once, more than once or not at all.

☐ **79.** It reduces triglycerides as well as total cholesterol.

☐ **80.** It is used for prophylaxis of atrial fibrillation.

☐ **81.** It may be used in left ventricular dysfunction where ACE (angiotensin-converting enzyme) inhibitors are not tolerated.

☐ **82.** It is contraindicated in patients on β blockers.

☐ **83.** It should be used for patients who cannot tolerate aspirin and have suffered a transient ischaemic attack (TIA) or ischaemic stroke.

☐ **84.** It often causes headache, flushing and postural hypotension.

☐ **85.** It should be used in combination with aspirin for 12 months after an acute non-ST-elevation myocardial infarction (NSTEMI).

☐ **86.** It should be considered in patients with heart failure already on an ACE inhibitor and thiazide.

☐ **87.** It may cause corneal microdeposits and phototoxicity.

☐ **88.** It may be safely used in young patients with hypertension and renal artery stenosis.

89. A 33-year-old marketing executive complains of palpitations at night. These come and go and, although he does not feel unwell with them, he gets a fluttering sensation in his chest for 30–60 seconds. He is otherwise well and takes no regular medication. His bloods and ECG are normal; however, a 24-hour ECG reveals short runs of atrial fibrillation. Which of the following statements about paroxysmal atrial fibrillation are true? Select one option only.

☐ A It affects approximately 10% of the population at some time in their lives

☐ B All patients should be anticoagulated because of risk of stroke

☐ C Digoxin is effective in this patient group

☐ D Lifestyle has little effect on symptoms

☐ E Patients with recurrent symptoms can use flecainide as a 'pill in the pocket' treatment

90. A 37-year-old woman complains of recurrent severe pain in the right upper quadrant after meals. On examination she is tender in the right upper quadrant on deep inspiration. Which one of the following statements is true?

☐ A If caused by gallstones the pain usually settles within a few minutes

☐ B When associated with jaundice the cause is usually malignant

☐ C Symptoms usually settle spontaneously with a change in diet

☐ D She should be referred for endoscopic retrograde cholecystopancreatography

☐ E A raised alkaline phosphatase (ALP) suggests that the diagnosis is gallstones

91. A 21-year-old who was started on antibiotics for tonsillitis 2 days ago presents with signs of a quinsy. Which of the following statements about this condition is true? Select one option only.

☐ A It is usually caused by infection with *Haemophilus influenzae* type b

☐ B It is an abscess within the tonsillar crypts

☐ C Earache, trismus and dysphagia are typical symptoms

☐ D It is usually bilateral

☐ E It should be treated by adding in metronidazole tablets

☐ F It does not recur

92. An 84-year-old man presents with a 12-month history of a painless swelling on the side of his face. It does not change with eating and is non-tender. On examination you find the appearance below.

What is the likely diagnosis?

- [ ] A Parotid adenoma
- [ ] B Salivary calculus
- [ ] C Mumps
- [ ] D Acute leukaemia
- [ ] E Acute parotitis

THEME: MANAGEMENT OF CHRONIC STABLE ASTHMA

Options

A   Check inhaler technique
B   Infliximab
C   Inhaled β_2 agonist as needed
D   Inhaled high-dose steroids
E   Inhaled regular dose steroids
F   Leukotriene receptor antagonist
G   Long-acting bronchodilator
H   Omalizumab
I   Oral theophylline
J   Regular steroids by mouth

PAPER 2

For each clinical scenario below, select the most appropriate therapeutic choice from the list of options. Each option may be used once, more than once or not at all.

93.   It is licensed for use in severe persistent allergic asthma with proven IgE-mediated sensitivity to inhaled allergens.

94.   This is add-on therapy in a patient using an inhaled β_2 agonist 5 days a week on average.

95.   It may be associated with increased morbidity and mortality.

96.   It has an additive effect with inhaled steroids.

97.   It should be considered at step 5 in the asthma management protocol.

98. A 35-year-old woman presents with steadily increasing deafness that is causing her to struggle to hear on the telephone. Which of the following statements about otosclerosis is true? Select one option only.

- ☐ A It causes a sensorineural deafness, worse in low frequencies
- ☐ B It typically presents in the fifth decade
- ☐ C Its incidence is rising
- ☐ D It often gets worse during pregnancy
- ☐ E Hearing aids are the only treatment
- ☐ F Only women are affected

99. A 25-year-old woman presents complaining of recurrent boils in her axillae. These come on for no obvious reason and she has had numerous courses of antibiotics over the last 5 years. She says that she is fed up and has had to stop shaving her armpits, which she finds very distressing. Which of the following statements about treatment of this condition is true? Select one option only.

- ☐ A Botox injections may reduce the frequency of attacks
- ☐ B Anhydrol forte may be helpful in place of antiperspirant
- ☐ C A low-dose combined oral contraceptive may be helpful
- ☐ D Long-term oral tetracycline is effective in reducing frequency of attacks
- ☐ E She should be referred at this point for surgical excision and skin grafting

100. A 73-year-old woman noticed a sudden popping sensation in her left arm. On examination her arm has the following appearance.

What treatment is required?

☐   A   Referral to physiotherapy for ultrasound therapy

☐   B   Referral to orthopaedics for repair

☐   C   Splinting of the arm

☐   D   Collar-and-cuff sling

☐   E   Steroid injection into the rotator cuff

☐   F   None

101. Which of the following are NOT features of epiglottitis? Select one option only.

☐   A   The patient is usually aged 2–6 years

☐   B   The patients is unwell and looks septic

☐   C   The voice is muffled

☐   D   There is increasing dysphagia

☐   E   There is drooling

☐   F   It is exclusively seen in children

102. A 32-year-old woman who has been suffering from SLE for 3 years wants to start a family, and comes to see you for advice on pregnancy and lupus. Which of the following statements is true about this subject? Select one option only.

- [ ] A Miscarriage rates are no higher in women with lupus than in the general population
- [ ] B The risk of pre-eclampsia is the same as for the general population
- [ ] C Some women with SLE have an increased risk of bearing a child with congenital heart block
- [ ] D Steroids are contraindicated as a treatment for flare-ups in pregnancy
- [ ] E Women should switch their medication to simple analgesia only from preconception to after delivery

103. A 36-year-old mother of two small children has been seeing the practice nurse for advice on weight loss. She has been to Weight Watchers™ and tried joining a gym, but to no avail. She would like some slimming pills. Her previous medical history includes hypertension, diagnosed during pregnancy, for which she now takes ramipril. Her BMI is 41. Which of the following statements about the NICE guidance of weight management is correct? Select one option only.

- [ ] A With a BMI > 30 sibutramine would be the most appropriate treatment for her
- [ ] B If effective, sibutramine can be used for up to 3 years, as long as weight loss is maintained
- [ ] C If she can lose 2 kg over a 4-week period, she would be eligible for a trial of orlistat
- [ ] D Orlistat is an appetite suppressant so would be ideal in someone who struggles to cope with a conventional low-caloric diet
- [ ] E Orlistat can be prescribed initially for 3 months, and continued as long as the person has lost 5% of his or her body mass

104. You see a 23-year-old man at the walk-in centre who has cut his knuckles on someone else's teeth during a pub fight the night before. On examination he has several puncture wounds over the knuckles and the hand is swollen. Which of the following statements about his management is NOT true? Select one option only.

- [ ] A He should be given co-amoxiclav 625 mg three times daily and advised to return for review the following day
- [ ] B The wound should be cleaned with saline and he should be advised about RICE for his soft tissue bruising
- [ ] C A radiograph should be taken of the hand to exclude underlying fracture or broken teeth
- [ ] D Consideration should be given to HIV testing
- [ ] E He should receive a tetanus booster

105. The local primary school has had an outbreak of nits (pediculosis capitis). Which of the following statements about the management of nits is NOT true? Select one option only.

- [ ] A Nits may be found in the pubic area
- [ ] B Resistance to insecticides is common
- [ ] C Fine tooth-combing and conditioning are the best treatment for nits
- [ ] D Nits can be seen only with a magnifying glass
- [ ] E Simethicone is an effective treatment

THEME: INTERVENTIONS TO IMPROVE HEALTH

Options

A   Caerphilly Study

B   EarlyBird 21 study

C   ExTraMATCH

D   Folic acid

E   High-dose vitamin E

F   HOPE-2

G   MAVIS trial

H   Selenium

I   Whitehall 2 study

For each of the statements below about recent research into exercise and lifestyle, indicate which option from the list is most appropriate. Each option may be used once, more than once or not at all.

☐ **106.** It showed that employees with chronic occupational stress had twice the risk of developing the metabolic syndrome than those without chronic stress.

☐ **107.** It found that exercise programmes in stable heart failure patients reduced hospital admissions and improved survival.

☐ **108.** It is associated with increased mortality.

☐ **109.** It showed that only a quarter of parents recognised that their child was overweight.

☐ **110.** It showed that regular vigorous exercise such as swimming or jogging in patients with no evidence of cardiovascular disease reduced the risk of premature death.

111. A 3-year-old girl presents with a rash on her face. She was previously well until she developed a flu-like illness 3 days ago. She has no eye or chest symptoms. Her face has the following appearance.

What is the diagnosis?

- [ ] A   Measles
- [ ] B   Rubella
- [ ] C   Shingles
- [ ] D   Parvovirus B19
- [ ] E   Chickenpox

THEME: PRESCRIPTION CHARGES

Options

A   Apply under low-income scheme

B   Automatically entitled to free prescriptions

C   Entitled to free NHS dental treatment

D   Entitled to free NHS sight tests

E   Entitled to free prescriptions on applying for an exemption certificate

F   Not entitled to free dental treatment

G   Not entitled to free NHS sight test

H   Not entitled to free prescriptions

I   Prescription pre-payment certificate

For each of the patients described below, select the most appropriate rule about health charges. Each option may be used once, more than once or not at all.

☐ **112.** **A 56-year-old businessman with diet-controlled diabetes who needs antibiotics.**

☐ **113.** **A 33-year-old woman who gave birth 9 months ago needs a dental crown.**

☐ **114.** **A 57-year-old accountant who takes thyroxine needs an eye test.**

☐ **115.** **An 18-year-old student who needs antibiotics.**

☐ **116.** **A 35-year-old person with newly diagnosed epilepsy taking phenytoin.**

117. A 76-year-old man presents with a rash on both legs for 2 years. It is itchy and he has been using E45. He has no previous history of note and is otherwise well. The rash is shown below.

What is the diagnosis?

- [ ] A   Asteatotic eczema
- [ ] B   Varicose eczema
- [ ] C   Pompholyx
- [ ] D   Psoriasis
- [ ] E   Contact dermatitis

THEME: EXAMINATION OF THE EYE

Options

A   Acute angle-closure glaucoma

B   Cataract

C   Chronic glaucoma

D   Corneal abrasion

E   Keratoconus

F   Optic atrophy

G   Recurrent uveitis

H   Retinoblastoma

For each of the scenarios described below, select the most appropriate diagnosis from the list of options. Each option may be used once, more than once or not at all.

☐   **118.   The red reflex appears white.**

☐   **119.   On fundoscopy the disc appears pale compared with the other eye.**

☐   **120.   The pupil is fixed but round.**

☐   **121.   The pupil is fixed but irregular.**

☐   **122.   The disc has a cupped appearance.**

123. A 5-year-old girl presents with warts on her eyelids. On examination she has firm umbilicated papules on her face and eyelids. Which of the following statements about molluscum contagiosum is NOT true? Select one option only.

- [ ] A It may be seen as a sexually transmitted infection
- [ ] B Secondary infection may cause lesions to become pustular
- [ ] C It should always be actively treated
- [ ] D Sufferers should use separate towels to prevent spread to other family members
- [ ] E Typically it resolves spontaneously over 3–18 months

124. A 21-year-old man presents with a painless swelling in his left lower eyelid for 3 months. On examination there is no erythema or discharge. Which of the following is the most likely diagnosis? Select one option only.

- [ ] A Basal cell carcinoma
- [ ] B Stye
- [ ] C Xanthelasma
- [ ] D Chalazion
- [ ] E Conjunctivitis

THEME: ANTIBIOTIC PRESCRIBING

Options

A Aciclovir

B Amoxicillin

C Augmentin (co-amoxiclav)

D Benzylpenicillin

E Cefradine

F Ciprofloxacin

G Chloramphenicol

H Erythromycin

I Flucloxacillin

J Fusidic acid

K Metronidazole

L Nitrofurantoin

M Phenoxymethylpenicillin

N Trimethoprim

For each infection described below, select the most appropriate antibiotic from the list of options. Each option may be used once, more than once or not at all.

☐ **125.** A 67-year-old woman who requires prophylaxis against recurrent urinary tract infections and has had a severe allergic reaction to Septrin (co-trimoxazole).

☐ **126.** A 21-year-old student who has been in close contact with a patient with meningococcal meningitis.

☐ **127.** A 4-year-old child with tonsillitis.

☐ **128.** A 35-year-old man with a chest infection who is allergic to penicillin.

☐ **129.** A 34-year-old veterinary nurse who has received a dog bite to the hand.

130. Which of the following statements about the management of diabetic ketoacidosis (DKA) is true? Select one option only.

☐ A Emergency treatment involves an immediate insulin injection and fluid rehydration

☐ B DKA usually has no prodromal phase

☐ C The respiratory rate is often reduced

☐ D Polydipsia often causes fluid overload and hyponatraemia

☐ E Initial treatment should include stat injection of intramuscular glucagons

131. A 21-year-old student presents with a 1-week history of tender lumps on his shins. He is otherwise fit and well and takes no regular medication. A photograph of his shins is shown below.

Which of the following statements about this condition is NOT true? Select one option only.

☐ A It may be caused by cat scratch disease

☐ B Patients should have a throat swab and chest radiograph as routine investigations

☐ C It may be caused by the oral contraceptive pill

☐ D Non-steroidal anti-inflammatory drugs (NSAIDs) may provide symptomatic relief

☐ E It is usually a sign of underlying malignancy

THEME: CHILD DEVELOPMENT

Options

A   3 months

B   5 months

C   5 years

D   8 weeks

E   10 months

F   18 months

G   30 months

For each of the developmental milestones below, select the most appropriate age from the list of options. Each option may be used once, more than once or not at all.

☐   **132.**   **Walks unsupported.**

☐   **133.**   **Uses single words appropriately.**

☐   **134.**   **Smiles responsively.**

☐   **135.**   **Able to sit unsupported.**

☐   **136.**   **Uses phrases.**

☐   **137.**   **Reaches for objects presented.**

☐   **138.**   **Maintains eye contact.**

139. With regard to drug treatments for rheumatological conditions, which of the following statements is true? Select one option only.

☐ A Infliximab is licensed for the prevention of recurrence in rheumatoid arthritis

☐ B Hydroxychloroquine will reduce pain, swelling and stiffness in systemic lupus erythematosus (SLE)

☐ C Penicillamine is given by intramuscular injection

☐ D Methotrexate produces immediate benefit in rheumatoid arthritis

☐ E Sulfasalazine has no effect on fertility, so it can be safely used in younger patients

140. A 53-year-old woman presents with 6 weeks of malaise and fatigue associated with swelling and erythema affecting her metacarpophalangeal joints in both hands. These are particularly stiff first thing in the morning. Which of the following is a likely diagnosis? Select one option only.

☐ A Primary nodal osteoarthritis

☐ B Rheumatoid arthritis

☐ C Reiter syndrome

☐ D Gout

☐ E Rheumatic fever

141. Which one of the following statements is true with regard to audit in primary care?

☐ A   Audit involves researching the effects of new treatment protocols

☐ B   Standards must be defined and agreed before an audit is carried out

☐ C   The 'audit cycle' refers to the continual need to refine our audit criteria

☐ D   The implementation of change is implicit in the audit cycle

☐ E   Audits should be doctor-led

142. Which of the following statements about the management of glue ear in a 27-month-old child is correct? Select one option only.

☐ A   All children with glue ear that persists for more than 3 months should have grommets fitted

☐ B   Oral amoxicillin will treat most cases of glue ear if used early

☑ C   Adenoidectomy at the time of grommet insertion significantly reduces the risk of recurrence

☐ D   Grommets are the only long-term solution to glue ear

☐ E   Glue ear causes sensorineural hearing loss

☐ F   Glue ear may be treated with cranial osteopathy

THEME: SHOULDER PROBLEMS

Options

A   Cervical spondylosis

B   Frozen shoulder

C   Osteoarthritis

D   Referred pain

E   Ruptured supraspinatus

F   Shoulder dystocia

G   Shoulder–hand syndrome

H   Subluxation of the glenohumeral joint

I   Supraspinatus tendonitis

For each of the cases described below select the most appropriate choice from the list of options. Each option may be used once, more than once or not at all.

☐   **143.**   A 19-year-old girl who is 5 weeks' pregnant presents with vaginal bleeding and pain in the tip of her left shoulder. On examination she has a full range of movement in the shoulder.

☐   **144.**   A 56-year-old man presents with several years of pain and reduced range of movement in his right shoulder. On examination there is limited range of movement and extensive crepitus.

☐   **145.**   A 67-year-old woman with a history of chronic neck pain complains of pain in her right shoulder with weakness in abduction. She also reports paraesthesiae in her arm at times.

☐   **146.**   A 45-year-old man is seen with a 12-week history of reduced range of movement in his left shoulder. This started without obvious cause and on examination you note that external rotation is particularly affected.

147. A 23-year-old man presents with pain and reduced range of movement in his left shoulder. He thinks that he may have fallen on to his shoulder the previous night after drinking, but cannot remember. On examination his shoulder looks flattened and, in addition to difficulty abducting the shoulder, he has a numb patch on the side of his humerus.

148. A 73-year-old woman attends the surgery complaining about a lesion on her hand that appeared 2 months ago and has rapidly grown in size. The lesion is shown below.

Which of the following statements about this lesion is true? Select one option only.

A   This lesion is likely to be a squamous cell carcinoma

B   This lesion is a ganglion and may be treated with needle aspiration

C   Biopsy is necessary to differentiate between a keratoacanthoma and an SCC

D   These lesions should always be treated because resolution is rare

E   Small lesions may be treated successfully with liquid nitrogen

F   These lesions are more common in men

THEME: MEDICAL RECORDS LEGISLATION

Options

A Access to Health Records Act

B Access to Medical Reports Act

C Children's Act

D Community Care Act

E Data Protection Act

F Freedom of Information Act

G Mental Health Act 1983

H Public Records Act

For each of the scenarios below, select one of the most appropriate Acts from the list of options.

☐ 149. It allows patients to see entries in their medical records made since 1991.

☐ 150. It allows patients to access and request alterations to be made to computer records.

☐ 151. It allows a charge of up to £10 to be made for access to records, plus copying expenses.

☐ 152. It assumes that a mother automatically has responsibility for a child.

☐ 153. It allows patients to attach a codicil to the record in question if he or she disagrees with it.

☐ 154. It allows doctors to withhold information from a patient's record that would be damaging to his or her mental health.

THEME: NHS INFORMATION TECHNOLOGY PROJECTS

Options

A   Choose and book

B   Connecting for Health

C   Electronic transfer of prescriptions

D   N3

E   PACS (Picture Archiving and Communications System)

For each of the descriptions below, select the most appropriate choice from the list of options. Each option may be used once, more than once or not at all.

☐ **155.** NHS IT stores and distributes radiological images.

☐ **156.** It provides indicative data on waiting times in different localities.

☐ **157.** This is the infrastructure for the NHS information technology network.

☐ **158.** It will allow patients access to their records via the internet.

☐ **159.** It aims to enable cross-referencing of medical records and drug data.

PAPER 2

160. A 67-year-old man who has been a lifelong smoker presents with haemoptysis, progressive shortness of breath and weight loss. His hands have the appearance shown below.

What is the probable underlying diagnosis? Select one option only.

- [ ] A   Inflammatory bowel disease
- [ ] B   Congenital heart disease
- [ ] C   Pneumonia
- [ ] D   Cystic fibrosis
- [ ] E   Lung cancer

161. A new mum comes to see you at the end of her tether. Her 4-week-old son has had awful colic every night for the last 2 weeks. He is otherwise well but she demands that something be done. On examination no abnormalities are found. Which of the following statements about colic is true? Select one option only.

- [ ] A   It is usually associated with vomiting at the end of an attack
- [ ] B   It occurs in 1% of infants
- [ ] C   It usually resolves over 1–2 weeks
- [ ] D   It may be helped with dicyclomine
- [ ] E   It may be helped with lactase added to feeds

THEME: GYNAECOLOGICAL MALIGNANCIES

Options

A   Cervical carcinoma

B   Cervical intraepithelial neoplasia

C   Choriocarcinoma

D   Endometrial carcinoma

E   Ovarian carcinoma

F   Vulval carcinoma

G   Vulval intraepithelial neoplasia

For each of the descriptions below, select the most appropriate diagnosis from the list of options. Each option may be used once, more than once or not at all.

- [ ] **162.** It tends to be multifocal.

- [ ] **163.** It causes postcoital bleeding.

- [ ] **164.** It is associated with raised β-hCG.

- [ ] **165.** It has a 30% 5-year survival rate.

- [ ] **166.** It is associated with diabetes.

167. A 29-year-old executive sales director with a history of varicose veins complains of perianal discomfort, discharge and occasional rectal bleeding. Which one of the following statements about his management is true?

- [ ] A Thrombosis of piles is associated with pain and fresh bleeding
- [ ] B Third-degree piles prolapse with defecation but are easily replaced
- [ ] C Blood is usually mixed in with the stool
- [ ] D Piles are always visible on external examination
- [ ] E Increased dietary fibre and fluids are an important part of treatment

168. You are referred a 3-month-old baby boy by the health visitor after his mother noticed that he is leaking urine from the middle of his penis. On examination there seems to be a small pit on the underside of the penis. Which of the following statements about this condition is true? Select one option only.

- [ ] A The condition is rare, with an incidence of 1:5000
- [ ] B It always presents in infancy
- [ ] C Surgery is always indicated
- [ ] D It is usually associated with other abnormalities of the urogenital tract
- [ ] E It may be a sign of female virilisation

THEME: HIRSUTISM

Options

A   Combined oral contraceptive

B   Cyproterone acetate

C   Dianette

D   Electrolysis

E   Finasteride

F   Metformin

G   Minoxidil

H   Referral

I   Spironolactone

J   Weight loss

For each of the patients described below, select the most appropriate therapy from the list of options. Each option may be used once, more than once or not at all.

169. A 22-year-old woman with excessive facial hair and irregular periods. Blood tests are normal.

170. A 47-year-old woman with hirsutism who has a history of DVT on the contraceptive pill and who has not found electrolysis or camouflage effective.

171. A 27-year-old woman of Mediterranean origin with normal periods who has a prominent hair on her upper lip only and is unable to take the pill.

172. An 18-year-old girl with hirsutism and acne, not responding to the combined oral contraceptive pill (COCP).

173. A 23-year-old woman who is hirsute with irregular periods and primary infertility.

THEME: DIZZINESS AND VERTIGO

Options

A   Acoustic neuroma

B   Benign paroxysmal positional vertigo

C   Cardiogenic syncope

D   Cervical vertigo

E   Hyperventilation

F   Menière's disease

G   Ramsay Hunt syndrome

H   Round window rupture

I   Migraine

J   Vestibular neuronitis

For each scenario described below, select the single most likely diagnosis from the list of options. Each option may be used once, more than once or not at all.

☐ **174.** Recurrent attacks of pressure in the ear are associated with tinnitus, deafness and vertigo.

☐ **175.** There is an acute onset of severe vertigo with vomiting, which usually settles over several days.

☐ **176.** It is associated with a sensation of light-headedness and palpitations before fainting.

☐ **177.** It is associated with vertigo only on moving the head in certain planes.

☐ **178.** Vertigo is accompanied by facial palsy and deafness.

179. A 63-year-old man requests a PSA (prostate-specific antigen) test to see if he has prostate cancer. Before testing you spend some time counselling him about the test and its use. Which of the following statements about PSA testing is true? Select one option only.

- ☐ A   The test is highly sensitive
- ☐ B   The test is highly specific
- ☐ C   A raised PSA may be caused by urinary infection
- ☐ D   PSA testing is a proven diagnostic test
- ☐ E   Anyone with a PSA > 4.0 mmol/l should be referred

180. A 29-year-old man registers at the practice, having just moved to the area. At his first consultation he admits that he has been injecting heroin for the last 8 months and would like help in stopping. Which one of the following statements about this area of practice is NOT true?

- ☐ A   He should be converted to a twice-daily maintenance dose of methadone and this should be gradually reduced
- ☐ B   He should be advised about the importance of safe sex
- ☐ C   GPs are not obliged under the terms of the GMS contract to provide substitution treatment for opiate dependency
- ☐ D   A treatment contract should be agreed with the patient that covers the responsibilities of each party
- ☐ E   A hierarchy of goals is recommended that will initially minimise harm and aim for eventual abstinence

181. A 19-year-old man presents complaining of an acute onset of breathlessness and pain in his left chest. He has no previous history of note. On examination he is tall and lean, and seems to be in good health. He has reduced air entry on the left side of his chest and is tachypoenic. Which of the following is the most likely diagnosis? Select one option only

- [ ] A Pleurisy
- [ ] B Pulmonary embolus
- [ ] C Panic attack
- [ ] D Pneumothorax
- [ ] E Bronchopneumonia

182. A 24-year-old girl who is about to go travelling for a year consults you for advice on antimalarials. Which of the following statements about prevention of malaria is true? Select one option only.

- [ ] A Malarone is taken weekly starting 1 week before travel until 4 weeks after return from a malaria region
- [ ] B Patients who are entitled to free prescriptions can get antimalarials on an FP10
- [ ] C As long as patients take antimalarials as prescribed they are at very low risk of catching malaria
- [ ] D Mefloquine is associated with neuropsychiatric side effects in up to 10% of patients
- [ ] E Doxycycline is associated with photosensitivity

183. You receive a letter of complaint from a patient. Which one of the following is a requirement relating to the practice response?

☐ A A written response must be received by the patient within 10 working days

☐ B The complaint must be acknowledged within 5 working days

☐ C The complaint needs to be considered only if it is received on paper

☐ D If the patient's concerns are not satisfied by the practice response, the patient can take the complaint to the Healthcare Commission

☐ E There is a time limit of 12 months for practice complaints

184. You are telephoned by the mother of a 15-year-old boy who is away on school camp. One of his classmates has just been diagnosed with mumps and his mother is concerned that he is at risk. Which of the following statements about mumps is true? Select one option only.

☐ A The incubation period is 7–10 days

☐ B Salivary gland swelling is pathognomonic and seen in all cases

☐ C Ten per cent of patients with mumps develop symptomatic meningeal involvement

☐ D Of postpubertal males 80% develop bilateral orchitis

☐ E Of those with orchitis 70% become infertile

THEME: CHEST PAIN

Options

A   Acute pericarditis

B   Angina

C   Aortic dissection

D   Costochondritis

E   Gastro-oesophageal reflux

F   Myocardial infarction

G   Panic attack

H   Pleurisy

I   Pneumothorax

J   Pulmonary embolus

For each clinical description below, select the most likely diagnosis from the list of options. Each option may be used once, more than once or not at all.

☐   **185.**   A crushing sharp pleuritic pain, relieved by leaning forwards.

☐   **186.**   A very sharp unilateral pleuritic pain with shortness of breath.

☐   **187.**   A tearing chest pain from the front of the chest through to the back.

☐   **188.**   An oppressive squeezing chest pain, radiating to the neck, which comes on at rest, and not relieved by nitrates.

☐   **189.**   A sharp pleuritic pain accompanied by shortness of breath and haemoptysis.

THEME: FEBRILE SEIZURES

190–197.

Options

A	> 15 minutes	G	Febrile
B	< 15 minutes	H	First episode
C	Admit	I	Paracetamol
D	Afebrile	J	Rash
E	Age < 18 months	K	Rectal diazepam
F	Age > 18 months	L	Recurrent episode

For each stage in the flowchart below, which describes the management of febrile seizures, select the most appropriate from the list of options. Each option may be used once, more than once or not at all.

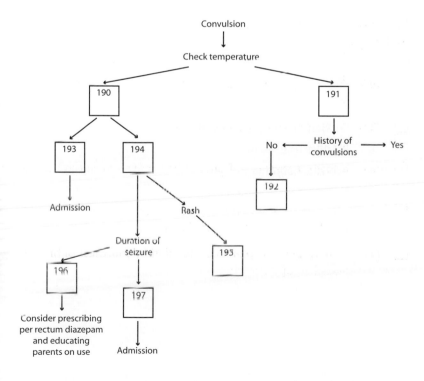

198. A 76-year-old woman complains of difficulty hearing and bilateral tinnitus. Her audiogram is shown below. What is the most likely diagnosis? Select one option only.

- [ ] A   Sudden-onset sensorineural hearing loss
- [ ] B   Presbyacusis
- [ ] C   Acoustic neuroma
- [ ] D   Noise-induced hearing loss
- [ ] E   Otosclerosis

199. Your local Primary Care Trust (PCT) is looking at the variation in emergency admission rates across the PCT area in an attempt to reduce referrals. They present the following data:

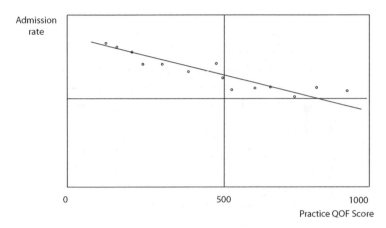

Which one of the following statements is true with regard to possible explanations for these results?

- [ ] A Practices with high QOF scores are more likely to be located in areas with high deprivation scores

- [ ] B Practices with high QOF scores might be making more earlier diagnoses, resulting in higher admission rates for elective treatment

- [ ] C Practices with high QOF scores might be exception reporting the most sick patients to inflate their QOF scores artificially

- [ ] D It is easier to obtain high QOF scores in areas of high morbidity where there are naturally high admission rates

- [ ] E Practices with high QOF scores have devolved much of their routine work to non-medical staff, who are better able to manage complex medical problems

200. A 65-year-old farmer presents with a 2-year history of a sore just below his eyelid. Which of the following statements about potential diagnoses is true? Select one option only.

☐ A   A rolled telangiectatic edge with central ulceration is characteristic of a SCC

☐ B   Basal cell carcinomas often have local lymph node involvement at diagnosis

☐ C   A rapidly growing lesion that forms a crater with a central plug is likely to be a keratoacanthoma

☐ D   Curettage and cautery are appropriate treatment for small SCCs

☐ E   A dermoid cyst can be excluded on histology only

Paper 2
Answers

1. **B:** **He should take warfarin for 6 months after discharge**

Although there are some data suggesting that warfarin may be stopped in this situation after 2 months, current recommendations are 6 months. Thrombophilia cannot be tested while on anticoagulants and it would be unwise to stop warfarin at this stage for testing.

2. **C:** **Check his FBC**

This child has symptoms of leukaemia, which is the most common malignant disease in children and often presents with muscle and joint pain. Signs of marrow failure include anaemia, frequent infections and thrombocytopenia, although blast activity may cause headache, fits and gum hypertrophy.

3. **I:** **Pamidronate**

Pamidronate or clodronate will reduce serum calcium levels.

4. **D:** **Dexamethasone**

Anorexia is a common symptom and usually responds to prednisolone or dexamethasone.

5. **B:** **Cholestyramine**

Pruritus caused by liver involvement may be treated with cholestyramine or Piriton (chlorpheniramine).

6. **A:** **Baclofen**

Baclofen or benzodiazepines help with muscle spasm.

7.   C: Chlorpromazine

Chlorpromazine is often helpful in hiccoughs, which may be caused by renal failure.

8.   E: Patient-initiated outpatient follow-up reduces outpatient visits by 38%

Taking low-dose steroids over 10 years increases mortality by 69% compared with patients not taking steroids. The FIN-RACo study (the FINnish RA Combination therapy study) showed that aggressive treatment of early rheumatoid arthritis (RA) with a combination of disease-modifying anti-rheumatic drugs (DMARDs) slows radiological progression of disease. Etanercept is effective, has a rapid onset of action (2 weeks) and is more effective in early RA than in established RA. The TICOR A (TIght COntrol for Rheumatoid Arthritis) trial showed significant benefits with monthly outpatient follow-up and aggressive use of joint injections. Where patients request appointments according to clinical need rather than according to an arbitrary timescale there are significant benefits for patients and the hospital.

9.   E: Breech presentation is a risk factor

Breech presentation and positive family history are risk factors. Ortolani testing involves attempting to relocate a dislocated hip whereas Barlow testing attempts to dislocate a hip. Ultrasound screening has a high pick-up rate but is associated with a high false-positive rate. Most children require splinting only.

10.   A: Topical glyceryl trinitrate (GTN)

This patient has symptoms suggestive of an anal fissure; where this is not settling with dietary changes or topical treatment, GTN or diltiazem application may be of benefit.

11.   C: Levomepromazine will help with agitation and nausea

Fentanyl or MST dose should be converted to 24-hour subcutaneous morphine dose according to the conversion chart in the BNF. Morphine is an excellent painkiller for all types of pain, but in less severe cases NSAIDs may be useful for bone pain. Morphine is the drug of choice for respiratory symptoms because it also reduces dyspnoea.

12.   A: Asbestosis

Asbestosis is a progressive lung fibrosis caused by inhalation of blue asbestos. It increases the risk of lung cancer 5-fold and in smokers by 55-fold. Industrial compensation is available. The prognosis is poor. Spirometry shows a restrictive defect; however, a chest radiograph may miss fibrosis and CT (computed tomography) may be more appropriate.

13.   C: Lazy eye may be caused by retinoblastoma

When testing for squint the affected eye takes up fixation when the good eye is covered. When the good eye is uncovered, the affected eye relaxes and fails to fixate. The good eye is unaffected when the bad eye is covered. Causes include anything that reduces the acuity in the affected eye, such as cataract, ptosis and retinoblastoma. The condition is not always obvious in infancy.

14.   B: GMS

GMS is nationally negotiated but has an element of local negotiation (LES).

15.   E: PMS plus

PMS plus projects usually involve an element of transfer of secondary care to primary care, eg taking over a local community hospital.

16.   C: LIFT

LIFT (Local Improvement Finance Trust) is a vehicle that allows PCTs to redevelop properties to address needs.

17.   F: Private contractor status

This work is negotiated between the PCT and individual practices.

18.   D: PMS

PMS Contracts included money for access and chronic disease management. Accordingly the maximum QOF scores were reduced.

19.   E: She should be treated with a permanent pacemaker

The diagnosis is complete heart block. She should be referred immediately for a pacemaker. The most common cause is ischaemic heart disease. If compromised, atropine 1 mg can be used.

20.   E: Vasectomy is reversible in only 50% of cases

The lifetime failure rate is less than 1:1000. Bruising is very common and the most common long-term complication is pain. It is usually performed under local anaesthetic and sterility should not be assumed until 3 months and two negative sperm counts have passed.

21.   E: Silver nitrate cautery may cause septal perforation

Most bleeds are anterior and unilateral with bleeding from Little's area, the plexus of capillaries derived ultimately from the internal and external carotid. The most common cause is probably idiopathic followed by iatrogenic, with aspirin and warfarin therapy being particular culprits. Bleeding points may be cauterised with silver nitrate but over-zealous or too frequent use of this may result in perforation of the nasal septum. Where pressure fails to settle the bleeding, Merocel packs are easily inserted by nurses or doctors and are extremely effective. BIPP packing is seldom used.

22. A: Dendritic ulcer

This is a typical history of a dendritic ulcer. The appearance could also be seen in corneal abrasion or corneal ulcer in a contact lens wearer, but not with this history. Treatment is with aciclovir five times a day.

23. D: Neuromuscular relaxants are the drug of choice in the Netherlands

Rates of physician-assisted suicide have fallen slightly since legalisation in the Netherlands. Physician-assisted suicide accounts for 1.7% of deaths in the Netherlands. The 'doctrine of double effect' refers to the use of a drug for its analgesic properties which also accelerates death as a side effect, eg diamorphine syringe drivers. It is legal to give the drug in this circumstance.

24. A: Dementia is usually associated with altered cognition and consciousness

Dementia does not affect consciousness. Where consciousness is affected, consider causes of delirium. Young patients may have metabolic defects, eg Wilson's disease or HIV.

25. B: Gilbert's syndrome

Isolated hyperbilirubinaemia is almost never of pathological significance. This can be demonstrated by taking a fasting bilirubin after an overnight fast.

26. F: Iatrogenic

Enzyme-inducing drugs and alcohol can elevate GGT levels.

27. H: Physiological

ALP may be elevated in adolescence, bone tumours and Paget's disease.

PAPER 2

28. **E:** **Hepatitis**

Acute hepatitis usually presents with a greatly elevated ALT.

29. **A:** **Gallstones**

LFTs usually return to normal after the obstruction has been removed.

30. **C:** **Topical metronidazole is effective**

Topical or oral metronidazole is often effective if regular cleaning with povidone–iodine is ineffective.

31. **E:** **This could be a presentation of a renal tumour**

Renal colic can be due to direct obstruction by tumour or bleeding from the tumour. Calcium levels can be raised and should be measured. Signs of infection should prompt admission. Stones are not usually visible on a plain film. An NSAID should be used unless contraindicated.

32. **E:** **Sildenafil**

Sildenafil may cause chromatopsia, usually green.

33. **A:** **All of them**

Patients who are predisposed to priapism should not take treatments for erectile dysfunction.

34. **C:** **MUSE**

MUSE is a transurethral system and should not be used in urethral stricture.

35.   F: Tadalafil

Tadalafil should be taken at least 30 minutes before sexual activity and the effect may persist for up to 36 hours.

36.   A: All of them

Patients with neurological disease, renal failure, diabetes, prostate cancer or who have had radical pelvic surgery qualify for impotence drugs on the NHS.

37.   D: The results should be treated with caution because of inclusion bias

Qualitative studies are notoriously prone to bias. This study has no standardised measure of depression scores at either the outset or the end, consists of self-reporting by patients who self-refer and pay for a treatment in which they presumably have faith, has no control group and relies on the use of only one therapist. It is therefore prone to inclusion bias, reporting bias and a strong placebo effect. The economic analysis is not valid because most patients with mild depression would not need drug treatment. The number needed to treat (NNT) cannot be calculated because there is no comparison group.

38.   A: Refer for barium enema

This patient has symptoms of a right-sided colonic cancer. Sigmoidoscopy will not visualise the area and barium enema, although the first-line investigation, may give a false-negative result. Raised ESR is consistent with cancer.

39.   A: Approximately 4000 people a year commit suicide in England and Wales

There is a bimodal social-class distribution, with middle classes being at lowest risk. Older divorced men who have just lost their jobs and live in towns are most likely to commit suicide. Overdose is the most common method, and violent attempts, such as hanging, are the most likely to succeed. There is a 1–2% risk of deliberate self-harmers committing suicide within 12 months.

40.   C: Edwards syndrome

Edwards syndrome is associated with heart abnormalities.

41.   B: Down syndrome

Patients with Down syndrome also frequently have congenital heart disease.

42.   D: Fragile X syndrome

Fragile X syndrome is associated with abnormalities of DNA structure and prenatal testing may be possible in females with affected relatives.

43.   E: Klinefelter syndrome

Klinefelter syndrome has the karyotype 47XXY and occurs in 1:1000 liveborn babies.

44.   I: Williams syndrome

Williams syndrome is inherited on chromosome 7 and is often associated with learning difficulties.

45.   A: Private fees can be set at whatever level the practice wishes

Private fees can be set on a free-market basis but practices should beware exploiting patients where they have no option to go elsewhere, eg for occupational medicals where their registered GP is required to complete a report. The Monopolies Commission banned the BMA from setting recommended fees some years ago. Private work is not covered by the GMS Contract. Private fees should be displayed prominently and patients made aware of these before services are provided.

46.   A: Ninety per cent of hip replacements last for more than 10 years

The infection rate is approximately 1%. Crossing the surgical leg over the non-surgical leg is associated with dislocation. The incidence of deep vein thrombosis (DVT) is 1.5% and of pulmonary embolus (PE) 1.1%. Hip resurfacing is superior to conventional arthroplasty for survival of the prosthesis and preservation of bone mineral density but is usually only indicated in early disease.

47.   A: Bereavement payment

This is payable to people under state pension age who are married or in a civil partnership.

48.   C: Child benefit

This is payable to all parents in the UK, regardless of income.

49.   F: Disability Living Allowance

DLA is payable to children and adults.

50.   E: DS1500

DS1500 allows a streamlined application for Attendance Allowance in those with a life expectancy of less than 6 months.

51.   B: Carers' Allowance

Carers' Allowance is paid to people on a low income who spend more than 35 hours a week caring for someone who receives DLA.

52.   A: Kawasaki's disease

This child has Kawasaki's disease, a febrile vasculitis affecting children. It may cause coronary artery aneurysms in a third of patients and has a mortality rate of around 3%. ECG changes are seen including arrhythmias and long QT interval. Treatment is with aspirin or intravenous immunoglobulin,

53.   E: Biventricular failure

This patient has signs of right- and left-sided heart failure. Cor pulmonale is right-sided heart failure secondary to pulmonary disease. The presence of a regular pulse precludes new-onset AF as a diagnosis.

54.   D: It may cause phimosis

Balanitis is usually caused by *Candida* species or coliforms. Topical antifungals and sometimes fusidic acid are often helpful. Recurrent attacks may cause phimosis and need circumcision. Fifty per cent of 6 year olds cannot fully retract their foreskin.

55.   C: Corticosteroids are a useful first-line therapy if used early

Corticosteroids may stimulate regrowth but 75% of patients recover spontaneously so first-line treatment should be reassurance and explanation. Autoimmune conditions such as vitiligo may be associated. Childhood onset and eyelash involvement are poor prognostic indicators.

56.   C: Of 2-week referrals, 99% are seen within 2 weeks

The Myocardial Infarction National Audit Project (MINAP) has shown consistent benefits in call-to-needle and arrival-to-needle times. The number of teenage pregnancies has been cut by less than 15% and in some areas is rising. Cancer mortality has fallen by 15% since 1995. A report from Asthma UK found that up to 10% of the difference in asthma admission rates between PCTs could be explained by performance in the QOF. The proportion of patients receiving thrombolysis within 30 minutes of arrival in hospital has risen from 39% to 80% since 2000.

57.   E: Scoliosis may be associated with deformity of the skull and ribcage

Of infants with scoliosis 50% will resolve spontaneously. Primary scoliosis often presents in adolescence where it is more common in girls. It is usually mid-thoracic and the curve is usually concave to the right. It may be associated with plagiocephaly in infants and prominence of the posterior rib cage in teenagers. Treatment where indicated usually involves insertion of rods.

58.   F: Septic abortion

She should be admitted for intravenous antibiotics and ERPC (evacuation of retained products of conception).

59.   D: Ectopic pregnancy

An empty uterus and a climbing or static quantitative β-hCG suggests a non-uterine pregnancy.

60.   B: Cervical incompetence

Cervical incompetence typically causes mid-trimester loss with few contractions.

61.   G: Threatened abortion

Of threatened abortions 75% settle spontaneously.

62.   D: Ectopic pregnancy

All women with abdominal pain should have a pregnancy test because there may be few gynaecological signs.

63.   D: Bronchiolitis

Bronchiolitis occurs in epidemics in winter, caused by respiratory syncytial virus. It is particularly severe in those under 6 months old and can be fatal. High-risk patients (eg congenital heart disease), those with apnoeas or tachypnoeas, and those with failure to feed should be admitted to hospital. Well children can often be managed at home.

64.   C: Employers must write to employees in advance of their retirement date and advise them of their rights to apply to work beyond this date

Age discrimination protects elderly and young people. Mandatory retirement cannot be lower than 65 years for men *and* women. The maximum qualifying length of service for benefits is 5 years. Dismissal on the basis of age is legal from 65 onwards, as long as it can be justified.

65. **C:** **The ESPIRIT trial showed that an aspirin and dipyridamole combination is effective in secondary prevention of ischaemic stroke and TIAs**

BHS guidelines recommend aspirin use in those with a 10-year risk > 20%. The ESPRIT trial found a significant reduction in mortality with no increase in bleeding compared with aspirin alone. The MATCH trial showed no benefit from adding clopidogrel to aspirin. Meta-analysis has shown self-monitoring of warfarin therapy to be safe and effective in selected patients. The CAPRIE trial showed clopidogrel to be more effective than aspirin for secondary prevention.

66. **E:** **If *Staphylococcus sp.* is suspected flucloxacillin should be added**

The first-line treatment for community-acquired pneumonia is amoxicillin at a dose of 500–1000 mg three times daily (BTS guidelines), which should cover intermediate resistant strains of *Strepcoccus pneumoniae*. In allergic individuals or where atypical pneumonia is suspected, a macrolide is appropriate. During flu outbreaks staphylococcal pneumonia has a high mortality and should be treated with flucloxacillin.

67. **C:** **Paroxetine can increase the period before ejaculation up to eight times longer than placebo**

Up to 31% of male respondents to surveys reported premature ejaculation. Clomipramine is useful when taken before intercourse or as a once-daily treatment, but has an adverse side-effect profile in many patients. Paroxetine once daily is the most effective treatment.

68. **D:** **Hepatitis C**

Hepatitis C often causes chronic active hepatitis; 90% of transmission is percutaneous.

69. **E:** **Hepatitis D**

Hepatitis D is endemic among hepatitis B carriers in the Mediterranean area.

70. **B:** **Hepatitis A**

Hepatitis A is endemic in less developed countries and is spread predominantly through food.

71. **B:** **Hepatitis A**

Hepatitis A seropositivity is high in psychiatric hospitals and similar institutions. Care workers should be immunised.

72. **C:** **Hepatitis B**

Hepatitis B causes chronic hepatitis in 1% of cases.

73. **E:** **Tight underwear**

The NICE guidelines advise that, although there is evidence that scrotal temperature can reduce sperm quality, there is no evidence that wearing looser-fitting underwear makes any difference. Caffeine consumption has not been shown to be harmful either.

74. **C:** **The ramipril should be stopped and specialist advice sought**

NICE guidance suggests that an increase of 50% in creatinine or a rise to > 200 µg/ml should prompt referral. Most cases are caused by occult renal artery stenosis which may cause secondary hypertension. Angiotensin receptor antagonists (ARBs) have the same effect and NICE recommend that both be started under specialist supervision if baseline creatinine > 150 µg/ml.

75.   **B:**   **Discuss his performance with other members of the practice team to see if there are other concerns**

This situation might have arisen for a number of reasons and it would be inappropriate to invoke disciplinary procedures at this stage. The behaviour may be a sign of burn-out or stress and this should be addressed sensitively by someone who he trusts. If these concerns are found to be genuine, referral might be appropriate if in-house procedures fail to bring about resolution. The Local Medical Committee provides invaluable support in this situation and should be considered before going outside the practice.

76.   **C:**   **It is typically triggered by particular head movements**

BPPV is rotatory vertigo brought on by head movements in a certain plane, eg lying back in a dentist's chair. It is not associated with any other neuro-otological symptoms and can be demonstrated with Hallpike testing, whereby torsional nystagmus is provoked after a latent period of 15–30 seconds. This fatigues with repeat testing. The presence of other neuro-otological symptoms should prompt further investigations to exclude alternative diagnoses, eg Menière's disease or cholesteatoma. Acoustic neuromas seldom cause vertigo.

77.   **D:**   **Malignant melanoma**

This lesion has the following features of melanoma: asymmetry, size > 6 mm, irregular edges or surface, and non-uniform pigmentation

78. **A:** **Patients can be screened for this condition using the SCOFF questionnaire**

Anorexia requires a BMI < 17.5 kg/m^2 and an inability to eat. Prevalence is 1–2% in women, much lower in men. Over a 4- to 8-year follow-up 2% of patients died and 65% achieved normal weight. The SCOFF questionnaire includes the following questions:

Do you make yourself **S**ick because you feel uncomfortably full?

Do you worry that you have lost **C**ontrol over how much you eat?

Have you recently lost more than **O**ne stone in a 3-month period?

Do you believe yourself to be **F**at when others say you are too thin?

Would you say that **F**ood dominates your life?

A score of ≥ 2 indicates a likely case of anorexia nervosa or bulimia.

79. **B:** **Atorvastatin**

80. **L:** **Sotalol**

Sotalol is effective in prophylaxis of AF and may be used while awaiting DC cardioversion to try to cardiovert patients chemically.

81. **N:** **Valsartan**

Angiotensin II receptor antagonists are licensed in heart failure and after myocardial infarction.

82. **O:** **Verapamil**

Verapamil should not be used in patients with bradycardias or heart block, or those who take β blockers.

83. C: Clopidogrel

NICE guidance suggests that the combination of aspirin and dipyridamole should be used as secondary prevention in patients who have had a TIA or ischaemic stroke.

84. H: Isosorbide mononitrate

85. C: Clopidogrel

86. M: Spironolactone

87. A: Amiodarone

Amiodarone has a long half-life and is associated with ophthalmic, dermatological and thyroid dysfunction.

88. G: Indapamide

ACE inhibitors and angiotensin II receptor antagonists are first-line treatment in young hypertensive patients, but where renal artery stenosis is present a thiazide is a better choice.

89. E: Patients with recurrent symptoms can use flecainide as a 'pill in the pocket' treatment

AF affects 0.4% of the general population, but incidence increases sharply with age. Patients should be anticoagulated if they have persistent prolonged attacks and are high risk, eg coexisting hypertension, smoking. Reductions in alcohol, caffeine, stress and smoking help to reduce the incidence of the condition. In patients with a structurally normal heart flecainide is effective as treatment.

PAPER 2

90.   E: A raised ALP suggests that the diagnosis is gallstones

Gallstones cause either a flatulent dyspepsia or biliary colic. Colic tends to be severe and can require treatment with pethidine injection. Pain usually comes 60–120 minutes after fatty meals and can last several hours. It is usually associated with raised ALP and stones can cause pancreatitis or obstructive jaundice. Where associated with weight loss, cancer should be considered in the differential diagnosis.

91.   C: Earache, trismus and dysphagia are typical symptoms

Most cases are caused by streptococcal infections, and the abscess is outside the tonsillar capsule close to the upper pole of the tonsil. The patient is usually unwell and unable to swallow fluids or solids. Intravenous fluids and intravenous broad-spectrum antibiotics, with interval tonsillectomy, are the usual management options.

92.   A: Parotid adenoma

The most common cause of smooth painless swelling is parotid adenoma. Alternative causes include metastatic lymph nodes or lymphoma. Acute parotitis, mumps and salivary calculi cause intermittent or short-lived symptoms.

93.   H: Omalizumab

Omalizumab (Xolair) is given by subcutaneous injection.

94.   E: Inhaled regular dose steroids

95.   G: Long-acting bronchodilator

Salmeterol and formoterol have been shown to be associated with increased admissions to hospital and increased mortality.

96.   F: Leukotriene receptor antagonist

Leukotriene receptor antagonists seem to be synergistic with inhaled steroids and these may be of particular benefit in patients with exercise-induced asthma or allergic rhinitis.

97.   J: Regular steroids by mouth

In regular oral steroid use, always consider the need for bisphosphonates.

98.   D: It often gets worse during pregnancy

Otosclerosis is an autosomal dominant disease with incomplete penetrance that affects 0.5–2% of the population, sex ratio 2 females:1 male, more common in white people. It tends to worsen during pregnancy, menstruation and the menopause. Most patients present before the age of 30. It causes a conductive hearing loss slightly worse at lower frequencies, often with a dip in the bone-conduction thresholds at 2 kHz. Stapedectomy is an effective treatment but there is a risk of hearing loss, so many patients choose to wear hearing aids instead. There is some evidence that the incidence is falling, thought to be a result of the use of fluoride in drinking water.

99.   D: Long-term oral tetracycline is effective in reducing frequency of attacks

Hidradenitis suppurativa is not a disease of apocrine glands, but rather an acne-like condition. Treatment options include short courses of antibiotics and oral steroids or local steroid injections. Long-term antibiotics may be useful and as a last resort some patients may require surgery. Dianette may be helpful in women because of the cyproterone acetate component.

100.   F: None

This patient has ruptured the long head of biceps, which produces a characteristic pop-eye appearance. No treatment is needed.

PAPER 2

101.   F: It is exclusively seen in children

Epiglottitis is usually seen in young children, but may be seen in adults, where the principal complaint is of severe pain on swallowing. The most common differential is croup, but children with epiglottitis are much sicker and should be admitted as an emergency before attempting to examine the child.

102.   C: Some women with SLE have an increased risk of bearing a child with congenital heart block

Women with anti-Ro antibodies have a 5% risk of having a child with congenital heart block. Miscarriage rates are higher particularly in patients with antiphospholipid antibodies. Pre-eclampsia and growth retardation are common especially in women with renal involvement. Preconceptual advice from a rheumatologist is essential and some drug switching may be necessary, eg to steroids.

103.   E: Orlistat can be prescribed initially for 3 months, and continued as long as the person has lost 5% of his or her body mass

Orlistat can be prescribed if BMI > 30 or BMI > 28 with risk factors. Sibutramine should be used only in patients who have not responded to a traditional weight management programme. It increases blood pressure significantly in up to 10% of patients.

104.   B: The wound should be cleaned with saline and he should be advised about RICE for his soft tissue bruising

The human mouth is full of anaerobes and aerobes that can rapidly cause severe illness. All patients in whom the skin is punctured should receive antibiotics and a tetanus booster, and those with any signs of spread should be admitted to either orthopaedics or plastic surgery according to the site of the bite. Always consider a foreign body as a cause of infection in traumatic wounds.

105. **D:** **Nits can be seen only with a magnifying glass**

Lice can be seen in the pubic area, eyelashes or scalp. They are easily visible either as lice or eggs. Resistance is common and where insecticides are used local prescribing guidelines should be followed to allow for rotation of drugs. Simethicone has recently been shown to be effective.

106. **I:** **Whitehall 2 study**

The Whitehall 2 study of 10 000 British civil servants found a dose-related effect even when confounders such as alcohol had been removed.

107. **C:** **ExTraMATCH**

This was a meta-analysis involving 801 stable patients.

108. **E:** **High-dose vitamin E**

Doses of vitamin E > 400 IU/day have been shown in a meta-analysis of 10 trials to increase mortality.

109. **B:** **EarlyBird 21 study**

The perception of children's weight was independent of socioeconomic grouping.

110. **A:** **Caerphilly Study**

This was not seen with light exercise.

111. **E:** **Chickenpox**

Chickenpox typically presents with a non-specific febrile illness followed by the development of a vesicular rash. Measles usually starts on the back of the neck and is also associated with conjunctival symptoms. Parvovirus B19 causes a slapped cheek appearance.

112.   H: Not entitled to free prescriptions

Patients with diabetes treated with drugs are entitled to free prescriptions.

113.   C: Entitled to free NHS dental treatment

Women who are pregnant and up to 12 months post partum are entitled to free dental treatment and NHS prescriptions.

114.   G: Not entitled to free NHS sight test

Myxoedema gives exemption from prescription charges not eye tests.

115.   B: Automatically entitled to free prescriptions

People aged 16, 17 or 18 and in full-time education are exempt from charges.

116.   E: Entitled to free prescriptions on applying for an exemption certificate

Those patients who need replacement therapy, or have medically treated diabetes, epilepsy or a fistula, are entitled to free prescriptions on applying and receiving an exemption certificate.

117.   B: Varicose eczema

Asteatotic eczema results from loss of lubricating fluid from the skin; it presents as a crazy paving pattern on the lower legs. Psoriasis causes thickened plaques of skin over flexor aspects, eg elbows. Pompholyx affects the soles of the feet and the palms of the hands.

118.   H: Retinoblastoma

Retinoblastoma is often diagnosed by loss of red reflex and has been picked up from family photos when one person has no red eye.

119.   F: Optic atrophy

Optic neuritis causes disc pallor; in the acute phase the disc may also be swollen.

120.   A: Acute angle-closure glaucoma

Unlike uveitis, the pupil is fixed but round.

121.   G: Recurrent uveitis

Recurrent uveitis causes adhesions around the periphery of the iris.

122.   C: Chronic glaucoma

The cup:disc ratio is used to monitor the progression of glaucoma.

123.   C: It should always be actively treated

Molluscum typically settles in time without active treatment. Where treatment is considered it should aim to produce minimal scarring. Several treatments have been tried including cryotherapy, imiquod and phenol expression.

124.   D: Chalazion

Chalazions are retention cysts in meibomian glands. They are similar in appearance to styes but lack signs of acute inflammation. Often settling spontaneously, ones that do not may be treated surgically. Infected chalazions are treated in the same way as styes.

PAPER 2

125.   L: Nitrofurantoin

Nitrofurantoin is the most appropriate choice in this case. Co-trimoxazole (Septrin) is a combination of trimethoprim and sulfamethoxazole.

126.   F: Ciprofloxacin

Ciprofloxacin is a useful alternative to rifampicin as prophylaxis.

127.   M: Phenoxymethylpenicillin

Phenoxymethylpenicillin is the first-line treatment for tonsillitis in patients who do not have penicillin allergy.

128.   H: Erythromycin

Erythromycin has a similar spectrum of activity to amoxicillin and also covers atypical pneumonia.

129.   C: Augmentin (co-amoxiclav)

All dog and cat bites or scratches should be treated with Augmentin (co-amoxiclav) or doxycycline and metronidazole if penicillin allergic.

130.   A: Emergency treatment involves an immediate insulin injection and fluid rehydration

DKA may follow a prodromal illness or present acutely as a consequence of an intercurrent illness. There is often abdominal pain and vomiting, and polydipsia with polyuria. Patients are often significantly dehydrated, although frequently they have an apparent hyperkalaemia on blood testing. Examination findings include tachypnoea and ketotic breath.

131.   **E:**   **It is usually a sign of underlying malignancy**

Common causes of erythema nodosum include streptococcal infections, sarcoidosis, infections and drugs. Treatment is conservative and aimed at the underlying cause.

132–138.

Ninety per cent of children achieve the developmental stage by the ages below. Failure to achieve one or more of these milestones by the age suggests that further assessment may be indicated.

132.   **F:**   18 months

133.   **F:**   18 months

134.   **D:**   8 weeks

135.   **E:**   10 months

136.   **G:**   30 months

137.   **B:**   5 months

138.   **A:**   3 months

139. **B:** **Hydroxychloroquine will reduce pain, swelling and stiffness in SLE**

Hydroxychloroquine is effective in SLE and RA. Infliximab is for use in active RA only. Sulfasalazine causes reversible effects on fertility. Methotrexate may take some weeks to become effective.

140. **B:** **Rheumatoid arthritis**

Primary nodal osteoarthritis affects the distal interphalangeal joints of the fingers. Reiter syndrome usually involves iritis or conjunctivitis. Gout would be unlikely to affect both sides simultaneously.

141. **D:** **The implementation of change is implicit in the audit cycle**

The audit cycle is the process of setting standards, measuring performance, diagnosing the problem, implementing change and then re-measuring. Standards can be 'soft', such as the number of complaints or 'hard', such as the number of patients treated to a blood pressure target.

142. **C:** **Adenoidectomy at the time of grommet insertion significantly reduces the risk of recurrence**

Long-term studies suggest that adenoidectomy at the time of grommets greatly reduces the risk of recurrence. Glue ear is not caused by bacterial infection; however, grommets are sometimes used to try to prevent recurrent otitis media. The major clinical significance of glue ear is that it can cause conductive hearing loss at critical stages in a child's development; most children have glue ear at some time in their lives, although very few go on to develop hearing impairment as a result. Treatment is reserved for those with demonstrable hearing loss that fails to resolve naturally. Alternatives to surgery include temporary hearing aids, but there is no evidence at the present time that dietary modification or osteopathy helps, although the natural tendency to resolution may be responsible for a powerful placebo effect.

143.   D: Referred pain

Pain in the shoulder may be a sign of diaphragmatic irritation, eg cholecystitis or ruptured ectopic.

144.   C: Osteoarthritis

Long-standing pain and reduced range of movement suggest osteoarthritis rather than rotator cuff and the history is too long for frozen shoulder. There is often prominent lipping of the joint.

145.   A: Cervical spondylosis

Cervical spondylosis may be present with or without neurological symptoms.

146.   B: Frozen shoulder

Frozen shoulder affects all movements but external rotation is particularly affected.

147.   H: Subluxation of the glenohumeral joint

This is a typical description of a dislocated shoulder.

148.   E: Small lesions may be treated successfully with liquid nitrogen

This is a myxoid cyst. These soft rubbery nodules are usually seen on the distal interphalangeal joints of fingers or toes. They usually arise after trauma and are 1.0–1.5 cm in diameter. They are not derived from the joint or tendon sheath, and are not ganglia or synovial cysts. They may cause a groove to develop in the nail. More common in women over 40, they often burst and treatment is indicated only for cosmetic reasons or discomfort. They may be treated with liquid nitrogen, intralesional steroid or excision, but often recur.

149.   **A:**   **Access to Health Records Act**

150.   **E:**   **Data Protection Act**

151.   **A:**   **Access to Health Records Act**

152.   **C:**   **Children's Act**

153.   **B:**   **Access to Medical Reports Act**

154.   **A:**   **Access to Health Records Act**

155.   **E:**   **PACS**

Picture Archiving and Communications Systems (PACS) capture, store and distribute radiological images around the NHS system.

156.   **A:**   **Choose and book**

Choose and book allows comparison of different services in a locality according to indicative waiting time.

157.   **D:**   **N3**

The N3 broadband network underpins the connectivity of Connecting for Health.

158.   **B:**   **Connecting for Health**

In time the government intends to keep patient records on the internet, which patients will be able to access.

159. C: Electronic transfer of prescriptions

The aim for electronic prescriptions is to reduce error by allowing cross-referencing of prescriptions with patient records.

160. E: Lung cancer

With a smoking history, clubbing and weight loss, cancer is the most likely diagnosis. Cystic fibrosis and congenital heart disease cause shortness of breath and clubbing but present earlier. Pneumonia would not normally cause clubbing; however, bronchiectasis may cause shortness of breath and clubbing.

161. E: It may be helped with lactase added to feeds

Colic is a disease of unknown origin but some evidence suggests that it may be caused by temporary lactose intolerance. It occurs in 20% of infants and usually lasts up to 3 months of age. Dicyclomine is contraindicated in those aged under 6 months. Vomiting suggests alternative diagnoses, eg constipation, Hirschsprung's disease.

162. G: Vulval intraepithelial neoplasia (VIN)

Unlike CIN, VIN tends to be multifocal and regular follow-up is needed even if the primary lesion is removed completely.

163. A: Cervical carcinoma

Cervical cancer tends to present with bleeding, usually postcoital but also intermenstrual or postmenopausal. A high index of suspicion is needed in these situations.

164.   C: Choriocarcinoma

Women who have a molar pregnancy are monitored for 2 years to detect choriocarcinoma. Rising β-hCG levels suggest that this has occurred, hence after a molar pregnancy patients are advised not to get pregnant for 2 years.

165.   E: Ovarian carcinoma

Ovarian cancer tends to be diagnosed late because of the non-specific nature of the symptoms.

166.   D: Endometrial carcinoma

Endometrial carcinoma is associated with diabetes and usually presents with postmenopausal bleeding.

167.   E: Increased dietary fibre and fluids are an important part of treatment

First-degree piles remain within the canal, second-degree piles prolapse but can be replaced, and third-degree piles are permanently prolapsed and can thrombose. Grade 1 piles are not visible on external examination or per rectum. Banding of piles can be done on an outpatient basis.

168.   E: It may be a sign of female virilisation

Crypto-orchidism and hypospadias raise the possibility of female virilisation. The condition is seen in 1:300 male births. Epispadias, where the opening is on the upper, dorsal side of the penis, may be associated with bladder abnormalities. Mild cases of hypospadias may present in adulthood.

169.   A: Combined oral contraceptive

In women with no biochemical evidence of hormonal imbalance a combined oral contraceptive is the best initial treatment.

170.   E: Finasteride

In women who are unable to take the COCP, or in whom it is not effective, finasteride may be effective. Adequate contraception is essential.

171.   D: Electrolysis

Cosmetic techniques should be considered for all women, particularly where hair is localised.

172.   C: Dianette

Dianette is licensed for the treatment of hirsutism and acne. It is preferable to cyproterone alone because adequate contraception is needed to prevent feminisation of a male fetus.

173.   H: Referral

This woman probably has polycystic ovary syndrome. Referral is indicated to optimise chances of conception and control symptoms.

174.   F: Menière's disease

This is a classic description of Menière's disease.

175.   J: Vestibular neuronitis

Vestibular neuronitis tends to produce severe vertigo, which often causes people to take to their beds for several days. It is thought to be viral.

176. **C: Cardiogenic syncope**

Vestibular disease causes rotatory vertigo. Light-headedness without vertigo is seldom caused by otological disease.

177. **B: Benign paroxysmal positional vertigo**

A benign paroxysmal positional vertigo causes maximal symptoms when the affected semicircular canal is stimulated more than the others.

178. **G: Ramsay Hunt syndrome**

Herpes zoster affecting the geniculate ganglion may cause facial nerve paralysis, vertigo and sensorineural deafness. It should be treated with aciclovir.

179. **C: A raised PSA may be caused by urinary infection**

PSA is neither highly specific nor sensitive. A significant number of people with prostate cancer are missed by PSA testing and many undergo prostate biopsy without having cancer confirmed. Old age, prostatic hyperplasia, infection and instrumentation can all elevate the PSA. There are age-specific cut-offs for elevated PSA.

180. **A: He should be converted to a twice-daily maintenance dose of methadone and this should be gradually reduced**

Methadone is given once daily and has a long half-life. Buprenorphine is safer in overdose and less addictive than methadone. Management of opiate abuse includes a holistic approach to lifestyle risk factors.

181.   D: Pneumothorax

Spontaneous pneumothorax is often idiopathic but, where recurrent, CT may demonstrate bullae. In this instance surgical pleurodesis may be indicated. In spontaneous pneumothorax cyanosis is rare and can often be treated with needle aspiration.

182.   E: Doxycycline is associated with photosensitivity

Malarone needs to be taken only from 2 days before entering a malaria zone until 1 week after leaving. It is taken daily. Antimalarials are available only on private prescription. Mefloquine causes neuropsychiatric side effects in less than 1% of patients. All patients should use insect repellents, long trousers and sleeves, and consider insect nets.

183.   A: A written response must be received by the patient within 10 working days

There is a time limit of 6 months for practice complaints. The complaint must be acknowledged within 2 working days. Complaints may be verbal, written or emailed to the practice. The Healthcare Commission deals with the *process* of the complaint, not the substance. There is a time limit of 6 months from the incident, but this can be extended, for example if a patient was too ill to complain. Out-of-hours complaints should be made to the relevant PCO (Primary Care Organisation).

184.   C: Ten per cent of patients with mumps develop symptomatic meningeal involvement

The incubation period is usually around 18 days. Of patients 70% develop salivary gland involvement, and infection is by droplets or fomites. Although 25% of post-pubertal males develop orchitis, it is unilateral in 80% and hence the risk of infertility is low.

185.   A: Acute pericarditis

Pericarditis shows typical saddle pattern on the ST segment on ECG.

186.   I: Pneumothorax

Pneumothorax is usually accompanied by tachypnoea and reduced breath sounds over the affected lung field.

187.   C: Aortic dissection

Aortic dissection is usually accompanied by weak asymmetrical pulses and new heart murmurs.

188.   F: Myocardial infarction

189.   J: Pulmonary embolus

There may be a pleural rub in pulmonary embolus but often the only sign is tachypnoea.

190.   G: Febrile

191.   D: Afebrile

192.   C: Admit

193.   E: Age < 18 months

194.   F: Age > 18 months

PAPER 2

195. **C:** Admit

196. **B:** < 15 minutes

197. **A:** > 15 minutes

198. **B:** Presbyacusis

A symmetrical high-frequency sensorineural loss is characteristic of presbyacusis. Bilateral tinnitus is not a sign of acoustic neuroma.

199. **B:** Practices with high QOF scores might be making more earlier diagnoses, resulting in greater admission rates for elective treatment

Practices with high QOF scores are more likely to be in areas of low deprivation. Exception reporting will inflate the QOF score but not affect the admission rate. Non-medical staff tend to be very good at rigid, protocol-led work, such as collecting data, but are less capable at managing complex problems.

200. **C:** A rapidly growing lesion that forms a crater with a central plug is likely to be a keratocanthoma

BCCs are locally invasive and have a characteristic rolled telangiectatic edge. SCCs spread via lymph nodes and need a histological diagnosis to differentiate from keratoacanthomas. Dermoid cysts are smooth and mobile. Curettage and cautery may be suitable for some very small BCCs in patients not fit for excision.

PAPER 2

Paper 3
Questions

Total time allowed is three hours. Indicate your answers clearly by putting a tick or cross in the box alongside each answer or by writing the appropriate letter alongside the appropriate answer.

THEME: RED EYE

1–5.

Options

A Acute glaucoma

B Conjunctivitis

C Corneal ulcer

D Episcleritis

E Subconjunctival haemorrhage

You are devising a treatment algorithm for a nurse practitioner to manage ophthalmological problems in a minor injury clinic. From the list of options complete the algorithm shown.

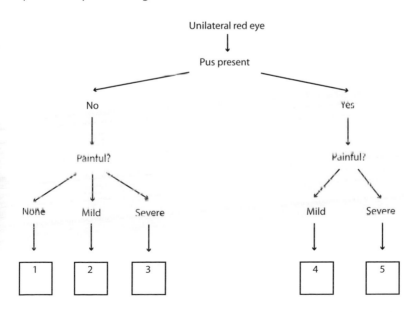

6. Which of the following statements about attention deficit hyperactivity disorder (ADHD) is true? Select one option only.

☐ A   Hyperkinetic behaviour is seen in 10% of children in the UK

☐ B   The diagnosis of ADHD is one of exclusion after other developmental conditions, eg dyslexia, have been excluded

☐ C   Good prognosis is associated with a supportive family

☐ D   Methylphenidate is effective in most patients

☐ E   Diet has no influence on ADHD

7. Which one of the following statements with regard to advance directives is true?

☐ A   Since October 2007 advance directives have had to be written rather than verbal

☐ B   Mental capacity is a prerequisite for completion of an advance directive

☐ C   Where a patient with a pre-existing advance directive becomes mentally incapacitated an advance directive is invalidated

☐ D   A competent adult can refuse treatment only in certain situations

☐ E   Any mentally competent person over the age of 16 can complete an advance directive

THEME: SCHOOL EXCLUSION AND COMMON ILLNESSES

Options

A   5 days

B   No exclusion necessary

C   Until 24 hours after symptoms have settled

D   Until lesions have crusted

E   Until treated

For each disease below, select the most appropriate exclusion period from the list of options. Each option may be used once, more than once or not at all.

- [ ] **8.** **Acute gastroenteritis in children.**
- [ ] **9.** **Impetigo.**
- [ ] **10.** **Scabies.**
- [ ] **11.** **Chickenpox.**
- [ ] **12.** **Scarlet fever.**
- [ ] **13.** **Threadworm.**

PAPER 3

14. A 34-year-old man is going on a charity trek to Kilimanjaro and comes to see you to ask for a prescription to stop him getting altitude sickness. Which of the following is the most effective prophylaxis? Select one option only.

☐ A   Dexamethasone

☐ B   Gingko biloba

☐ C   Acetazolamide

☐ D   Coca extract

☐ E   Sildenafil

15. A 33-year-old man has had the lesions in the figure since childhood. He also has macular patches on his arms and legs.

What is the diagnosis?

☐ A   Multiple lipomas

☐ B   Neurofibromatosis

☐ C   Dercum's disease

☐ D   Gouty tophi

☐ E   Rheumatoid nodules

16. A 9-year-old boy is brought in by his mother with a 3-month history of abdominal pain that frequently causes him to miss school. Examination is normal. Which one of the following statements is true with regard to the management of this problem?

☐ A   Normal weight gain and growth are reassuring signs

☐ B   Positive serological testing for *Helicobacter pylori* is strongly associated with chronic abdominal pain

☐ C   All patients should have baseline blood tests carried out

☐ D   Symptoms settle within 3 weeks in 95% of patients with functional abdominal pain

☐ E   Chronic abdominal pain is no more common in children of parents who have suffered anxiety than in those who have not

17. A 3-year-old boy, who was treated 5 days ago for tonsillitis, is brought in by his mother with puffiness around his eyes over the last 3 days. He seems well in himself and his mother is concerned that he may have hayfever. On examination he has some oedema around his ankles where his socks have been, but is otherwise well. Dipstick testing of his urine reveals protein 4+ and blood 1+. What is the single most likely diagnosis?

☐ A   Nephrotic syndrome

☐ B   Angio-oedema

☐ C   Wilms' tumour

☐ D   Urinary tract infection

☐ E   Haemolytic–uraemic syndrome

PAPER 3

THEME: THE REGULATION OF DOCTORS

Options

A   Appraisal

B   Graduation

C   None of the above

D   Recertification

E   Registration

F   Renewal

G   Revalidation

For each description below of the processes in medical regulation, select the most appropriate from the list of options. Each option may be used once, more than once or not at all.

- [ ] **18.** It aims to identify and address development needs.

- [ ] **19.** It requires the doctor to show the results of appraisals.

- [ ] **20.** It is a contractual obligation for GPs.

- [ ] **21.** It will require submission of material to the General Medical Council.

- [ ] **22.** Only doctors who see patients will need to complete this process.

- [ ] **23.** It will be administered by the appropriate Royal College.

- [ ] **24.** It may include knowledge tests.

- [ ] **25.** It is based on the GMC document Good Medical Practice.

26. A 46-year-old woman presents with sharp pain radiating into the toes with walking. Examination reveals a tender spot between the third and fourth metatarsals. Which of the following is the most likely diagnosis? Select one option only.

- [ ] A Morton's neuroma
- [ ] B Gout
- [ ] C Bunions
- [ ] D Plantar fasciitis
- [ ] E Hammer toe

27. With regard to painkillers in palliative care, which of the following correctly describes painkillers in order of potency, with weakest first and strongest last? Select one option only.

- [ ] A Codeine, tramadol, morphine, oxycodone, diamorphine
- [ ] B Tramadol, codeine, oxycodone, morphine, diamorphine
- [ ] C Codeine, oxycodone, tramadol, diamorphine, morphine
- [ ] D Codeine, tramadol, oxycodone, morphine, diamorphine
- [ ] E Oxycodone, codeine, tramadol, morphine, diamorphine

28. A 29-year-old woman presents with a facial nerve palsy. Which of the following statements is true about this condition? Select one option only.

- [ ] A Bell's palsy is usually caused by herpes zoster
- [ ] B It is always the result of local facial nerve damage
- [ ] C Of patients with a facial nerve palsy 90% recover complete facial nerve function
- [ ] D Bell's palsy is associated with altered facial sensation and taste
- [ ] E Treatment for facial nerve palsy involves a watch-and-wait policy
- [ ] F Antivirals have no place in the management of facial nerve palsy

29. A 67-year-old man presents with sudden painless loss of vision in one eye. Which of the following would be consistent with a diagnosis of central retinal artery occlusion? Select one option only.

☐ A Fundoscopy reveals a bright-red spot at the fovea

☐ B Pupil on the affected side reacts normally to light

☐ C Retina appears engorged on fundoscopy

☐ D Visual field loss always affects the entire visual field

☐ E Acuity is usually well preserved initially

30. A 53-year-old woman complains of persistent chest infections. On further questioning she reports that she has a constant cough, produces large quantities of phlegm every day and that this can be precipitated by change in posture. She occasionally gets bad breath and haemoptysis. Her previous medical history is unremarkable except for whooping cough as a child. On examination she has coarse crepitations in both midzones. Which of the following is the most likely diagnosis?

☐ A Bronchopneumonia

☐ B Bronchiolitis

☐ C Extrinsic allergic bronchiolitis

☐ D Bronchiectasis

☐ E Kartagener syndrome

31. A 29-year-old care worker complains of 3 days of profuse diarrhoea, fever and abdominal cramps. You send a stool specimen for culture and the result confirms campylobacter infection. Which of the following statements about this infection is true? Select one answer only.

- [ ] A It seldom persists for more than 72 hours
- [ ] B It may cause septicaemia
- [ ] C It should be treated with loperamide
- [ ] D It is usually acquired through eating chicken
- [ ] E It is a normal commensal in the human bowel

32. A 37-year-old man with no previous medical history of note complains of a cough and shortness of breath over several weeks since returning from a holiday in Spain. He initially attributed this to a cough caught on holiday but has now noticed ankle swelling. On examination he has crepitations in both bases, a third heart sound and a displaced apex beat. Which of the following is the most likely diagnosis? Select one option only.

- [ ] A Pulmonary embolus
- [ ] B Atypical pneumonia
- [ ] C Cardiomyopathy
- [ ] D Rheumatic heart disease
- [ ] E Pericarditis

PAPER 3

243

33. **Which of the following statements about risk factors for child abuse is correct? Select one option only.**

☐ A   Prematurity is a risk factor for child abuse

☐ B   Carers with physical disabilities are a risk factor

☐ C   Parents who have been abused in childhood are more likely to become abusers themselves

☐ D   The first-born child is at greater risk than later siblings

☐ E   The majority of deaths from physical abuse occur before the age of 5 years

☐ F   All of the above

34. **A 54-year-old woman presents with a florid rash on her arms after a day spent gardening. She did not use any pesticides or weedkillers, but spent the day cutting back weeds. The rash affects only sun-exposed areas. She is otherwise well and takes no regular medication. The rash is shown below.**

Which of the following is a possible diagnosis?

☐ A   Phytophotodermatitis

☐ B   Actinic prurigo

☐ C   Chronic actinic dermatosis

☐ D   Solar urticaria

☐ E   Drug-induced photodermatitis

35. Rising levels of antimicrobial resistance in your area has prompted the local medical community to look at strategies to reduce the levels of antibiotic prescribing in the area. Which one of the following statements about this problem is true?

☐ A Diagnostic and treatment algorithms can reduce antibiotic prescription rates for nursing homes

☐ B MRSA rates are mostly the result of use of antibiotics in farming and are consequently no different in areas of high antibiotic prescribing

☐ C Deferred scripts for simple upper respiratory tract infections have been shown to reduce the number of prescriptions filled by up to 20%

☐ D Studies have shown that patients are concerned about levels of antibiotic resistance

☐ E Parents are more likely to fill deferred scripts for their children than for themselves

36. You see a 24-year-old woman with painful lesions on her labia. On examination she has genital herpes. Which one of the following statements about the management of this condition is true?

☐ A In women the lesions usually occur in the perianal area

☐ B The first attack is usually mild, with severity increasing with recurrent attacks

☐ C Healing in primary herpes takes 5–7 days

☐ D Prompt use of aciclovir will eradicate the virus, preventing recurrent attacks

☐ E Regular antiviral medication can reduce transmission to sexual partners

PAPER 3

THEME: FUNDOSCOPY

Options

A

B

C

D

E

For each patient described below, select the fundus image that you would expect to see. Each option may be used once, more than once or not at all.

- [ ] **37.** A 67-year-old man complains of general malaise, pain on eating and reduced vision.

- [ ] **38.** A 72-year-old patient with diabetes who attends for a routine diabetic check.

- [ ] **39.** A 25-year old woman with recurrent episodes of photopsia followed by visual loss and severe headache.

- [ ] **40.** A 49-year-old man presents with acute onset of visual loss in the inferior portion of his visual field.

- [ ] **41.** A 77-year-old woman complains of increasing difficulty with reading and reports that she has noticed that straight lines appear curved.

42. A 33-year-old woman has just been diagnosed with coeliac disease. She comes to see you to discuss the diagnosis. Which one of the following statements about coeliac disease is true?

- [ ] A Two-thirds of affected patients are undiagnosed
- [ ] B Eighty per cent of patients present with gastrointestinal symptoms
- [ ] C Failure to stick to a low-gluten diet causes diarrhoea, but has no long-term complications
- [ ] D The disease is usually an autoimmune phenomenon triggered by infection
- [ ] E Eighty per cent of patients are able to stick to a gluten-free diet

43. Your practice manager suggests that you adopt a routine policy of copying letters to patients. Which one of the following statements relating to this policy is true?

- [ ] A Letters about patients should be sent only to the patient, not to carers of adult patients
- [ ] B There are no circumstances in which letters should not be copied
- [ ] C Copying letters has been shown to help inform patients and improve their ability to make treatment decisions
- [ ] D It should be assumed that patients wish to receive copies of letters unless they explicitly decline
- [ ] E The costs of copying letters are the responsibility of the patient

44. **You practise in an area of high deprivation. Which one of the following statements is true with regard to deprivation and health?**

☐ A   Deprivation is linked to diabetic eye disease

☐ B   Deprivation in general practice is measured by the ponderal index

☐ C   Deprivation scores account for a significant proportion of variation in out-of-hours activity

☐ D   High deprivation scores are not associated with high referral rates

☐ E   The global sum in the GMS Contract does not take account of deprivation levels

45. **One of your patients with severe osteoarthritis of the hip attends for his medication review. He has been taking non-steroidal anti-inflammatory drugs (NSAIDs) for some years but is concerned by recent media speculation about the long-term safety of these drugs. Which one of the following statements about this class of drug is true?**

☐ A   COX-2 inhibitors have been shown to be associated with significantly lower rates of gastrointestinal haemorrhage compared with conventional NSAIDs

☐ B   Patients taking COX-2 inhibitors have been shown to have double the risk of myocardial infarction

☐ C   Topical NSAIDs are no more effective than placebo in the short term at reducing pain and stiffness

☐ D   NSAIDs can trigger liver failure

☐ E   Co-prescription of ranitidine with NSAIDs is of proved efficacy in reducing the risk of gastrointestinal bleeding

THEME: SEIZURES

Options

A   Febrile seizure

B   Grand mal epilepsy

C   Jacksonian seizure

D   Petit mal epilepsy

E   Pseudoseizure

F   Reflex anoxic seizure

G   Temporal lobe epilepsy

H   Vasovagal syncope

For each scenario descried below, select the most appropriate diagnosis from the list of options. Each option can be used once, more than once or not at all.

☐ **46.** A 2-year-old child is seen with recurrent episodes of becoming pale and limp, and holding his breath. This is usually provoked by pain or surprise and he sometimes has a seizure before making a spontaneous recovery.

☐ **47.** A 10-month-old girl who has been below par for 2 days is noted by her mother to have a fever. Shortly after giving her paracetamol, she has a grand mal seizure that lasts for 30 seconds. After this she is initially drowsy but soon recovers. She has no focal neurological signs.

☐ **48.** A 7-year-old girl seems to daydream frequently and has no recollection afterwards. When asked to hyperventilate she becomes vacant for a few seconds. She is otherwise well. Examination shows no other abnormalities.

☐ **49.** A 34-year-old man with a history of seizures develops myoclonic convulsions that move up the affected limb, resulting in a generalised seizure.

☐ **50.** A 28-year-old unemployed man presents with a 3-minute episode of myoclonic jerking. Afterwards he quickly recovers but has no knowledge of what happened. He has no incontinence and does not bite his tongue.

PAPER 3

51. A 21-year-old has been sent in by his new partner to get himself screened for *Chlamydia sp.* Which of the following symptoms may be seen in chlamydia infection in men? Select one option only.

☐ A Arthritis
☐ B Urethritis
☐ C Asymptomatic
☐ D Epididymitis
☐ E Proctitis
☐ F All of the above

52. Which of the following is not a symptom of cholesteatoma? Select one of the following.

☐ A Dizziness
☐ B Otorrhoea
☐ C Deafness
☐ D Facial nerve palsy
☐ E Tinnitus
☐ F Rhinorrhoea

PAPER 3

THEME: BREAST CANCER

Options

A   Malmö Mammographic Screening Trial

B   MARIBS trial

C   Million Women Study

D   Women's Health Initiative

For each of the trial findings below, select the trial title from the list of options. Each option may be used once, more than once or not at all.

☐ **53.**   It showed that MRI is almost twice as sensitive at picking up breast cancer in high-risk women.

☐ **54.**   It showed no increase in incidence of breast cancer in those taking conjugated oestrogens.

☐ **55.**   It found a significantly increased rate of false-positive mammography results in HRT users.

☐ **56.**   It demonstrated a 10% rate of over-diagnosis of breast cancer.

☐ **57.**   It found that low body mass index, previous breast surgery and use of HRT led to increased recall and therefore reduced specificity of mammography.

58. You are asked to do a new baby check on a 3-day-old girl born at home after an uneventful pregnancy. The labour was normal and the baby has been fine until today, when she was noted to be slightly blue around the lips on feeding, recovering quickly. On examination there is a systolic murmur and you are unable to feel pulses in the legs. Which of the following is a likely diagnosis? Select one option only.

- [ ] A   Coarctation of the aorta
- [ ] B   Patent ductus arteriosus
- [ ] C   Transient tachypnoea of the newborn
- [ ] D   Fallot's tetralogy
- [ ] E   Ventricular septal defect

59. A 5-year-old boy has been suffering from constipation and soiling for many months and his mother feels that something needs to be done now that he is starting school. He was born after a normal delivery and had no problems until the age of 2. On examination he is well and the only abnormality of note is a loaded colon. Which of the following statements about constipation is true? Select one option only.

- [ ] A   Constipation in children may be a sign of systemic disease
- [ ] B   The parents can be reassured that he will grow out of his symptoms
- [ ] C   Hirschsprung's disease always presents in the neonatal period
- [ ] D   The parents should be trained in the use of enemas to treat any recurrence early
- [ ] E   Stimulant laxatives are contraindicated in children

60. A 3-year-old boy has just been discharged from hospital with a diagnosis of epilepsy. His parents bring him to see you to discuss the diagnosis and provide more information about the condition. Which of the following statements is true about epilepsy? Select one option only.

- [ ] A   In over 50% of cases of seizure, an underlying cause can be identified
- [ ] B   20% of patients are able to stop taking anticonvulsants within 2 years without recurrence
- [ ] C   There is a 25% risk of an epileptic parent passing on epilepsy to offspring
- [ ] D   The child should not swim alone
- [ ] E   As long as seizures are controlled he will be able to drive when he reaches the appropriate age

61. Which of the following statements about the medical management of ophthalmic disease is NOT true? Select one option only.

- [ ] A   Raised intraocular pressure (IOP) does not always require medication
- [ ] B   Photodynamic therapy will treat a minority of cases with macular degeneration
- [ ] C   Topical steroids in prolonged use may cause glaucoma
- [ ] D   Arc eye can be treated with cyclopentolate
- [ ] E   Patients with corneal abrasion should be given topical anaesthesia to use until the abrasion heals
- [ ] F   Latanoprost eye drops may cause colour changes in the iris

62. A 4-year-old girl is brought in by her mother, who reports that she has stopped growing. She was born at term after an uneventful pregnancy and her height and weight were on the 50th centile. On examination she appears well but her height and weight are both now on the 9th centile. Which of the following statements about failure to thrive is not true? Select one option only.

☐ A   It always has an organic basis

☐ B   Where it results from coeliac disease, it is usually associated with diarrhoea

☐ C   It may be caused by hyperthyroidism

☐ D   It may be caused by urinary tract infection

☐ E   Where caused by growth hormone deficiency it is usually apparent only from 6–12 months

63. Your next patient is a 76-year-old man with glaucoma. Which of the following statements about glaucoma is true? Select one option only.

☐ A   Glaucoma is usually asymptomatic

☐ B   Patients with raised IOP but no signs of glaucoma can be reassured

☐ C   It affects up to 2% of the population

☐ D   Treatment aims to reduce the IOP and reverse any loss of visual field

☐ F   It is a disease of middle-aged and elderly individuals

PAPER 3

64. A 63-year-old man who is normally fit and well on no regular medication presents with an acutely swollen, red and painful left knee. On examination he is afebrile and aspiration of the knee effusion reveals slightly turbid fluid. On microscopy birefringent calcium pyrophosphate crystals are seen. Which of the following statements about this condition is true? Select one option only.

- [ ] A The most likely diagnosis is septic arthritis
- [ ] B The patient is suffering from pseudogout
- [ ] C This condition may be a result of warfarin therapy
- [ ] D Radiographs of the knee aid diagnosis
- [ ] E He is suffering from gout

65. You practise in an area with a high African–Caribbean population, a number of whom have haemoglobinopathies. Which of the following statements about these conditions is true? Select one option only.

- [ ] A Most homozygous carriers of the sickle gene are asymptomatic
- [ ] B Sickle cell crises may be precipitated by infection
- [ ] C Stroke is rare in sickle cell patients
- [ ] D Patients should be given vitamin C supplements
- [ ] E During pregnancy crises are less common as a result of increased plasma volume

66. A 67-year-old woman is sent to see you by her optician who is concerned about the appearance of her eye, noted during a routine check-up.

Which of the following is the most appropriate management of this condition?

- [ ] A Betnesol eye drops
- [ ] B Ketorolac eye drops
- [ ] C Reassurance
- [ ] D Artificial tears
- [ ] E Excision
- [ ] F Topical aciclovir

67. Which one of the following drugs is contraindicated in pregnancy?

☐ A Fluconazole
☐ B Penicillin V
☐ C Codeine phosphate
☐ D Cefradine
☐ E Insulin

68. A 35-year-old woman complains of several years of increasingly painful periods, together with more recent difficulties with deep dyspareunia. She has been trying for a baby for 2 years without success. Which one of the following statements about her management is true?

☐ A Her symptoms are likely to have a strong psychological component as a result of her infertility and this should be addressed as part of her overall management
☐ B Norethisterone will help with her period pains
☐ C She should be referred for an ultrasound examination of her pelvis
☐ D Lack of specific signs on examination suggests that her dyspareunia is psychological
☐ E Non-steroidal agents are often effective during exacerbations of pain

PAPER 3

THEME: MENSTRUAL DISORDERS

Options

A   Endometriosis

B   Intermenstrual bleeding

C   Menorrhagia

D   Metrorrhagia

E   Primary amenorrhoea

F   Secondary amenorrhoea

For each of the descriptions below, select the most appropriate diagnosis from the list of options. Each option may be used once, more than once or not at all.

☐ 69.   Irregular acyclical bleeding in a 46-year-old woman.

☐ 70.   First-line treatment should be tranexamic acid.

☐ 71.   It may be a sign of chromosomal disorder.

☐ 72.   In 40% of patients this is the result of weight loss.

☐ 73.   It is commonly seen in women taking the contraceptive pill.

PAPER 3

74. **Which one of the following statements about NHS expert patient programmes is true?**

☐ A   There is a statutory requirement for primary care trusts (PCTs) to set up expert patient programmes

☐ B   Expert patient programmes have been shown to reduce medication use

☐ C   The Dose Adjustment for Normal Eating (DAFNE) project brought about improved satisfaction with treatment but no effect on blood glucose levels

☐ D   Participation in expert patient programmes empowers patients and increases attendance at accident and emergency departments in patients with sickle cell disease

☐ E   Expert patient programmes have been shown to be cost-effective

75. **A disgruntled former employee makes an application under the Freedom of Information Act to see your practice financial records. Which one of the following statements about this issue is correct?**

☐ A   The practice must disclose the incomes of individual partners in a given financial year

☐ B   The practice can refuse to comply if the prime motive is malicious

☐ C   The practice must comply with a request within 14 working days

☐ D   Data that fall under the auspices of the Data Protection Act are exempt

☐ E   The Freedom of Information Act enshrines the rights of patients to access their medical records

THEME: CHRONIC OBSTRUCTIVE AIRWAY DISEASE (COAD)

Options

A   Carbocysteine

B   Domiciliary oxygen

C   Inhaled low-dose steroids

D   Long-acting antimuscarinic bronchodilator

E   Long-acting theophylline

F   Oral steroids

G   Short-acting β_2 agonist

H   Short-acting antimuscarinic bronchodilator

I   Smoking cessation

For each statement about the management of COAD, select the most appropriate from the list of options. Each option may be used once, more than once or not at all.

☐ **76.** **It is proven to reduce the progressive decline in lung function.**

☐ **77.** **It is indicated in patients with persistent hypoxaemia.**

☐ **78.** **It may be effective in reducing the number of exacerbations in patients with COAD and chronic productive cough.**

☐ **79.** **A trial of this drug should be considered in patients with mild-to-moderate obstruction.**

☐ **80.** **Management should be considered in patients with persistent symptoms despite a regular inhaled antimuscarinic bronchodilator.**

THEME: ARRHYTHMIAS

Options

A   Atrial fibrillation

B   Atrial flutter

C   Complete heart block

D   First-degree heart block

E   Second-degree Mobitz type 1 (Wenckeback) heart block

F   Sinus arrhythmia

G   Supraventricular tachycardia

H   Torsade de pointes

I   Ventricular ectopics

J   Ventricular tachycardia

K   Wolf–Parkinson–White syndrome

PAPER 3

For each ECG description below, select from the list of options the one that best suits the description. Each option may be used once, more than once or not at all.

☐   **81.**   **No discrete P waves are seen on the ECG; QRS complexes are irregularly spaced.**

☐   **82.**   **P waves and QRS complexes are seen separately but are not coordinated. The rate is around 40.**

☐   **83.**   **ECG shows a short PR interval and an upward slanting of the QRS complex.**

☐   **84.**   **QRS complexes and P waves are normal in appearance but the rate increases and decreases across the rhythm strip.**

☐   **85.**   **Intermittent broad QRS complexes are seen with prolonged pause before the next normal P wave.**

THEME: FALLS IN ELDERLY PEOPLE

Options

A   Bisphosphonates

B   Calcium

C   Calcium/vitamin D_3

D   Cawsley–Cookthorne exercises

E   Exercise programmes

F   Hip protectors

G   Hormone replacement therapy

H   Parathyroid hormone injections

I   Strontium

J   Tibolone

K   Raloxifene

L   Vitamin D

For each of the statements below about falls in elderly people, select the most appropriate from the list of options. Each option may be used once, more than once or not at all.

86.   It is recommended in NICE guidance for all postmenopausal women on treatment for osteoporosis.

87.   It is recommended in NICE guidance for primary prevention of fracture in patients with osteoporosis who are intolerant of bisphosphonates.

88.   It has been shown in a Cochrane study to reduce fracture rate.

89.   It has been shown in meta-analysis to reduce falls by 20% with a number needed to treat of 15.

90.   It has been proven to increase bone mineral density in the lumbar spine, trochanter and femoral neck.

91. **Which of the following statements about NICE guidance on heart failure is true? Select one option only.**

☐ A All patients should be considered for a cardioselective β blocker as a first-line treatment

☐ B Thiazide diuretics have no role in managing chronic heart failure

☐ C Angiotensin-converting enzyme (ACE) inhibitors are first-line treatment for heart failure with evidence of left ventricular systolic dysfunction

☐ D Functional status should be formally assessed and documented for all patients with NYHA class 3 or 4 heart failure

☐ E β Blockers have no contraindications and can be used safely in all patients with heart failure

92. **One of your patients has advanced bowel cancer. His wife has come to see you to discuss his care. You have referred them to the local hospice nurses. Which of the following statements about hospice nurses is true? Select one option only.**

☐ A Hospice nurses provide day-to-day nursing care

☐ B Hospice nurses are on call to help in a crisis, eg provide night sitters

☐ C Hospice nurses are all extended prescribers and can initiate analgesic therapy

☐ D Hospice nurses provide counselling services for patients and families

☐ E Hospice nursing services in England are funded entirely through charitable donation

93. A 53-year-old man has recently been diagnosed with hypertension. He has done some research on the internet and is keen to avoid medication. Which of the following statements about non-pharmacological interventions is true? Select one option only.

☐ A Reducing dietary salt has a negligible effect on blood pressure

☐ B Blood pressure will fall with exercise but it must be high intensity and for at least 3 hours a week

☐ C Drinking less than 28 units a week in men has no effect on blood pressure

☐ D Weight loss of 1 kg will reduce blood pressure by 1–2 mmHg

☐ E All patients should adopt a high-fibre diet

94. A 45-year-old man who has recently started a new relationship complains of low libido. On further questioning he admits to feeling lethargic and weak, and has noticed that he has less stubble than previously. He takes no regular medication and is otherwise well, and does not suffer from headaches. Which of the following would be the most appropriate investigation in this situation? Select one option only.

☐ A MRI of the brain

☐ B Semen analysis

☐ C Depression screening

☐ D Short Synacthen test

☐ E FSH (follicle-stimulating hormone) and testosterone levels

PAPER 3

95. An 82-year-old man with a history of hypertension controlled on bendroflumethiazide presents with 3 months of weakness in his hands, which has deteriorated to the point where he has to hold a cup of tea with two hands. On examination he has wasting and fasciculation of his hands but no sensory symptoms. His tongue appears wasted and fasciculates. He chokes on occasions when swallowing fluids. Which of the following is the most likely diagnosis? Select one option only.

- [ ] A   Multiple sclerosis
- [ ] B   Motor neurone disease
- [ ] C   Myasthenia gravis
- [ ] D   Guillain–Barré disease
- [ ] E   Parkinsonism

96. A 41-year-old woman with painful swollen metacarpophalangeal joints on both hands for the last 3 weeks presents in surgery. Which of the following is the most appropriate investigation at this time? Select one option only.

- [ ] A   Autoantibodies
- [ ] B   HLA-B27 testing
- [ ] C   Plain radiograph
- [ ] D   Total IgE levels
- [ ] E   CRP (C-reactive protein) and ESR (erythrocyte sedimentation rate)

THEME: PRESCRIPTIONS FOR DRUGS

Options

A   Claim cost of drug back from the Department of Health

B   Claim dispensing fee

C   Claim an item of service fee

D   Claim under personally administered items

E   Covered by the appropriate direct enhanced service

F   Issue prescription on FP10 for the named patient

G   Write a prescription for pharmacist to dispense before
     starting treatment

For each of the situations described below, select the most appropriate
action from the list of options. Each option may be used once, more than
once, or not at all.

- [ ] **97.** **A 76-year-old man attends for his first goserelin (Zoladex)
  injection since joining the practice.**

- [ ] **98.** **A 23-year-old man has cut his eyebrow playing rugby. It is
  closed by the practice nurse using Steri-Strips.**

- [ ] **99.** **On a visit to a 67-year-old man with 24 hours of vomiting,
  you give him an intramuscular injection of Stemetil
  (prochlorperazine).**

- [ ] **100.** **A 70 year-old man with terminal cancer is to start a
  morphine pump. The district nurses will set this up but
  needs the appropriate drugs.**

- [ ] **101.** **A 25-year-old patient with diabetes attends for an
  influenza immunisation.**

102. A 38-year-old woman presents with a painful lesion on her eyelid of 2 days' duration. The appearance is shown below. Which of the following statements about this condition is correct? Select one option only.

- [ ] A   This is a chalazion and should settle in time
- [ ] B   This should be treated with chloramphenicol eyedrops
- [ ] C   This lesion is a basal cell carcinoma and should be referred urgently to plastic surgery
- [ ] D   This is a periorbital cellulitis and management should be directed at the underlying sinus infection
- [ ] E   This is a superficial infection and should be treated with anti-staphylococcal antibiotics

103. One of your partners announces that he would like to become a GPwSI in dermatology. This provokes heated discussion among the partners. Which one of the following statements about GPwSIs is true?

- [ ] A There is a nationally agreed pay scale
- [ ] B Separate indemnity insurance is needed for this work
- [ ] C GpwSI services have been shown to be more efficient than hospital services
- [ ] D PCTs have the final say in deciding whether a candidate is sufficiently qualified
- [ ] E Funding for training is available from within the GMSC

104. A 57-year-old man presents after a fall with an acutely swollen knee and difficulty bending the joint. He takes no regular medication and is otherwise fit and well, although a little overweight. Which one of the following statements about his management is true?

- [ ] A He should be treated for a probable septic arthritis with antibiotics and reviewed in 1 week
- [ ] B The presence of blood on aspiration requires referral to exclude intra-articular fracture
- [ ] C If haemarthrosis is confirmed he should be screened for haemophilia
- [ ] D It does not cause permanent joint damage
- [ ] E The joint should not be splinted because this prevents mobilisation

PAPER 3

105. A number of concerns have been raised recently in the media about the safety of hormone replacement therapy (HRT). Which one of the following statements about current evidence is true?

- [ ] A   Topical HRT is more effective than systemic HRT for the prevention of recurrent urinary tract infections
- [ ] B   1 in 100 woman taking combined HRT for 5 years will develop ovarian cancer as a result
- [ ] C   Use of combined HRT is associated with breast cancer with a number needed to harm of 10 000
- [ ] D   Use of combined HRT increases the risk of venous thromboembolism by 25%
- [ ] E   Use of combined HRT increases the risk of endometrial cancer significantly

106. Which one of the following statements about the National Clinical Assessment Authority (NCAA) is true?

- [ ] A   The NCAA is responsible for the performance of doctors
- [ ] B   The NCAA is a disciplinary body only
- [ ] C   The average completion time for an NCAA assessment is 8 weeks
- [ ] D   Women are less likely to be reported to the NCAA than men
- [ ] E   Non-white dentists are over-represented in patients referred to the NCAA

107. A 72-year-old man with no previous medical history of note presents after experiencing indigestion the previous night, which woke him up. He feels slightly better now. Examination reveals some tenderness in his epigastrium. His ECG is shown below (heart rate 67/minute, QT interval 428 ms).

Heart Rate: 67 bpm

QT Interval: 428 ms

Which one of the following statements about this case is true?

- [ ] A He should be given an antacid and reviewed the following day
- [ ] B Bloods should be taken for cardiac enzymes and he should be reviewed the following day
- [ ] C He should be given aspirin and admitted under the medical take
- [ ] D He should be referred for upper gastrointestinal endoscopy
- [ ] E He should be admitted under the on-call surgeon

108. Which one of the following statements about osteoarthritis is true?

- [ ] A Topical non-steroidal preparations are effective in relieving pain
- [ ] B Taping is an effective long-term therapy for osteoarthritis of the knee
- [ ] C Meta-analyses have shown that intra-articular steroid injections are not effective in comparison with saline injections
- [ ] D Physical exercise should be avoided because it often exacerbates osteoarthritis
- [ ] E Acupuncture has not been proved to be beneficial for pain or function

109. A 12-year-old girl is seen complaining of nocturnal enuresis. This has been going on since she was potty trained and happens on average once or twice a week. She has tried fluid restriction and frequent waking but to no effect. Which of the following statements about this condition is true? Select one option only.

- [ ] A The condition is more common in girls than boys, affecting 5% of 13-year-old girls
- [ ] B She can be reassured that no further tests or treatments are necessary and that she will grow out of the condition in time
- [ ] C All patients should have their urine tested
- [ ] D Desmopressin is an effective long-term treatment
- [ ] E Imipramine generally provides a lasting cure

110. A rather embarrassed 17-year-old boy is seen at the out-of-hours centre complaining of dysuria and discharge from his penis. This started about a week earlier and is increasingly uncomfortable. He is normally fit and well. You send a urethral swab for microscopy and culture and a midstream urine. The results come back showing a few pus cells in his urine but no growth on either culture. What is the most likely diagnosis? Select one option only.

- [ ] A   Gonorrhoea
- [ ] B   Chronic prostatitis
- [ ] C   Non-specific urethritis
- [ ] D   Urinary tract infection
- [ ] E   Balanitis xerotica et obliterans

111. Which one of the following statements about care of elderly people in the UK is true?

- [ ] A   Cholinesterase inhibitors can reverse the progress of dementia if given early enough in the course of the disease
- [ ] B   Hip protectors are effective and compliance is generally good
- [ ] C   Most elderly people receiving care get it from trained carers
- [ ] D   Of the over-65 age group, 30% will fall in any given year
- [ ] E   Sedative hypnotics are safe and effective in elderly people

THEME: HEADACHES

Options

A   Analgesic overuse headache

B   Carbon monoxide poisoning

C   Chronic daily headache

D   Chronic paroxysmal hemicrania

E   Cluster headache

F   Migraine

G   Raised intracranial pressure

H   Severe headache of sudden onset

I   Tension-type headache

For each scenario described below, select the most appropriate diagnosis from the list of options. Each option may be used once, more than once or not at all.

☐ **112.** A 34-year-old woman with recurrent attacks of severe headache affecting one side of the head only. These last less than 45 minutes and settle with non-steroidal drugs.

☐ **113.** A 23-year-old man who has been taking co-codamol for recurrent 'migraine' most days for the last 3 months. He describes bilateral pressure in his temples that does not limit activity.

☐ **114.** A 27-year-old man complains of recurrent severe headaches that he describes as the worst headaches that he can imagine. They have been occurring every day for the last week. He gets associated watering of his right eye.

☐ **115.** A 24-year-old woman presents with an acute onset of severe headache. She has no neck stiffness or altered conscious level and examination reveals normal fundi.

☐ **116.** A 19-year-old student living in digs complains of nausea, headache and lethargy over several weeks. On examination he has cherry-red lips and is confused.

THEME: HYPERTENSION TRIALS

Options

A   Anglo-Scandinavian Cardiac Outcomes Trial: Blood Pressure-Lowering Arm (ASCOT)

B   Antihypertensive and Lipid Lowering Treatment to Prevent Heart Attack Trial (ALLHAT)

C   British Hypertension Society guidelines for hypertension management

D   Hypertension Optimal Treatment (HOT) trial

E   Losartan Intervention for Endpoint Reduction (LIFE)

F   NICE guidelines for hypertension management

G   Study on Cognition and Prognosis in the Elderly (SCOPE)

H   Swedish Trial in Old Patients with Hypertension-2 (STOP-2)

For each description below, select the most appropriate trial from the list of options. Each option may be used once, more than once or not at all.

117.   It demonstrated an optimal blood pressure target of 139/83 for cardiovascular event reduction.

118.   It demonstrated the superiority of amlodipine and perindopril in reducing myocardial infarction.

119.   It sets treatment targets of 140/85 or 130/80 for people with diabetes.

120.   It advises that β blockers should not be used as first-line treatments.

121.   it showed a 42% relative risk reduction in the risk of stroke for patients treated with candesartan.

122.   It recommends routine screening for hypertension at 5-yearly intervals.

123. Which of the following statements about peanut allergy is true? Select one option only.

- [ ] A The prevalence of nut allergy in children is 20%
- [ ] B Of patients with peanut allergy 50% are allergic to other nuts
- [ ] C Most children with nut allergy will grow out of the condition by adulthood
- [ ] D Skin-prick tests are the gold standard for identifying true nut allergy
- [ ] E Sodium cromoglicate is an effective prophylactic therapy

124. A 3-year-old with left-sided earache is brought in by his mother. Which of the following statements about the management of acute otitis media is correct? Select one statement only.

- [ ] A Prompt use of antibiotics results in rapid resolution of symptoms
- [ ] B Decongestants help to open the eustachian tube, relieving the pressure on the drum
- [ ] C Ciprofloxacin is active against *Pseudomonas* spp. and is an effective first-line treatment in this patient
- [ ] D Regular analgesics and rest are the most effective initial treatment
- [ ] E Untreated otitis media inevitably results in glue ear

125. A 56-year-old woman presents with a chronic rash on her face that she tends to cover with heavy applications of make-up. She has no medical history of note but does get recurrent conjunctivitis and itchy eyes. On examination she has papules and pustules over her nose and forehead. What is the likely diagnosis? Select one option only.

☐ A   Systemic lupus erythematosus

☐ B   Acne vulgaris

☐ C   Acne rosacea

☐ D   Dermatitis herpetiformis

☐ E   Allergic contact dermatitis

126. An 18-year-old girl presents with a sore throat. On examination you find the appearance below.

What is the significance of this condition?

☐ A   It is a sign of lymphoid hyperplasia in the ring of Waldeyer

☐ B   It is a sign of antrochoanal polyps

☐ C   It may indicate a cleft palate

☐ D   It is a consequence of recurrent tonsillitis

☐ E   It is never of any significance

PAPER 3

127. A 35-year-old woman who has just returned from a holiday in Thailand attends the local walk-in centre complaining of sudden-onset pleuritic chest pain, breathlessness and coughing up blood-stained phlegm. She had a dry cough and sore throat while on holiday but is otherwise well. She takes the contraceptive pill but no other medication and has no previous medical history of note. Which of the following statements about her management is true? Select one option only.

- [ ] A A fever of 37.5°C suggests an infective cause rather than pulmonary embolism
- [ ] B An elevated D-dimer is a highly specific sign of thromboembolism
- [ ] C ST or T-wave abnormalities on an ECG suggest a myocardial infarction
- [ ] D A normal D-dimer excludes thromboembolism with 95% sensitivity
- [ ] E Pulmonary emboli always cause chest pain

128. A 61-year-old woman complains that her periods have started again after 4 years off HRT. She is otherwise well apart from tablet-controlled diabetes and asthma. Examination of her abdomen and vaginal examination are unremarkable. Which of the following actions would be appropriate? Select one option only.

- [ ] A Refer for sigmoidoscopy to exclude piles as a cause of bleeding
- [ ] B Carry out a cervical smear
- [ ] C Refer under the 2-week rule to gynaecology
- [ ] D Refer for an ultrasound scan of the uterus
- [ ] E Refer routinely to gynaecology outpatients
- [ ] F Send a midstream urine to exclude renal tract causes

129. A 5-week-old baby boy is brought in by his mother with 'projectile vomiting'. This started about 1 week ago and has been steadily worsening. He is otherwise well and seems to be ravenously hungry after each vomit. He is otherwise well but has started to lose weight. Which of the following statements about this condition is true? Select one option only.

- [ ] A In pyloric stenosis a pyloric mass is always palpable
- [ ] B Gastro-oesophageal reflux can cause these symptoms
- [ ] C These symptoms are always suggestive of organic disease
- [ ] D Where a child is lethargic and off feeds, pyloric stenosis is almost always the cause
- [ ] E Gastroenteritis is a common cause of these symptoms

130. A 41-year-old man with a history of gallstones presents with sudden onset of upper abdominal pain radiating through to the back and associated with vomiting. On examination he has upper abdominal tenderness. Which one of the following is a possible diagnosis?

- [ ] A Acute pancreatitis
- [ ] B Hiatus hernia
- [ ] C Chronic pancreatitis
- [ ] D Gastroenteritis
- [ ] E Abdominal aortic aneurysm

131. Which one of the following interventions is NOT useful in treating premenstrual tension?

- [ ] A Fluoxetine
- [ ] B Norethisterone
- [ ] C Agnus castis
- [ ] D Spironolactone
- [ ] E Evening primrose oil

PAPER 3

THEME: INCONTINENCE

Options

A   Cystocele

B   Neurological incontinence

C   Overflow incontinence

D   Stress incontinence

E   Urethral caruncle

F   Urge incontinence

G   Urinary tract infection

H   Vesicocolic fistula

I   Vesicovaginal fistula

For each of the patients described below, select the most appropriate diagnosis from the list of options. Each option may be used once, more than once or not at all.

☐   **132.   An elderly woman with diabetes and peripheral neuropathy has had difficulty passing urine for some time. She now presents with persistent urinary dribbling. On examination her bladder is palpable.**

☐   **133.   A 74-year-old woman with a history of diverticular disease has noticed bubbles of air in her urine.**

☐   **134.   A 66-year-old woman with no previous history of note complains of several months of difficulty with urination. When she needs to go, she has to go quickly, but sadly she does not often make it and is incontinent.**

☐   **135.   A 47-year-old woman who has had four children, all by vaginal delivery, complains of leakage on coughing. On examination she has a small degree of uterine descent only.**

☐   **136.   A 7-year-old girl who has previously been continent develops nocturnal enuresis and incontinence of urine.**

THEME: LEARNING DISABILITY

Options

A   Attention deficit hyperactivity disorder (ADHD)

B   Autism

C   Cerebral palsy

D   Developmental aphasia

E   Dyslexia

F   Dyspraxia

G   Fragile X syndrome

H   None of the above

For each of the descriptions of children with learning difficulties below, select the most appropriate diagnosis from the list of options. Each option may be used once, more than once or not at all.

137.   A child of 7 with normal development in maths and non-verbal tasks is assessed as having verbal skills at the level of a 4 year old.

138.   A child of 8 with poor hand–eye coordination is unable to ride a bicycle without stabilisers and noted by his parents to be accident prone. His development is otherwise normal.

139.   A 30-month-old child who had normal development up to 18 months appears to be indifferent to his surroundings, has no interest in toys and does not play with other children. He has only four words and is prone to temper tantrums.

140.   This is often associated with dyslexia.

141.   A 24-month-old girl with poor balance, shaky movements when trying to feed herself and impaired speech development.

142. A 67-year-old woman presents with a 4-week history of spots on her fingers and toes. She reports a history of 'arthritis' but has not consulted a doctor about this. Examination reveals the following appearance of her hands.

Which of the following is the most likely diagnosis? Select one option only.

- [ ] A   Vasculitis
- [ ] B   Splinter haemorrhages
- [ ] C   Idiopathic thrombocytopenic purpura
- [ ] D   Rheumatoid arthritis
- [ ] E   Giant cell arteritis

143. A 33-year-old woman presents with a rash on her arms and trunk. She is otherwise well and has no other symptoms. She takes no regular medications. On examination she has a target-like rash with central pallor. Which of the following is NOT a cause of this rash? Select one option only.

- [ ] A Aspirin
- [ ] B Vitamin deficiency
- [ ] C Mycoplasma infection
- [ ] D Ulcerative colitis
- [ ] E Herpes zoster

144. A 35-year-old patient is persistently aggressive and abusive and the practice manager would like to remove the patient from the practice list. Which one of the following statements about this process is true?

- [ ] A The patient should receive a letter explaining the action that is being taken
- [ ] B The letter must give the specific reasons for removal
- [ ] C The removal takes place with immediate effect
- [ ] D The most common reason for removal from a doctor's list is violence or aggressive behaviour
- [ ] E If a member of a household is removed from the list, other members living at the same address should also be removed

145. You are asked to visit a 79-year-old man living in a residential home who has been unable to pass urine for the last 12 hours. On arrival he has a tender bladder, palpable to his umbilicus, and you catheterise him immediately. Which of the following statements about urinary retention is true? Select one option only.

☐ A   Acute retention may result from constipation

☐ B   It is seen only in men

☐ C   It is always the result of obstruction at the prostate

☐ D   It should be treated with a suprapubic catheter if there is a coexistent urinary tract infection

☐ E   It is always painful

☐ F   All of the above

146. Which of the following is NOT a cause of rickets? Select one option only.

☐ A   Chronic renal failure

☐ B   Fat malabsorption

☐ C   Anticonvulsant medication

☐ D   Hyperparathyroidism

☐ E   Dietary lack of vitamin D_3

147. A 23-year-old student presents to the walk-in centre complaining of intense itching on his fingers, wrists and arms. He says that this is worse at night and after showering. On examination he has extensive scratch marks and papules with raised white lines in the skin. He has no previous medical history of note and takes no regular medication. Which of the following is the most likely diagnosis? Select one option only.

☐ A   Nodular prurigo

☐ B   Pemphigus

☐ C   Dermatitis artefacta

☐ D   Pompholyx

☐ E   Scabies

THEME: THE GMS2 CONTRACT

Options

A   Direct enhanced service

B   Global sum

C   Local enhanced service

D   Minimum Practice Income Guarantee

E   Non-GMS NHS work

F   Private work

G   Quality and Outcomes Framework

For each of the descriptions below, select the most appropriate term from the list of options. Each option may be used once, more than once or not at all.

☐ **148.** Insurance medicals.

☐ **149.** A scheme whereby the local PCT pays practices £3 for each choose and book referral and a lump sum if they meet a target number of referrals.

☐ **150.** Sport diving medicals.

☐ **151.** Community hospital work.

☐ **152.** Includes a component for staff pension and national insurance costs.

☐ **153.** A scheme whereby GPs are paid to manage goserelin (Zoladex) injections.

☐ **154.** An optional performance-related pay scheme.

THEME: NOSOCOMIAL INFECTIONS

Options

A   *Candida albicans*

B   *Clostridium difficile*

C   Methicillin-resistant *Staphylococcus aureus* (MRSA)

D   Norwalk virus

E   *Pseudomonas aeruginosa*

F   *Staphylococcus aureus*

G   *Staphylococcus epidermidis*

H   Vancomycin-resistant enterococci

For each description of a nosocomial infection, select the most appropriate organism from the list of options. Each option may be used once, more than once or not at all.

- [ ] **155.** It is often seen in those with pre-existing lung disease.
- [ ] **156.** It causes a viral gastroenteritis with watery diarrhoea, vomiting and myalgia lasting up to 48 hours.
- [ ] **157.** It is often seen in blood cultures from relatively well patients with intravenous devices.
- [ ] **158.** It is often acquired through contact with animals; this pathogen rarely causes illness in healthy patients but may be seen in dialysis and transplant units or in patients who are fed by nasogastric tube.
- [ ] **159.** It is becoming increasingly sensitive to trimethoprim.

160. A 35-year-old asylum seeker registers at your practice. At his new patient check he reports 6 months of weight loss, night sweats and a cough with haemopytsis at times. On examination he has erythema nodosum and reduced air entry in his right mid zone, with dullness to percussion over this area. He has no previous history of note and has no risk factors for HIV. Which of the following is a likely diagnosis? Select one option only.

- ☐ A   Tuberculosis
- ☐ B   *Pneumocystis carinii* pneumonia
- ☐ C   Bronchopneumonia
- ☐ D   Lung cancer
- ☐ E   Sarcoidosis

161. A 17-year-old student experiences diarrhoea that fails to settle after 3 days. She is passing stools eight or nine times a day and there is blood and mucus mixed in with the stool. On examination she has generalised abdominal tenderness, particularly over the descending colon. Which of the following is the single most likely diagnosis? Select one option only.

- ☐ A   Ulcerative colitis
- ☐ B   Diverticulitis
- ☐ C   Tubular adenoma
- ☐ D   Gastroenteritis
- ☐ E   Crohn's disease

THEME: DISEASE OF THE OUTER EAR

Options

A   Basal cell carcinoma

B   Cauliflower ear

C   Chondrodermatitis nodularis helices

D   Ear wax

E   Eczema

F   Furunculosis

G   Foreign body

H   Otitis media

I   Subchondral haematoma

For each scenario described below, select the single most likely diagnosis. Each option may be used once, more than once or not at all.

☐   **162.   Associated with blunt trauma to the ear, this must be treated promptly to prevent long-term deformity.**

☐   **163.   If severely affected, it may cause deafness and tinnitus, although seldom painful.**

☐   **164.   It is usually seen in children or people with a learning disability.**

☐   **165.   It is associated with extreme tenderness.**

☐   **166.   It is a tender papule affecting the helix that is chronic.**

167. A 19-year-old man comes to see you to get a medical form signed to allow him to undertake a recreational scuba-diving course. Which one of the following conditions would NOT allow scuba-diving without expert assessment?

☐ A   Mild asthma brought on by exertion only

☐ B   Previous anterior cruciate repair

☐ C   Severe eczema

☐ D   Previous history of depression

☐ E   Colour blindness

168. A 67-year-old woman presents with a lump in the front of her neck. She thinks that this has been present for only a few months. She has no other symptoms and takes no regular medication. On examination there is a smooth non-tender lump that moves on swallowing. Which of the following statements about this patient is correct? Select one option only.

☐ A   Thyroid function tests (TFTs) should be performed. If they are normal no further action is necessary at this time. They should, however, be repeated on a regular basis because she will probably become clinically hypothyroid at some stage

☐ B   If thyroid function shows a raised TSH (thyroid-stimulating hormone) she should be started on thyroxine and have TFTs repeated in 3 months to assess effect

☐ C   She should be referred under the 2-week rule

☐ D   She is in the acute phase of Hashimoto's thyroiditis and can be reassured

☐ E   If she is clinically euthyroid this is most probably a physiological goitre

PAPER 3

THEME: PSYCHIATRIC DRUGS

Options

A	Amisulpiride	G	Lithium
B	Carbamazepine	H	Mirtazepine
C	Citalopram	I	Moclobemide
D	Dothiepin	J	Paroxetine
E	Fluoxetine	K	Risperidone
F	Haloperidol	L	Venlafaxine

For each description below, select the most appropriate drug from the list of options. Each option may be used once, more than once or not at all.

☐ **169.** It should not be used by patients taking methyldopa.

☐ **170.** It is associated with risk of stroke in elderly people.

☐ **171.** It may increase IOP.

☐ **172.** It should not be used in patients with a history of arrhythmia.

☐ **173.** It requires regular monitoring of renal function.

174. A 48-year-old man with poorly controlled type 2 diabetes presents with sudden onset of visual loss. Examination of his eye reveals loss of red reflex, acuity of 6/24 in the affected eye (6/6 in the good eye) and blood in the posterior chamber of the eye. Which of the following is the most likely diagnosis? Select one option only.

☐ A Vitreous detachment

☐ B Branch retinal vein occlusion

☐ C Central retinal artery occlusion

☐ D Commotio retinae

☐ E Vitreous haemorrhage

THEME: RENAL DISEASE

Options

A   Glomerulonephritis

B   Goodpasture syndrome

C   Hydronephrosis

D   Nephritic syndrome

E   Nephrotic syndrome

F   Polycystic kidney disease

G   Renal osteodystrophy

H   Renal tubular acidosis

I   Uraemia

For each disease described below, select the most appropriate diagnosis from the list of options. Each option may be used once, more than once or not at all.

☐   **175.   It is characterised by haematuria, uraemia and oedema.**

☐   **176.   It is characterised by proteinuria and oedema with normal urea and creatinine.**

☐   **177.   It is inherited as either a recessive or dominant form.**

☐   **178.   It is seen in a patient with symptoms of glomerulonephritis and haemoptysis.**

☐   **179.   It is a combination of secondary hyperparathyroidism, osteomalacia and vitamin D deficiency.**

180. With regard to the 'stages of change' process of recovery from addiction, which one of the following statements is true?

- [ ] A   In the pre-contemplative phase, people are aware that they have a problem but don't feel able to consider the possibility of change
- [ ] B   Most patients move steadily through the stages of pre-contemplation, contemplation, preparation, action, maintenance
- [ ] C   The stages of change theory applies only to patients with no organic injury
- [ ] D   The action phase involves changing behaviour only
- [ ] E   Where a patient relapses, further treatment attempts using this model are unlikely to be successful

181. An 87-year-old man complains that he always has to have his ears syringed. Which of the following statements about ear wax is true? Select one option only.

- [ ] A   Repeated wax accumulation suggests local ear disease
- [ ] B   Wax impaction is asymptomatic
- [ ] C   Wax impaction may be the result of hearing aid use
- [ ] D   Syringing may be safely carried out in any patient with wax impaction
- [ ] E   It may be safely treated with Hopi candles
- [ ] F   All races produce similar ear wax

THEME: SKIN LESIONS

Options

A   Amelanotic melanoma

B   Basal cell carcinoma

C   Bowen's disease

D   Epithelioma

E   Hamartoma

F   Keratoacanthoma

G   Malignant melanoma

H   Neurofibroma

I   Pyogenic granuloma

J   Squamous cell carcinoma

For each description below, select the most appropriate diagnosis from the list of options. Each option may be used once, more than once or not at all.

☐   **182. It typically has a pearly rim with surface telangiectasia.**

☐   **183. This is an indurated lesion that is rapidly growing and has a central ulcer.**

☐   **184. This is a lesion that developed after a minor injury, rapidly growing over 2 weeks with a fleshy appearance.**

☐   **185. This is a rubbery nodular lesion on the flexor aspect of the arm, present for several years and with numerous other similar lesions.**

☐   **186. Recurrence has been shown to be prevented by use of sunscreen.**

THEME: THYROID FUNCTION TESTS

187–191.

Options

A   Autoimmune thyroiditis

B   Euthyroid

C   Hyperthyroidism

D   Hypothyroidism

E   Hypopituitarism

F   Sick euthyroidism

G   Subclinical hyperthyroidism

H   Subclinical hypothyroidism

For each of the sets of thyroid tests below, select the most appropriate diagnosis from the list of options. Each option may be used once, more than once or not at all.

Thyroid function tests

☐   **187.** $\Downarrow$ TSH $\Downarrow$ T$_4$ $\Downarrow$ T$_3$

☐   **188.** $\Rightarrow$ TSH $\Rightarrow$ T$_4$ $\Downarrow$ T$_3$

☐   **189.** $\Uparrow$ TSH $\Rightarrow$ T$_4$ $\Rightarrow$ T$_3$

☐   **190.** $\Downarrow$ TSH $\Uparrow$ T$_4$ $\Uparrow$ T$_3$

☐   **191.** $\Uparrow$ TSH $\Downarrow$ T$_4$ $\Downarrow$ T$_3$

$\Downarrow$, **low level,** $\Uparrow$, **elevated level,** $\Rightarrow$, **normal level.**

192. A rather anxious mother has brought her child in to see you having discovered a lump in his abdomen while drying him after a bath. On examination he has a mass in his left upper quadrant. You manage to obtain some urine and this is positive on dipstick testing for blood. He is otherwise well. What is the likely diagnosis? Select one option only.

- [ ] A Hydronephrosis
- [ ] B Hepatoblastoma
- [ ] C Wilms' tumour
- [ ] D Constipation
- [ ] E Splenomegaly

193. Which one of the following statements about immunisation is true?

- [ ] A BCG immunisation is no longer routinely given to children born in the UK
- [ ] B Hepatitis B immunisation is part of the routine childhood immunisation strategy in the UK
- [ ] C The Sabin polio vaccine is now used routinely in the UK
- [ ] D Low uptake of MMR since the autism scare has resulted in increased cases of mumps in university students whose parents refused to have them immunised as children
- [ ] E Varicella immunisation has been shown to be effective in preventing chickenpox only

THEME: VAGINAL DISCHARGE

Options

A   Atrophic vaginitis

B   Bacterial vaginosis

C   Cervical erosion

D   Candidiasis

E   Endometritis

F   Gonorrhoea

G   Physiological

PAPER 3

For each of the clinical scenarios described below, select the most appropriate diagnosis from the list of options. Each option may be used once, more than once or not at all.

☐ **194.** A 23-year-old woman presents with itching, soreness and mild dyspareunia. On examination there is a white exudate on a background of erythematous mucosa.

☐ **195.** A 34-year-old woman who had a normal delivery 4 weeks ago presents with low-grade fever, a purulent vaginal discharge and low abdominal pain.

☐ **196.** A 26-year-old woman complains of an increase in vaginal discharge in the middle of her cycle. There is no odour and no itch, although the discharge does stain slightly.

☐ **197.** A 36-year-old woman has become aware of a fishy vaginal discharge with some associated itch.

☐ **198.** A 67-year-old woman has recently started a new relationship. She has noticed a blood-stained discharge and dyspareunia. She is otherwise well and has no systemic symptoms.

199. A meta-analysis of studies for a new drug is presented below:

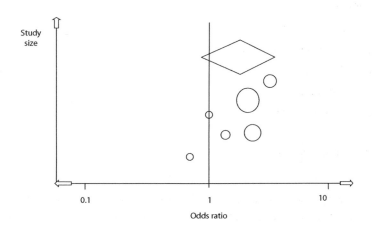

Which of the following statements about the data is true? Select one option.

◻ A The studies all suggest a positive benefit from the drug

◻ B The meta-analysis suggests an unequivocal favourable effect

◻ C The 95% confidence intervals for the meta-analysis cross the line of no effect

◻ D The odds ratio for the meta-analysis is 1

◻ E An odds ratio of 3 implies that the intervention is 30% more likely to result in a positive outcome

200. You attend a meeting organised by the local PCT to look into setting up exercise classes to help people lose weight. One of the local public health consultants presents the following data from a trial that showed the benefits of increased exercise:

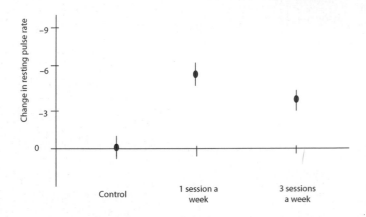

Which one of the following statements about these data is true?

☐ A   The data show a linear relationship between frequency of exercise and physical fitness

☐ B   The data show a definite benefit for exercise in reducing weight

☐ C   The drop-off in benefit with increased exercise might be a result of patient drop-out, eg resulting from injury

☐ D   Change in resting pulse rate is a valid surrogate marker for weight loss

☐ E   The confidence intervals suggest that there is no definitive benefit for either group

Paper 3
Answers

1.   **E: Subconjunctival haemorrhage**

2.   **D: Episcleritis**

3.   **A: Acute glaucoma**

4.   **B: Conjunctivitis**

5.   **C: Corneal ulcer**

6.   **D: Methylphenidate is effective in most patients**

Hyperkinetic behaviour is seen in 0.5–1% of children in the UK. In the USA a broader definition has led to the diagnosis being made in 10% of children. The condition is often associated with dyslexia and dyspraxia. Methylphenidate can cause abdominal pain, disturbed sleep and growth retardation. Some children with hyperkinetic behaviour react to certain foods.

7.   **B: Mental capacity is a prerequisite for completion of an advance directive**

Advance directives may be written or verbal, but if there are certain situations where specific conditions are set out, they must be in writing. Advance directives are written at a time of mental competency to be used when the patient is no longer mentally competent (eg dysphasic or comatose). Competent adults can refuse treatment in any situation as long as they understand the implications of this. The minimum age is 18.

8.   **C:**   Until 24 hours after symptoms have settled

9.   **D:**   Until lesions have crusted

10.   **E:**   Until treated

11.   **A:**   5 days

12.   **A:**   5 days

13.   **B:**   No exclusion necessary

14.   **C:**   Acetazolamide

Acetazolamide is effective in prevention and treatment of altitude sickness. Dexamethasone is effective in treatment but the side-effect profile makes it unsuitable for prophylaxis. Sildenafil is an effective treatment for high-altitude pulmonary oedema and there is some evidence that it is effective in increasing exercise tolerance at altitude.

15.   **B:**   Neurofibromatosis

This patient has neurofibromatosis, an autosomal dominant condition associated with bilateral acoustic neuromas, café-au-lait patches and multiple neurofibromas.

16.   A: Normal weight gain and growth are reassuring signs

A review in the *BMJ* in 2007 found no difference in incidence of positive serology between controls and cases for coeliac disease or *H. pylori* antibodies. Cognitive–behavioural therapy aimed at the family is beneficial. Children with chronic abdominal pain in childhood are more likely to develop irritable bowel syndrome as adults. Only patients with red flag symptoms need further investigation. 30% of children suffer persistent abdominal pain.

17.   A: Nephrotic syndrome

The finding of heavy proteinuria with oedema suggests nephrotic syndrome. This may follow an acute glomerulonephritis but is often idiopathic. Children should be admitted initially for investigation and fluid balance; however, 90% respond to steroids. After discharge the parents need to monitor the urine for protein but the prognosis for most children is good.

18.   A: Appraisal

The preparation of a personal development plan is crucial to the appraisal process.

19.   G: Revalidation

Revalidation is envisaged to take place once every 5 years.

20.   A: Appraisal

Appraisals are a contractual obligation under the GMS Contract.

PAPER 3

21.   G: Revalidation

22.   G: Revalidation

Revalidation is required to see patients. People who wish to remain on the medical register but not see patients, eg researchers, do not need to undertake this process.

23.   D: Recertification

Recertification will be the responsibility of individual Royal Colleges.

24.   D: Recertification

Recertification is expected to involve some or all of patient feedback, knowledge tests or simulation tests.

25.   A: Appraisal

26.   A: Morton's neuroma

This is the typical location for Morton's neuroma, usually arising from the common digital nerve. Treatment is with local steroid/anaesthetic injection or excision if persistent.

27.   A: Codeine, tramadol, morphine, oxycodone, diamorphine

28.   D: Bell's palsy is associated with altered facial sensation and taste

Facial nerve palsy may be caused by injury from the CNS to the terminal branches and causes include: tumour, Guillain–Barré syndrome and sarcoidosis. Peripheral causes include herpes zoster (Ramsay Hunt syndrome), which requires prompt treatment with aciclovir, middle-ear infection and trauma, usually iatrogenic during middle-ear or parotid surgery. Recovery depends on cause, with only 60% of Ramsay Hunt syndrome patients making a complete recovery. Bell's palsy is an idiopathic facial nerve palsy and is thus a diagnosis of exclusion.

29.   A: Fundoscopy reveals a bright-red spot at the fovea

Fundoscopy reveals a pale opaque retina with narrow thread-like arteries. The fovea has a cherry-red appearance. The pupil reacts poorly to light and the visual field loss may be segmental or total depending on the site of the obstruction.

30.   D: Bronchiectasis

Bronchiectasis is a persistent dilatation of the bronchi resulting in persistent infection. It may be seen as part of a syndrome (situs invertus, sinusitis and bronchiectasis), after infections or obstruction or in defective host defences. It is treated with physiotherapy and antibiotics and, if resistant to treatment, surgery may be considered.

31.   D: It is usually acquired through eating chicken

Campylobacter sp. is the most common notified cause of diarrhoea in the UK. It often settles spontaneously in under 5 days but may persist for 3–4 weeks. It may rarely cause Reiter syndrome or arthritis. Where treated ciprofloxacin or erythromycin should be used.

32.   C: Cardiomyopathy

Cardiomyopathy usually presents with signs of heart failure and/or arrhythmias, of which AF is the most common. It may be hereditary or acquired and Coxsackievirus is a common culprit. The history is too long for a pulmonary embolism and atypical pneumonia would not normally be associated with signs of heart failure. Most patients are managed with β blockers and ACE inhibitors.

33.   F: All of the above

Risk factors for child abuse can be considered as child factors, eg disability or prematurity, family, eg poor housing, and carer factors, eg history of drug abuse.

34.   A: Phytophotodermatitis

This is a phototoxic response to psoralens released by plants. It resembles a contact dermatitis and is usually seen on the arms and legs. Drugs such as doxycycline may also cause a photosensitive rash. Actinic prurigo and chronic actinic dermatosis are chronic conditions.

35.   A: Diagnostic and treatment algorithms can reduce antibiotic prescription rates for nursing homes

A study in the *BMJ* in 2005 showed that rigid adherence to algorithms could reduce prescription rates. Antibiotic resistance levels are significantly higher in areas of high primary care antibiotic prescribing. Little et al. have carried out a number of studies of deferred prescriptions in primary care with good results. Patients' attitudes studied as part of the deferred script trials suggest that patients are more concerned about giving antibiotics to their children than about levels of antibiotic resistance. Deferred scripts for simple upper respiratory tract infections have been shown to reduce the number of prescriptions filled by up to two-thirds

36.   **E:**   **Regular antiviral medication can reduce transmission to sexual partners**

The first attack is usually the most severe. Women usually develop lesions on the cervix, vulva and vagina, men on the prepuce. Healing usually takes 2–4 weeks in primary herpes and 10 days in recurrent attacks. A trial in the *New England Journal of Medicine* in 2004 found that daily use of valaciclovir reduced transmission by 75% between discordant couples. Attacks in immunocompromised patients tend to be longer and more severe.

37.   **A:**   **Acute ischaemic optic neuritis**

Temporal arteritis causes an acute ischaemic optic neuritis.

38.   **E:**   **Peripheral diabetic retinopathy**

This photograph shows peripheral diabetic retinopathy and maculopathy.

39.   **D:**   **Normal retina**

This is a description of migraine. The retina is normal.

40.   **C:**   **Retinal detachment**

This photograph shows a retinal tear and detachment.

41.   **B:**   **Dry ARMD**

This photo shows dry age-related macular degeneration.

PAPER 3

42.   A: Two-thirds of affected patients are undiagnosed

Most patients present with non-specific symptoms such as fatigue or anaemia. At least 45% of patients fail to adhere to the diet and risk lymphoma, osteoporosis and infertility. Many cases are familial. Gluten-free products are available on prescription.

43.   C: Copying letters has been shown to help inform patients and improve their ability to make treatment decisions

Consent to copying of letters should be recorded in the patient's record. The general principle of informed consent applies to copying letters. Where adults have carers, letters should be copied to carers where appropriate, for example detailing medication changes.

44.   A: Deprivation is linked to diabetic eye disease

Deprivation is most strongly associated with diabetic eye disease, bronchitis and emphysema. Indices commonly used are those of Jarman and Townsend and high scores are associated with increased referral rates, consultation rates and visiting rates.

45.   B: Patients taking COX-2 inhibitors have been shown to have double the risk of myocardial infarction (MI)

A review of current data in *Drugs and Therapeutics Bulletin* in 2005 found little evidence to support the use of COX-2 inhibitors as first-line treatment. A meta-analysis published in the *BMJ* in 2006 found a doubling of risk of MI in people taking COX-2s and also in people on high-dose ibuprofen and diclofenac. A paper in *Heart* in 2006 found a 30% increase in risk of admission with heart failure after NSAID use. Topical NSAIDs have been shown to be effective at 2 weeks and topical diclofenac might be effective in the longer term (*BMJ* 2004). Misoprostol has been shown to be effective in preventing gastrointestinal bleeds but a report in the *BMJ* in 2006 suggested that H2-receptor antagonists and proton-pump inhibitors are not effective.

PAPER 3

46. F: Reflex anoxic seizure

Reflex anoxic seizure usually needs explanation and reassurance only. The child usually grows out of the condition. If there are any unusual features referral may be necessary.

47. A: Febrile seizure

Febrile seizures are common between 6 months and 5 years, affecting 4% of children; 30% of sufferers have another convulsion but only 1% go on to develop epilepsy. First episodes should be admitted to exclude meningitis. Parents should be advised how to manage seizures.

48. D: Petit mal epilepsy

Petit mal epilepsy can be precipitated by hyperventilation. It has a good prognosis.

49. C: Jacksonian seizure

Jacksonian seizures start as focal seizures, which may spread to become generalised.

50. E: Pseudoseizure

Pseudoseizures do not have the usual features of epilepsy such as post-ictal confusion and drowsiness or incontinence. There is often secondary gain.

51. F: All of the above

Infection in men may produce any of these symptoms, which are often transient and mild and contribute to the high prevalence rates in the community. In women cervicitis and pelvic inflammatory disease are seen, in addition to urethritis and arthritis.

PAPER 3

52.   F: Rhinorrhoea

Cholesteatoma may cause local symptoms, most commonly smelly otorrhoea and transient dizziness, but may also cause tinnitus and deafness as a result of ossicular disruption and toxin damage to the acoustic nerve. Spread into the middle-ear cleft may damage the facial nerve or cause brain abscess.

53.   B: MARIBS trial

The MARIBS trial found that MRI detected 77% of cancers found whereas mammography detected only 40%. Mammography was slightly more specific, however.

54.   D: Women's Health Initiative

There was an increase in biopsy rate but no increase in cancer diagnosis over a 7-year follow-up.

55.   C: Million Women Study

A 64% increase in false-positive mammography results has been reported in present and past HRT users.

56.   A: Malmö Mammographic Screening Trial

Some 15 years after the trial ended it has been estimated that 10% of cancers diagnosed would never have presented clinically.

57.   C: Million Women Study

These influences, but not the contraceptive pill, increased mammographic density.

PAPER 3

58.   **A: Coarctation of the aorta**

Coarctation usually presents between day 2 and day 6 with symptoms of heart failure as the ductus arteriosus closes. Femoral pulses may not be felt and there is usually a systolic murmur. The patient should be admitted for definitive treatment.

59.   **A: Constipation in children may be a sign of systemic disease**

Hypothyroidism, polyuria and prune-belly syndrome may all cause constipation. Hirschsprung's disease may present in older children if there is a small segment affected. Enemas often cause emotional and physical trauma and the child should be admitted if this is considered necessary. Stimulant laxatives may be needed long term; the first-line treatment should, however, be increased fibre and lactulose.

60.   **E: As long as seizures are controlled he will be able to drive when he reaches the appropriate age**

Driving is not affected if epilepsy is controlled for group 1 entitlement and for group 2 if the person has been seizure free and off medication for at least 10 years. Sixty per cent of cases are idiopathic. Other causes include structural, metabolic and infective origins. Seventy per cent of patients are successfully controlled with drugs, of whom 50% can eventually stop their medication. The risk of epilepsy in the offspring of an affected parent is about 3%. The risk of congenital abnormalities in children whose mothers have epilepsy is 2.5–7.5%.

PAPER 3

61. **E:** **Patients with corneal abrasion should be given topical anaesthesia to use until the abrasion heals**

Topical anaesthesia should never be given to patients to use after discharge because of risk of further trauma to an anaesthetised eye. Exudative macular degeneration may be suitable for treatment with photodynamic therapy. These patients are, however, a minority. Up to 2% of the adult population have raised IOP without signs of glaucoma. These require surveillance but no medication. Latanoprost eye drops also cause eyelashes to grow, which may result in significant asymmetry if used on only one side.

62. **A:** **It always has an organic basis**

Failure to thrive may be a sign of problems in the maternal relationship. This can be identified by admitting to hospital and monitoring weight gain and calorie intake. Neonatal hyperthyroidism is usually a result of transplacental transfer of thyroid stimulating antibodies. It is therefore usually transient but where it persists may cause failure to thrive. Any chronic infection can cause failure to thrive and a urinary tract infection should always be excluded.

63. **C:** **It affects up to 2% of the population**

Glaucoma is usually painless but does cause deterioration in visual fields, affecting peripheral sensitivity and progressing to tunnel vision. Up to 2% of adults have an IOP > 21 mmHg without signs of glaucoma. They require lifelong follow-up. Congenital glaucoma must be recognised early to prevent irreversible damage. Treatment of all types of glaucoma aims to prevent further damage, not reverse existing damage.

64.   B: The patient is suffering from pseudogout

This is a typical history of pseudogout. In an acute monoarthritis affecting a large joint, microscopy of the effusion will differentiate infection, bleeding and crystal arthopathy with urate or calcium pyrophosphate crystals. Radiographs rarely aid diagnosis, but in pseudogout may show chondrocalcinosis.

65.   B: Sickle cell crises may be precipitated by infection

Heterozygous patients are carriers and are usually asymptomatic; homozygotes have severe haemolytic anaemia and frequent crises. Folic acid 5 mg a day should be given to sickle cell patients. Pregnancy, and in particular delivery, are especially hazardous.

66.   E: Excision

This is a pterygium. It has grown across the limbus onto the cornea and is obstructing vision. Betnesol is a treatment for iritis or severe episcleritis, ketorolac a treatment for mild episcleritis or inflamed pingueculae and aciclovir a treatment for dendritic ulcers.

67.   A: Fluconazole

Fluconazole has caused multiple malformations in animal studies.

68.   E: Non-steroidal agents are often effective during exacerbations of pain

She has endometriosis and early referral for laparoscopy is essential to maximise her chances of conception. Medical and surgical therapies have been shown to improve fertility. There is often a psychological element but this is always secondary to the endometriosis, and education and support for the patient and her partner will often help in this regard.

PAPER 3

69.   D: Metrorrhagia

Metrorrhagia is usually seen in perimenopausal women. Treatment is aimed at the underlying cause.

70.   C: Menorrhagia

Tranexamic acid is the most effective first-line treatment for menorrhagia.

71.   E: Primary amenorrhoea

Primary amenorrhoea may be a sign of gonadal dysgenesis or genetic abnormality. Causes also include imperforate hymen and transverse vaginal septum, but this is actually cryptomenorrhoea because menstruation is taking place proximal to the obstruction.

72.   F: Secondary amenorrhoea

Other common causes of secondary amenorrhoea include polycystic ovaries, hyperprolactinaemia and hypothyroidism.

73.   B: Intermenstrual bleeding

Switching to a triphasic pill will often help.

74.   B: Expert patient programmes have been shown to reduce medication use

Expert patients are more likely than other patients to make effective use of available health services The DAFNE study brought about significant reductions in blood glucose levels. All of the pilot projects so far have shown objective and subjective benefits.

75.   D: Data that fall under the auspices of the Data Protection Act are exempt

Commercially sensitive information and personal information are exempt, because they are covered by the Data Protection Act. Practices have 20 working days in which to respond. They cannot refuse a request on grounds of motive.

76.   I: Smoking cessation

Smoking cessation is essential in all patients if their decline in forced expiratory volume in 1 second is to be slowed.

77.   B: Domiciliary oxygen

Long-term oxygen therapy is indicated in patients with a $Pao_2 < 7.3$ kPa on two separate occasions or with complications, eg polycythaemia. It must be used for at least 15 hours a day.

78.   A: Carbocysteine

Mucolytics should be trialled for 4 weeks and discontinued if there is no benefit. They may cause gastrointestinal bleeds.

79.   F: Oral steroids

Mild-to-moderate obstruction may be caused by asthma so a trial of high-dose inhaled steroids or oral steroids is recommended.

80.   D: Long-acting antimuscarinic bronchodilator

Tiotropium or alternatively a long-acting, inhaled β_2 agonist is indicated in this group.

PAPER 3

81.   **A:**   **Atrial fibrillation**

82.   **C:**   **Complete heart block**

83.   **K:**   **Wolff–Parkinson–White syndrome**

84.   **F:**   **Sinus arrhythmia**

85.   **I:**   **Ventricular ectopics**

86.   **C:**   **Calcium/vitamin D_3**

Unless clinicians are positive oral intake is adequate.

87.   **I:**   **Strontium**

Strontium rather than raloxifene is recommended in this situation.

88.   **L:**   **Vitamin D**

Vitamin D, but not calcium, has been shown to reduce fracture rate. Calcium alone increases bone mineral density but does not reduce fractures.

89.   **L:**   **Vitamin D**

A meta-analysis in the *Journal of American Medical Association* in 2004 confirmed this finding, thought to be caused by enhanced muscle function.

90.   A: Bisphosphonates

Bisphosphonates tend to be well tolerated. The effect wanes with time after discontinuation.

91.   C: ACE inhibitors are first-line treatment for heart failure with evidence of left ventricular systolic dysfunction

β Blockers should be added in to patients already on ACE inhibitors but should be considered for all patients. Functional status should be monitored for all patients.

92.   D: Hospice nurses provide counselling services for patients and families

Hospice nurses provide a supportive role rather than hands-on nursing. The Macmillan charity may fund night sitters in some cases.

93.   D: Weight loss of 1 kg will reduce blood pressure by 1–2 mmHg

There is a linear relationship between obesity and blood pressure. Drinking more than 3 units a day increases the prevalence of blood pressure threefold. A meta-analysis of the effect of exercise found a statistically significant effect on BP with even low intensity exercise. Increasing dietary fibre is helpful in patients who have a very-low-fibre diet.

94.   E: FSH and testosterone levels

This clinical presentation suggests hypogonadism. Oligospermia is a consequence of hypogonadism. The investigations should be aimed at determining whether hypogonadism exists and whether it is primary or secondary. Where radiological investigations are used, CT is usually more appropriate. Depression screening is useful in erectile dysfunction but this patient has signs of hormonal deficiency.

95.   B: Motor neurone disease

Motor neurone disease often presents with fairly minor symptoms, often in the hands. There are no sensory symptoms and the eyes are never affected. A mixture of upper and motor neurone signs are seen and 25% of patients have bulbar signs.

96.   E: CRP and ESR

In the acute phase of a joint swelling the most appropriate tests are measurement of CRP and ESR, which would point to an inflammatory arthritis and allow monitoring of response. A plain radiograph may be useful if there is diagnostic doubt or osteomyelitis is suspected. Autoantibodies are often misleading and seldom add anything useful to the management at this time. HLA-B27 may be appropriate in Reiter syndrome or ankylosing spondylitis, but these do not usually present in this way. IgE levels are used in allergic disease.

97.   B: Claim dispensing fee

Most injections can be purchased by the practice and a dispensing fee claimed.

98.   F: Issue prescription on FP10 for the named patient

99.   A: Claim cost of drug back from the Department of Health

It is illegal to restock a doctor's bag with a prescription for a named patient. The cost can be claimed back from the Department of Health, but most practitioners feel that the effort is not worth the refund.

100.   G: Write a prescription for pharmacist to dispense before starting treatment

101. C: Claim an item of service fee

Immunisations are covered by the appropriate item of service fee. Most practices also negotiate bulk discounts and make considerable profit on these.

102. E: This is a superficial infection and should be treated with anti-staphylococcal antibiotics

A chalazion is in the eyelid, rather than the eyebrow. Chloramphenicol will treat local eye infections such as conjunctivitis. A BCC has a central ulcer with surrounding pearly telangiectatic border. Periorbital cellulitis originates from the sinuses in most cases but causes a diffuse cellulitis with later proptosis and loss of colour vision.

103. D: PCTs have a final say in deciding whether a candidate is sufficiently qualified

Individuals and their trusts decide the level of pay in an area. Most indemnity policies will cover GPwSI work but candidates should check before starting work. GpwSI work lies wholly outside the GMS Contract, but funding might be available through practice-based commissioning. A paper looking at dermatology clinics found no cost savings but that the service was popular with patients.

104. B: The presence of blood on aspiration requires referral to exclude intra-articular fracture

Haemarthrosis is often seen in patients with haemophilia but it would be unusual to present for the first time at this age. Haemarthrosis after trauma can be associated with ligamentous injury or fracture. A removable splint is helpful and passive exercises should start after 48 hours. There is no consensus on joint aspiration.

PAPER 3

105.   A: Topical HRT is more effective than systemic HRT for the prevention of recurrent UTIs

The Million Women Study provided extensive evidence of risks associated with HRT. Use of combined HRT increases the risk of ovarian cancer by 1 in 2500 users. After 5 years of HRT use there was an absolute increase of 1% in the incidence of breast cancer, giving an NNH of 100. The increase in relative risk of thromboembolism is 300–400%, but the absolute risk was less than 1% after 5 years of use. Use of combined HRT increases the risk of ischaemic stroke by 1%, an NNH of 100. It does not increase the risk of haemorrhagic stroke. Meta-analysis of 22 trials found no evidence of weight gain. Use of unopposed oestrogen can cause endometrial cancer.

106.   D: Women are less likely to be reported to the NCAA than men

The NCAA was originally set up to include doctors only but since 2003 has covered salaried dentists as well. The NCAA is an educational body that sets out to improve standards of performance in the NHS. The average assessment period is 24 weeks. Non-white doctors, but not non-white dentists, are over-represented.

107.   C: He should be given aspirin and admitted under the medical take

The ECG shows an inferior MI. This can be a difficult diagnosis and is often misinterpreted as indigestion by patient and doctor alike.

108.   A: Topical non-steroidal preparations are effective in relieving pain

An article in the *BMJ* in 2004 summarised the evidence for managing osteoarthritis. Taping is effective in the short term and both physical training and endurance training are helpful. Steroid injections are effective, with an odds ratio of 1.6 compared with placebo. Glucosamine reduces the radiological rate of joint-space loss compared with placebo.

109.   C: All patients should have their urine tested

Nocturnal enuresis is more common in boys and may persist to adulthood. All patients should be assessed to exclude chronic renal impairment, diabetes mellitus and diabetes insipidus. Desmopressin may be useful for short-term use but is not considered safe long term. Imipramine provides short-term benefit but relapse is common and the side-effect profile is unfavourable for long-term use in children.

110.   C: Non-specific urethritis

Chronic prostatitis usually causes perineal pain. Gonorrhoea causes a thick mucoid discharge that is often evident on examination. A UTI would be evident on culture of a midstream urine (MSU). Balanitis xerotica et obliterans causes chronic thickening and depigmentation of the glans.

111.   D: Of the over-65 age group, 30% will fall in any given year

Hip protectors are effective but compliance is poor. Sedatives are more likely to cause harm than good by a factor of 2. There are over 6 million informal carers in the UK often providing more than 50 hours of care a week. Cholinesterase inhibitors are only weakly effective in slowing progression of dementia.

112.   D: Chronic paroxysmal hemicrania

This can be treated with prophylactic NSAIDs. It may be confused with cluster headaches, but these are more migrainous and often associated with other signs, eg watering of the eye.

113.   A: Analgesic overuse headache

Analgesic overuse headache is found in patients taking analgesics on more than 15 days per month for at least 3 months. It responds to withdrawal but may take some weeks.

PAPER 3

114.   E: Cluster headache

These may be treated acutely with triptans or ergotamine. Prophylaxis with lithium or verapamil may be effective.

115.   H: Severe headache of sudden onset

Patients with sudden-onset severe headache should be considered for admission to rule out subarachnoid haemorrhage.

116.   B: Carbon monoxide poisoning

Carbon monoxide poisoning should be considered in patients with unexplained headache. The condition may be fatal, but usually responds well to hyperbaric oxygen.

117.   D: HOT trial

118.   A: ASCOT

119.   C: BHS guidelines for hypertension management

120.   F: NICE guidelines for hypertension management

121.   G: SCOPE

122.   C: BHS guidelines for hypertension management

123.   B: Of patients with peanut allergy 50% are allergic to other nuts

The prevalence of nut allergy has been estimated at 0.3–7.5%. Almonds are the most frequently cross-reacting nut. Skin-prick testing is positive in 50–70% of those with confirmed nut allergy and are useful in excluding allergy, but less so in confirming it. The RAST (radioallergosorbent test) is less sensitive. There are no proven treatments other than avoidance and use of an EpiPen for severe reactions.

124.   D: Regular analgesics and rest are the most effective initial treatment

Acute otitis media may be viral or bacterial. The mainstay of treatment is analgesia rest and fluids. Studies have shown that antibiotics may be safely deferred at the initial consultation as long as there are no systemic signs, with instructions to return if symptoms fail to settle. Ciprofloxacin is contraindicated in children. Amoxicillin or erythromycin is the most appropriate antibiotic in most patients. Decongestants have no role in treating otitis media. Forty per cent of patients develop a middle-ear effusion, but in only 10% does this persist > 3 months.

125.   C: Acne rosacea

Acne rosacea is a common inflammatory condition that is often associated with facial flushing and secondary eye involvement. The pustules and papules distinguish it from dermatitis and SLE. Treatment usually involves prolonged treatment with tetracyclines.

126.   C: It may indicate a cleft palate

A bifid uvula may be a sign of a submucosal cleft palate. This is particularly relevant if adenoidectomy is contemplated because adenoidal overgrowth may compensate for a cleft palate, and adenoid removal therefore results in nasal escape.

PAPER 3

127.   D: A normal D-dimer excludes thromboembolism with 95% sensitivity

D-dimer is sensitive but not specific. A mild neutrophilia and fever are common in pulmonary embolism (PE), as are signs of right heart strain on ECG. Massive PE causes the S1 Q3 T3 pattern of changes. PE should be suspected in sudden-onset breathlessness, shock and cardiac arrest.

128.   C: Refer under the 2-week rule to gynaecology

Postmenopausal bleeding should be assumed to be cancer until proved otherwise. It is associated with diabetes and should be referred under the 2-week rule.

129.   B: Gastro-oesophageal reflux can cause these symptoms

These symptoms are classically attributed to pyloric stenosis but the differential diagnosis includes reflux, overfeeding and sepsis. A child who is off feeds and lethargic should be investigated for sepsis. The child with pyloric stenosis or reflux is usually well. New parents often report projectile vomiting but pathology is seldom found.

130.   A: Acute pancreatitis

Abdominal aortic aneurysm usually presents with pain and shock without vomiting; a pulsatile mass is felt in the abdomen. Chronic pancreatitis usually causes chronic pain and vomiting.

131.   E: Evening primrose oil

There is no strong evidence of anything other than placebo benefit for evening primrose oil. Goserelin is effective but the side-effects outweigh the benefits. Selective serotonin release inhibitors (SSRIs) are the most effective treatment for mood problems, although spironolactone helps with bloating.

132.   C: Overflow incontinence

Diabetic neuropathy may cause retention with overflow.

133.   H: Vesicocolic fistula

Bubbles of air or faecal matter is usually a sign of a fistula between the bladder and bowel. Other causes include carcinoma and radiotherapy.

134.   F: Urge incontinence

Urge incontinence is often made worse by a coexistent urinary tract infection (UTI) and may be treated with anticholinergics or bladder training.

135.   D: Stress incontinence

Genuine stress incontinence can be treated with support, eg ring pessaries where there is significant prolapse. Where this fails surgery should be considered.

136.   G: UTI

Children who develop nocturnal enuresis or incontinence should have a UTI excluded.

137.   D: Developmental aphasia

Developmental aphasia can affect the ability to find, understand and express words. Patients will often say that they know the word but cannot remember it.

138.   F: Dyspraxia

Dyspraxia usually causes problems with fine motor and gross motor skills.

139.   B: Autism

Autism represents a spectrum of disorders but all patients seem to have a lack of engagement with the environment and other people.

140.   F: Dyspraxia

There is a considerable overlap of dyslexia, dyspraxia and ADHD.

141.   C: Cerebral palsy

Cerebral palsy is broadly classified as spastic, athetoid or ataxic.

142.   A: Vasculitis

This photograph shows a vasculitic rash of the digits, which suggests small vessel disease; with a history of arthritis it suggests connective disease, eg SLE. Giant cell arteritis affects large vessels, eg temporal arteritis.

143.   E: Herpes zoster

This is a typical description of erythema multiforme and may be associated with genital and mouth ulcers with fever in Stevens–Johnson syndrome. Other causes include drugs, infection, vitamin deficiency, pregnancy and inflammatory bowel disease.

144.   A: The patient should receive a letter explaining the action that is being taken

Every year, 75 000 patients are removed from GP lists in England. Removal takes place 8 days after a letter has been sent to the PCT. Only 2% of removals were for violence or aggression. It might be appropriate to remove other members of the household, such as where they require home visits and a violent family member lives in the home, but this is seldom necessary. The letter to the patient does not need to be explicit if this is not appropriate; instead, it can cite an irretrievable breakdown in the doctor–patient relationship.

145.   A: Acute retention may result from constipation

Urinary retention may be acute or chronic. Acute retention is usually painful and may be precipitated by a UTI or constipation. Obstruction may also be caused by clot or stones obstructing the bladder outlet or urethra. It may also be seen in a retroverted uterus, cystocele or genital herpes.

146.   D: Hyperparathyroidism

Rickets may be caused by inadequate intake of sunlight, vitamin D and fat, eg in coeliac disease, inadequate metabolism, eg induction of hepatic enzymes by anticonvulsants, or end-organ resistance. Hypoparathyroidism causes rickets, and nephrotic syndrome causes loss of vitamin D-binding protein.

147.   E: Scabies

Scabies is caused by *Sarcoptes scabei*, a mite that causes irritation as it burrows under the skin. It is acquired through person-to-person contact and can live off the host for only up to 36 hours. It causes intense itching and this may persist for 2–3 weeks after treatment, because the hypersensitivity to the mites and their allergens continues.

148.   F: Private work

Insurance medicals are not covered by the GMS contract and are paid for by the insurer.

149.   C: Local enhanced services

Local enhanced services are designed to address local needs and are negotiated by individual PCTs and their practices.

150.   F: Private work

151.   E: Non-GMS NHS work

Community hospital contracts are not covered by the GMS contract and are negotiated locally between GPs and PCTs, often on a price per day scheme.

152.   B: Global sum

Previous allowances were rolled up into the global sum.

153.   A: Direct enhanced services (DESs)

Goserelin (Zoladex) injections and immunosuppressant drugs are covered by DESs.

154.   G: Quality and Outcomes Framework (QOF)

The QOF scheme is voluntary, although virtually every practice in the country has signed up.

155.   E: *Pseudomonas aeruginosa*

Pseudomonas is common in patients with bronchiectasis or cystic fibrosis.

156.   D: Norwalk virus

The Norwalk virus is highly infectious with an incubation period of 48 hours. Large outbreaks have occurred on cruise ships.

157.   G: *Staphylococcus epidermidis*

Coagulase-negative staphylococci are rarely harmful.

158.   H: Vancomycin-resistant enterococci (VREs)

VREs are thought to have arisen as a result of feeding vancomycin-related antibiotics to livestock to increase meat yield.

159.   C: MRSA

MRSA is increasingly sensitive to co-trimoxazole (Septrin) and other older antibiotics.

160.   A: Tuberculosis (TB)

Pulmonary TB is increasingly common in migrant and homeless individuals. It typically affects the lungs but may affect virtually any organ. Migrant individuals should be screened at port of entry, but illegal immigrants often slip through the net. The disease may be asymptomatic and a high index of suspicion is necessary in patients with any chronic respiratory or systemic symptoms.

PAPER 3

161.   A: Ulcerative colitis

Crohn's disease often presents in a similar way but usually has signs of inflammation elsewhere, eg perianal sepsis and right iliac fossa signs. Diverticulitis affects older patients.

162.   I: Subchondral haematoma

A subchondral haematoma should be drained promptly to prevent avascular necrosis and the development of a cauliflower ear.

163.   D: Ear wax

When completely occluding the external auditory meatus, wax may cause deafness and tinnitus.

164.   G: Foreign body

Children often put beads or food in their ears. This may initially go unnoticed but eventually results in a purulent discharge.

165.   F: Furunculosis

Furunculosis is often extremely tender at the point of maximal inflammation, with pain reproduced by moving the tragus. Deafness is rare.

166.   C: Chondrodermatitis nodularis helices

Chondrodermatitis nodularis causes tenderness over the helix in men and antihelix in women. BCCs tend to be painless.

167. A: Mild asthma brought on by exertion only

Asthma, particularly brought on by exertion, is a contraindication to diving. Referral to a diving physician is warranted, however, to carry out exercise spirometry because many patients are misdiagnosed or grow out of their asthma. Guidelines on exclusions from diving can be found at www.uksdmc.co.uk. A history of spontaneous pneumothorax is a contraindication because of the risk of asymptomatic pleural blebs.

168. C: She should be referred under the 2-week rule

This presentation is typical of thyroid cancer and should be referred under the 2-week rule. Associated signs include lymphadenopathy, stridor, hoarseness and dysphagia.

169. I: Moclobemide

Monoamine oxidase inhibitors (MAOIs) react with tyramine in the diet, methyldopa and cold remedies. They should not be used together with tricyclic depressants and at least 2 weeks should pass between use of an MAOI and a tricyclic depressant.

170. K: Risperidone

Haloperidol is the drug of choice for agitation in elderly people.

171. D: Dothiepin

Tricyclic depressants increase IOP and should be used with caution in these patients.

172. L: Venlafaxine

Venlafaxine may prolong the QT interval.

173. G: Lithium

Reduction in renal function may cause lithium toxicity and these patients should have regular measurement of lithium levels and renal function.

174. E: Vitreous haemorrhage

This is a typical description of vitreous haemorrhage. The blood is often seen as a cloud in the vitreous and may be an early sign of retinal detachment. It is most commonly seen in patients with diabetic retinopathy.

175. D: Nephritic syndrome

This is caused by acute glomerular inflammation.

176. E: Nephrotic syndrome

The predominant feature of nephrotic syndrome is protein loss and hypoalbuminaemia is common.

177. F: Polycystic kidney disease

Adult polycystic kidney disease is inherited as an autosomal dominant trait. Infantile polycystic kidney disease is recessive.

178. B: Goodpasture syndrome

This is a vasculitis characterised by anti-glomerular basement membrane antibodies.

179. G: Renal osteodystrophy

Renal osteodystrophy is seen in patients with renal failure and may be a result of aluminium poisoning.

180.   C: The stages of change theory applies only to patients with no organic injury

Once a patient has successfully been in the action phase for 6 months, they move into the maintenance phase. The process through these stages is often a spiral or rebound process. Action involves behavioural and environmental changes, such as the avoidanace of provoking situations (eg parties where drugs are available).

181.   C: Wax impaction may be the result of hearing aid use

Wax is found in two forms: wet wax in white people and those of African origin and dry wax in Chinese people. As patients age, wax becomes dryer and harder to shed naturally. Anything that upsets normal wax transport may cause impaction, from thick hairs to hearing aid moulds. It may cause a feeling of obstruction, deafness or cough. Hopi candles may cause burns. Patients with recurrent otitis externa or perforations should not be syringed.

182.   B: Basal cell carcinoma

BCCs are slow growing and locally invasive.

183.   J: Squamous cell carcinoma

Rapidly growing lesions with these features are often SCCs and should be referred under the 2-week rule.

184.   I: Pyogenic granuloma

Pyogenic granulomas may have central ulceration and may need biopsy to be distinguished from SCCs.

185.   H: Neurofibroma

Neurofibromas usually run in families and present as rubbery lesions all over the body.

PAPER 3

186.   J: Squamous cell carcinoma

Studies suggest that recurrence of SCCs may be reduced by use of sunscreen. BCCs, however, do not show this characteristic.

187.   E: Hypopituitarism

A low TSH in hypothyroidism suggests that hypopituitarism may be the cause.

188.   F: Sick euthyroidism

Low T_3 (triiodothyronine) with normal TSH and T_4 (thyroxine) is sometimes seen in intercurrent illness or with certain medications, eg amiodarone.

189.   H: Subclinical hypothyroidism

Raised TSH with normal T_4 and T_3 results from subclinical hypothyroidism. If thyroid antibodies are present, 5% will become hypothyroid each year.

190.   C: Hyperthyroidism

Hyperthyroidism should be diagnosed only if T_4 is raised; low TSH alone can result from intercurrent illness.

191.   D: Hypothyroidism

192.   C: Wilms' tumour

Wilms' tumour accounts for 50% of tumours in infants. It may present with abdominal pain, a mass or haematuria. Hepatoblastoma is right sided. Splenomegaly would not normally be associated with haematuria. The prognosis is generally good with a 80% 5-year survival rate for stage 1 tumours.

193.   A: BCG immunisation is no longer routinely given to children born in the UK

BCG immunisation is now given to infants only in communities with an incidence of TB > 1/2500. A paper in the *New England Journal of Medicine* in 2005 showed a 51% reduction in incidence of zoster and a 67% reduction in neuralgia when varicella vaccine was given to those aged over 60. Hepatitis B immunisation is only given to at-risk infants. Polio is now given as an inactive vaccine rather than live. The increase in mumps in university students is a result of their not receiving the vaccine because they are too old but not having caught mumps naturally.

194.   D: Candidiasis

Candidiasis may be recurrent and if this is the case diabetes should be excluded.

195.   E: Endometritis

Endometritis can occur in patients after a miscarriage, termination or post partum.

196.   G: Physiological

Physiological discharge may increase during pregnancy, at certain stages of the cycle and during sexual arousal.

197.   B: Bacterial vaginosis

Bacterial vaginosis has a characteristic smell but may be symptomless. It can be treated with clindamycin or metronidazole.

198.   A: Atrophic vaginitis

Atrophic vaginitis can be treated with topical HRT or lubrication.

199.   C: The 95% CIs for the meta-analysis cross the line of no effect

The diamond represents the pooled studies. The borders of the diamond represent the 95% confidence intervals. An odds ratio of 3 suggests that the event is three times more likely.

200.   C: The drop-off in benefit with increased exercise might be a result of patient drop-out, eg resulting from injury

These data relate to a fall in resting pulse with participation in exercise programmes. Resting pulse rate is a valid surrogate marker for fitness, but not for weight loss. Increasing fitness can lead to weight loss if combined with dietary change, but alone it has not been shown to lead to weight reduction in moderate exercise – appropriate data for this discussion would measure weight loss with participation in an exercise programme.

Paper 4
Questions

Total time allowed is three hours. Indicate your answers clearly by putting a tick or cross in the box alongside each answer or by writing the appropriate letter alongside the appropriate answer.

1. **A 23-year-old woman returns from a season as a holiday rep in Greece and is horrified to discover that she has perineal warts. Which of the following statements is true about this condition? Select one option only.**

   ☐ A   Carriers are always symptomatic

   ☐ B   Perianal warts are always associated with anal intercourse

   ☐ C   Warts usually improve during pregnancy

   ☐ D   Vaginal warts in pregnancy are an indication for caesarean section to prevent transmission to the baby

   ☐ E   Condom use may reduce the risk of transmission

2. **A 74-year-old man with diabetes mentions at his diabetic annual review that he has been getting increasing pain in his calves on walking over the last 6 months, such that he can now only walk 50 metres without stopping. On examination he has poor peripheral pulses and sluggish capillary return. You refer him to a vascular surgeon but in the meantime decide to treat him medically to try to improve his quality of life. Which of the following statements about management is NOT true? Select one option only.**

   ☐ A   Ramipril may improve walking distance

   ☐ B   Phosphodiesterase inhibitors are licensed for use in mild-to-moderate claudication

   ☐ C   Warfarin will prevent thrombotic occlusion of stenotic arteries

   ☐ D   People with diabetes should aim for an HbA1c < 6.5%

   ☐ E   Smoking cessation is the single biggest modifiable risk factor

PAPER 4

THEME: ABDOMINAL PAIN IN CHILDHOOD

Options

A   Acute appendicitis

B   Constipation

C   Diabetic ketoacidosis

D   Henoch–Schönlein purpura

E   Hydronephrosis

F   Infantile colic

G   Inguinal hernia

H   Intussusception

I   Meckel's diverticulum

J   Mesenteric adenitis

K   Otitis media

L   Pneumonia

M   Testicular torsion

N   Torsion of testicular appendage

PAPER 4

For each of the descriptions below, select the most likely diagnosis from the list of options. Each option may be used once, more than once or not at all.

☐ 3.   A 7-month-old child with paroxysmal colicky pain and pallor. During attacks he draws his legs up and has vomiting and diarrhoea. On examination the abdomen is distended. His nappy has blood-stained mucus.

☐ 4.   A 9-year-old boy complains of 2 days of abdominal pain that is aggravated by movement, increasing in severity and accompanied by a low-grade fever. On examination there is tenderness in the right iliac fossa.

☐ 5.   A 3-week-old baby with recurrent episodes of paroxysmal screaming accompanied by drawing up of the knees. The attacks occur in the evening and last 2–3 hours. The child is otherwise well.

6. A normally fit and well 12-month-old child presents with rectal bleeding.

7. A 7-year-old girl presents with abdominal pain, fever and shortness of breath. Examination of her abdomen reveals generalised abdominal tenderness but no peritonism.

8. A 6-year-old girl with 3 days of abdominal pain, a rash on her buttocks and arthralgia. Examination reveals microscopic haematuria.

9. A 13-year-old boy presents with a 3-week history of malaise, abdominal pain, weight loss, frequency of urination and thirst. He has generalised abdominal tenderness.

10. A 12-year-old boy complains of increasing abdominal pain over several days. On examination he has a swollen tender scrotum.

11. A 73-year-old woman in a nursing home. who has recently been treated with amoxicillin for an upper respiratory tract infection, develops fever, profuse watery diarrhoea and dehydration. Which of the following statements about management is NOT true? Select one option only.

A Her amoxicillin should be changed to ciprofloxacin

B She should be moved to a single room

C She should have a stool specimen sent for culture

D She should be treated with vancomycin

E She should be barrier nursed

12. You are playing squash with your 55-year-old senior partner when he screams out and collapses to the floor clutching his left ankle. After some minutes he is able to stand but cannot easily move his foot. Which one of the following statements about his injury is true?

- [ ] A Achilles tendonitis usually presents in this way
- [ ] B A partial tear will usually show no signs on examination other than tenderness and a swelling in the mid-tendon
- [ ] C Fusiform swelling in the midpoint of the tendon together with foot movement on squeezing the calf suggest Achilles tendonitis
- [ ] D Complete ruptures should always be treated surgically
- [ ] E Partial tears should always be treated because of the risk of developing a full tear

13. A 19-year-old student presents with cold fingers and toes. She tells you that every time she gets cold her fingers go white, then purple and then return to normal. She is otherwise well and takes no regular medication. Which of the following statements about this condition is true? Select one option only.

- [ ] A All cases should be referred to exclude significant pathology
- [ ] B It is a contraindication to the combined oral contraceptive pill
- [ ] C It is more common in men
- [ ] D Is usually caused by cryoglobulins precipitating at low temperatures
- [ ] E It may be associated with oesophageal disease

14. Which of the following statements about dry eyes is true? Select one option only.

- [ ] A Stenger's test involves placing blotting paper between the lower lid and the eyeball to measure objectively the quantity of tears produced
- [ ] B It is usually a result of nasolacrimal obstruction
- [ ] C It is usually aggravated by cold air
- [ ] D It can be effectively treated with topical antibiotics
- [ ] E It may be associated with autoimmune disease

15. A newly wed couple attend for preconceptual advice. The husband had a brother who died from cystic fibrosis and they are concerned that they may have an affected child. Which of the following statements about their risks of passing cystic fibrosis on to their children is true? Select one option only.

- [ ] A If they are both carriers they have a 50% risk of having an affected child
- [ ] B If he is not a carrier they have a 0% risk of passing on the gene to their offspring
- [ ] C If he is a carrier and she is not there is a 50% risk of offspring being carriers
- [ ] D As long as she is not a carrier there is no risk of the gene being passed on to their offspring
- [ ] E Cystic fibrosis is inherited as an autosomal dominant trait

16. A 2-year-old girl is brought to the GP out-of-hours centre suffering from croup. She is febrile, has a respiratory rate of 24 and a croupy cough. There is no intercostal recession. Which of the following is the most appropriate treatment for her? Select one answer only.

☐ A   Inhaling humidified air

☐ B   Intramuscular hydrocortisone

☐ C   Nebulised salbutamol

☐ D   Nebulised epinephrine (adrenaline)

☐ E   Oral dexamethasone

17. A 67-year-old man presents complaining of general malaise and unilateral reduced vision. Fundoscopy shows the appearance below. What is the diagnosis?

☐ A   Age-related macular degeneration

☐ B   Retinal detachment

☐ C   Retinal vein thrombosis

☐ D   Ischaemic optic neuropathy

☐ E   Vitreous haemorrhage

18. A 57-year-old man who is a smoker presents with increasing shortness of breath over 4 weeks. On examination he has reduced air entry at the left base, with dullness to percussion and bronchial breathing heard above the area. You diagnose a pleural effusion. Which of the following statements about pleural effusion is NOT true? Select one option only.

☐ A Pleural effusions are always visible on chest radiograph

☐ B Unilateral pleural effusion may be an early sign of heart failure

☐ C It may result from ascites

☐ D It may result from liver disease

☐ E It may result from infection

19. A 37-year-old new mother has come to discuss the diagnosis of Down syndrome in her newborn son. She is particularly concerned about implications for future children. Which of the following statements about Down syndrome is true? Select one option only.

☐ A Most Down syndrome infants are born to women over the age of 35

☐ B Down syndrome is an autosomal dominant trait

☐ C Of children with Down syndrome 99% survive to adulthood

☐ D Where only one parent carries a translocation, the recurrence risk is < 1/1000

☐ E None of the above

☐ F All of the above

20. You are asked to give a short talk to the local Women's Institute on the prevention of stroke and healthy living. Which of the following statements about risk factors for stroke is NOT true? Select one option only.

☐ A High-fat diet is a major modifiable risk factor for stroke

☐ B High blood pressure doubles the risk of stroke in women and quadruples the risk in men

☐ C Reducing dietary salt will decrease blood pressure and increase efficacy of antihypertensives

☐ D Smoking is the single biggest risk factor for stroke

☐ E Alcohol consumption is a risk factor only when the weekly consumption exceeds 50 units in men and 42 units in women

21. On a Monday morning you see a 21-year-old man who has a broken nose from a fight the previous Saturday night. Which of the following statements is true about the management of a fractured nose? Select one option only.

☐ A The patient should be referred immediately to the on-call ENT team for manipulation under anaesthetic

☐ B Clear rhinorrhoea is common and of no consequence

☐ C As a result of soft tissue swelling, radiological imaging is essential in confirming the diagnosis

☐ D Septal haematomas are common and usually resolve spontaneously

☐ E Manipulation under anaesthetic is best performed 5–7 days after injury

THEME: PAINFUL LEGS

Options

A   Cellulitis

B   Chronic venous insufficiency

C   Deep vein thrombosis

D   Gout

E   Intermittent claudication

F   Lymphoedema

G   Raynaud's phenomenon

H   Ruptured Baker's cyst

I   Superficial thrombophlebitis

J   Thrombophlebitis obliterans

For each description below, select the most appropriate diagnosis from the list of options. Each option may be used once, more than once or not at all.

☐ 22.   A 75-year-old woman with a 9-month history of non-pitting oedema and erythema in both legs.

☐ 23.   A 54-year-old man with longstanding varicose veins complains of acute-onset erythema, tenderness and swelling on the side of his calf. He is afebrile.

☐ 24.   A 79-year-old patient with diabetes and calf pain worse on walking. The leg is erythematous when sitting but blanches on elevation.

☐ 25.   A 54-year-old woman on HRT complains of pain in her right calf for 3 days. The calf is diffusely red and tender. She has no fever.

☐ 26.   A 56-year-old man with rheumatoid arthritis presents with painful swelling behind his knee. On examination he has tenderness and erythema in the popliteal fossa.

PAPER 4

27. **Which one of the following statements about ageism in medicine is true?**

☐ A GPs are equally likely to ask about smoking and alcohol in patients aged 55 and patients aged 75

☐ B GPs are less likely than cardiologists to treat patients differently according to age

☐ C NICE guidelines on social value judgements justify discrimination on the basis of age in some situations

☐ D Research data on novel treatments always includes data from geriatric patients

☐ E The National Service Framework for Older People supports discrimination in certain circumstances

28. **A 27-year-old man presents concerned that he is going bald. There is a strong family history of premature balding and on examination he has hair loss over the vertex. Which of the following statements about management of hair loss is true? Select one option only.**

☐ A Minoxidil provides an effective and lasting treatment

☐ B Finasteride is safe and effective

☐ C Depot testosterone injection will reverse baldness and provide long-term benefit

☐ D Pyrithione zinc shampoo, if used regularly, will slow hair loss

☐ E Cyproterone acetate is a safe and effective treatment for male pattern baldness

PAPER 4

29. While working at the local GP out-of-hours service, you see a 34-year-old man with a history of epilepsy since childhood who had a seizure earlier. While waiting to be seen he has another seizure and subsequently develops status epilepticus. Which of the following is NOT an appropriate action in this situation? Select one option only.

☐ A   ABC of resuscitation
☐ B   Check blood glucose
☐ C   High-flow oxygen
☐ D   Intravenous lorazepam
☐ E   Intramuscular phenytoin

30. A 5-year-old girl is seen with her mother. The mother reports that for the last few weeks she has been persistently scratching her bottom, particularly at night. The mother has noticed some scratch marks around her anus but nothing else. She is otherwise well and takes no regular medications. What is the most likely diagnosis? Select one option only.

☐ A   Threadworm infestation
☐ B   Psychological pruritus
☐ C   Hookworm infestation
☐ D   Tapeworm infestation
☐ E   Eczema

PAPER 4

31. Which of the following statements about dyslexia is NOT true? Select one option only.

- [ ] A Dyslexia can be defined as performance in literary skills that is 2 years behind expected at a certain age
- [ ] B It may be seen in association with dyspraxia
- [ ] C It may be associated with low self-esteem
- [ ] D It may be hereditary
- [ ] E Children with dyslexia do not qualify for a 'Statement of Special Educational Needs'

32. A 7-year-old girl has been asked to see you by her teachers who are concerned that she seems to be daydreaming a lot. On closer questioning her parents admit that recently she has been having episodes where she goes blank for a few seconds at a time and does not seem to recall the event afterwards. On examination she is physically well. Which of the following statements about this condition is true? Select one option only.

- [ ] A The absences can often be triggered by hyperventilation
- [ ] B Patients may go on to develop generalised seizures
- [ ] C EEG will show a characteristic pattern
- [ ] D Prognosis depends on IQ
- [ ] E All of the above

33. A 76-year-old man is seen for a routine blood pressure follow-up and you notice this lesion on his face.

Which of the following is the most appropriate management of this case?

☐ A   Cryotherapy

☐ B   Topical 5FU (5-fluorouracil) cream with hydrocortisone for rash

☐ C   Curettage and cautery

☐ D   Topical diclofenac

☐ E   Excision

34. Which of the following statements about risk factors for ischaemic heart disease is true? Select one option only.

☐ A Smoking increases the risk of developing ischaemic heart disease by 50

☐ B Data from the Framingham project suggest that hypercholesterolaemia is the most significant risk factor after smoking

☐ C Statins are indicated in people with diabetes only after the age of 45 or if total cholesterol > 5.4

☐ D The progesterone-only contraceptive pill is contraindicated in patients with risk factors for ischaemic heart disease

☐ E Diabetes increases the risk of developing ischaemic heart disease by 200–300%

35. A 33-year-old woman presents with a 3-month history of weight loss, sweating, increased appetite and palpitations. She also reports that her periods have become irregular but has no previous history of note. On examination you note a fine tremor and a resting pulse rate of 110. Which of the following is the most likely diagnosis? Select one option only.

☐ A Hypothyroidism

☐ B New-onset type 1 diabetes mellitus

☐ C Carcinoid syndrome

☐ D Polycystic ovarian syndrome

☐ E Hyperthyroidism

THEME: CONSULTATION MODELS

Options

A   Biomedical model

B   Byrne and Long

C   Cambridge–Calgary

D   Health belief model

E   Helman's folk model

F   Neighbour's model

G   Pendleton

H   Triaxial RCGP model

For each of the descriptions of consultation models below, select the most appropriate answer from the list of options. Each option may be used once, more than once or not at all.

☐ **36.** **It suggests that the decision to consult depends on general interest in health, patient's ideas about his own vulnerability, a cost–benefit analysis and trigger factors.**

☐ **37.** **It includes the formation of a contingency plan and acknowledges the needs of the doctor.**

☐ **38.** **It highlights the need for doctors to address patient problems in social, physical and psychological terms.**

☐ **39.** **It emphasised the importance of maintaining a positive relationship with the patient.**

☐ **40.** **It acknowledges the process by which patients seek answers to six questions.**

PAPER 4

41. **With regard to risk factors for heart failure, which of the following statements is true? Select one option only.**

☐ A   Arrhythmias are a risk factor for chronic heart failure

☐ B   Essential hypertension is a risk factor for acute heart failure

☐ C   Acute myocardial infarction is a risk factor for acute heart failure

☐ D   Mitral stenosis is a common cause of acute heart failure in developing countries

☐ E   The most common cause for chronic heart failure in elderly people in the UK is diabetes

42. **Which of the following statements about benefits in palliative care are true? Select one option only.**

☐ A   The report on a DS1500 should include the diagnosis, regardless of whether or not the patient knows it

☐ B   No fee is payable from the Benefits Agency, but practitioners may charge the patient

☐ C   The DS1500 is used when the patient's life expectancy is less than 12 months

☐ D   The DS1500 can be applied for only by the patient named in the form

☐ E   An exact prognosis needs to be given

PAPER 4

43. With regard to the risk of pandemic influenza, which one of the following statements is true?

☐ A   H5N3 is the strain of avian flu that is most dangerous for humans

☐ B   Avian influenza is spread by contaminated droppings and respiratory secretions

☐ C   The incubation period is 7 days

☐ D   Infectivity lasts up to 21 days

☐ E   Tamiflu is highly effective against avian influenza

44. You are asked to give a talk to the local practice nurse group about the latest developments in the prevention of cervical cancer. Which one of the following statements is true?

☐ A   Cervical cancer is the most common cancer in women

☐ B   Cervical cytology is an objective process that is free from operator error

☐ C   The incidence of cervical cancer has fallen by 12% since 1988

☐ D   Cervical smears have a number needed to screen of 1000 to prevent one death

☐ E   Screening takes place at 5-yearly intervals to age 50

PAPER 4

45. Understanding the role of bereavement in palliative care is important in helping patients and their carers to cope. Which of the following statements lists the correct order of the stages of bereavement? Select one option only.

- [ ] A   Denial, shock, depression, anger/guilt, acceptance
- [ ] B   Shock, denial, depression, anger/guilt, acceptance
- [ ] C   Shock, anger/guilt, depression, denial, acceptance
- [ ] D   Shock, denial, anger/guilt, depression, acceptance
- [ ] E   Shock, denial, anger/guilt, acceptance, depression

46. While working at the out-of-hours centre, you see a 44-year-old woman with sudden-onset unilateral sensorineural deafness. Which of the following statements about this condition is correct? Select one option only.

- [ ] A   This condition should be treated as an emergency and the patient referred to the on-call team
- [ ] B   Early high-dose steroids have proved to be effective in restoring hearing
- [ ] C   The presence of accompanying vertigo is suggestive of a viral labyrinthitis and has a good prognosis
- [ ] D   Recovery usually takes place within 48 hours
- [ ] E   A high-frequency loss has a better prognosis than a low-frequency one

47. A 45-year-old man presents with a 9-month history of difficulty straightening his middle finger on one hand. On examination he has a palpable nodule on the palm of his hand.

Which of the following is the most effective first-line treatment for this condition? Select one option only.

☐ A Physiotherapy
☐ B Watchful waiting
☐ C Surgical exploration
☐ D Local steroid injection
☐ E Splinting

48. A 35-year-old man who has just got off a plane from a skiing trip to Bulgaria comes to see you about his painful swollen knee, sustained in a fall 2 days ago. He has not consulted a doctor yet because he does not speak Bulgarian. Which one of the following statements about the assessment of a knee injury is true?

- [ ] A Excessive forward movement of the tibia suggests a posterior cruciate tear
- [ ] B Excessive valgus movement of the knee suggests a lateral collateral ligament tear
- [ ] C Excessive forward movement of the tibia suggests an anterior cruciate tear
- [ ] D Excessive valgus movement of the knee suggests a lateral collateral ligament tear
- [ ] E Sagging of the tibia when the knee is flexed suggests a patellar tendon tear

49. Which one of the following pairs of drugs interact and therefore cannot be given together?

- [ ] A Penicillin and clavulanic acid
- [ ] B Hydrochlorothiazide and atenolol
- [ ] C Fluvastatin and erythromycin
- [ ] D St John's wort and phenytoin
- [ ] E Amlodipine and atenolol

50. A 43-year-old man with a history of mild asthma only presents with an acute onset of sharp chest pain, localised to the sixth rib area anteriorly, eased by leaning forwards. He reports that the pain radiates into his left arm. On examination he has a rub heard at the left sternal edge and an ECG shows saddle-shaped ST elevation throughout, with no ST depression. Which of the following statements is true? Select one option only.

☐ A He should be treated with thrombolysis if there are no contraindications

☐ B He should be treated with intramuscular opiate analgesia and admitted for observation and serial cardiac enzymes

☐ C He should be treated with a non-steroidal anti-inflammatory drug (NSAID) and if pain resolves can be discharged

☐ D He should be given tinzaparin and referred for a ventilation–perfusion scan

☐ E He should be given a proton pump inhibitor and discharged

51. One of your patients comes to see you after an outpatient appointment where he was told that he has diabetes insipidus. He is understandably concerned and wishes to discuss the diagnosis and implications. Which of the following statements about diabetes insipidus is NOT true? Select one option only.

☐ A It is caused by excess secretion of antidiuretic hormone by the pituitary

☐ B Patients usually present with polydipsia and polyuria

☐ C Mild cases may be treated with adequate oral fluid replacement

☐ D Moderate-to-severe cases are treated with desmopressin

☐ E Psychogenic polydipsia can be differentiated from diabetes insipidus with a water deprivation test

PAPER 4

52. A 77-year-old man presents with recurrent pain and swelling in his hands. On examination you note the following appearance of his hands.

Which of the following statements is true about this condition?

- [ ] A The appearance is the result of pus below the skin and should be incised
- [ ] B This condition is most commonly caused by dietary factors
- [ ] C This appearance reflects acute inflammation and usually returns to normal between attacks
- [ ] D Biopsy of the mass is essential to confirm diagnosis
- [ ] E It may be iatrogenic

53. An 82-year-old man is seen accompanied by his visiting daughter who has noticed an ulcer on his left ankle. He is not sure how long it has been there. His previous medical history includes ischaemic heart disease and prostatism. He admits that the ulcer has been rather painful, particularly at night. On examination he has a punched-out ulcer on his foot with pallor around the area. Which of the following is a likely diagnosis? Select one option only.

- A   Venous ulcer
- B   Vasculitic ulcer
- C   Varicose ulcer
- D   Dendritic ulcer
- E   Arterial ulcer

54. A 63-year-old man presents with sudden-onset tingling and burning pain in the right cheek. The pain is short-lived but recurrent and started after cleaning his teeth. He has no other symptoms and is usually well. He had a similar episode 2 years previously that resolved spontaneously after 1–2 days. Which of the following diagnoses is likely in this case?

- A   Trigeminal neuralgia
- B   Glossopharyngeal neuralgia
- C   Ramsay Hunt syndrome
- D   Atypical facial pain
- E   Acoustic neuroma

PAPER 4

THEME: DRUGS FOR DEMENTIA

Options

A Amitriptyline

B Aspirin

C Diazepam

D Donepezil

E Fluoxetine

F Galantamine

G Gingko

H Haloperidol

I Memantine

J Risperidone

K Zopiclone

For each of the descriptions listed below, select the most appropriate drug from the list of options. Each option may be used once, more than once or not at all.

☐ **55.** When used for agitation it is associated with excess risk of cardiovascular mortality.

☐ **56.** It is useful for daytime agitation.

☐ **57.** It is the first choice for depression in patients with dementia.

☐ **58.** It has been shown to be effective at slowing decline in memory with a number needed to treat of 7.

☐ **59.** It is used for moderate-to-severe dementia, and has positive effects on cognitive scores, global scores and function.

60. A 64-year-old woman presents with early morning stiffness in her shoulders and hips. Blood tests show a raised ESR. Which of the following statements about polymyalgia rheumatica is true? Select one option only.

- [ ] A   Objective assessment of muscle power reveals weakness in the upper limbs but not the lower limbs
- [ ] B   Systemic symptoms are rare
- [ ] C   The sex ratio is 10 females:1 male
- [ ] D   Most patients can stop treatment within 6 months
- [ ] E   Methotrexate can be used as a steroid-sparing agent

61. A 27-year-old man presents with recurrent itchy ears. Which of the following statements about this condition is correct? Select one option only.

- [ ] A   Otitis externa is caused by inflammation of the skin of the internal auditory meatus
- [ ] B   It is always bacterial in origin
- [ ] C   It may be precipitated by over zealous use of cotton buds
- [ ] D   Use of aminoglycoside antibiotics is absolutely contraindicated unless a perforation can be definitely excluded
- [ ] E   Systemic complications are common
- [ ] F   If adequately treated is unlikely to recur

PAPER 4

THEME: DERMATOLOGICAL TREATMENTS

Options

A	Benzoyl peroxide	H	Isotretinoin
B	Betamethasone ointment	I	Methotrexate
		J	Oral steroids
C	Calcipotriol	K	PUVA
D	Dairy-free diet	L	Selenium sulphide shampoo
E	Diprosalic ointment	
F	Emollients	M	Tacrolimus
G	Hydrocortisone ointment	N	Topical clindamycin

For each statement below, select the most appropriate treatment from the list of options. Each option may be used once, more than once or not at all.

☐ **62.** It is a first-line treatment for acne rosacea.

☐ **63.** A 53-year-old woman who has had severe eczema affecting her hands for many years. The only thing that helps is Elocon. She has started to develop thinning of the skin and telangiectasia.

☐ **64.** A 2-year-old girl with persistently dry skin on her legs. She has not had any previous treatment.

☐ **65.** A 17-year-old girl with acne. She has not previously tried any medication.

☐ **66.** A 23-year-old man with localised plaque psoriasis. He has previously tried emollients with no effect.

67. You see a 40-year-old ex-soldier who wishes to claim compensation for hearing loss he feels is due to his service in the armed forces. Which of the following statements about noise-induced hearing loss is true? Select one option only.

☐ A Examination of the tympanic membranes shows a characteristic appearance

☐ B It is always bilateral and symmetrical

☐ C It is an inevitable consequence of noise exposure without ear protection

☐ D Audiograms typically show a dip at 1–2 kHz

☐ E Health and safety legislation sets out specific duties on the employer-dependent on levels of noise exposure

☐ F It is untreatable

68. A 76-year-old man comes in with his daughter after having been seen in the stroke clinic following a transient ischaemic attack (TIA) 1 week previously. He has made a complete recovery and has started on aspirin, ramipril and simvastatin for secondary prevention. He is particularly concerned about driving because his wife cannot drive and he is the main carer for her. Which of the following statements is true? Select one option only.

☐ A He may drive after 3 months if there are no recurrences

☐ B He should notify the DVLA and his insurance company

☐ C Patients with multiple TIAs occurring over a short period of time should refrain from driving until 3 months after attacks have ceased

☐ D Seizures occurring at the time of TIA require the driver to cease driving for 2 years

☐ E Patients with proven carotid artery stenosis should not drive until this has been surgically repaired

PAPER 4

THEME: DIABETES TRIALS

Options

A   DCCT

B   DREAM

C   HOPE

D   HPS

E   MICRO-HOPE

F   NICE guidelines

G   UK PDS

For each of the study descriptions below, select the appropriate trial from the list of options. Each option may be used once, more than once or not at all.

☐ **69.** It demonstrated the importance of tight blood pressure control in reducing stroke and heart failure.

☐ **70.** The use of ramipril was associated with a reduction in myocardial infarction of 22%.

☐ **71.** It demonstrated a reduction in incidence of type 2 diabetes with rosiglitazone.

☐ **72.** Ramipril use reduces the risks of developing nephropathy.

☐ **73.** It demonstrated a reduction in all-cause mortality.

74. A 73-year-old woman complains of increasing problems knitting which she thinks is due to arthritis in her fingers. She has hypertension only and is otherwise well. On examination she has hard, non-tender swellings on her fingers with the appearance shown in the photograph below.

What is the cause of the lesions? Select one option only.

- [ ] A Primary nodal osteoarthritis
- [ ] B Seropositive arthritis
- [ ] C Psoriatic arthopathy
- [ ] D Gout
- [ ] E Myxoid cyst

75. A 56-year-old man who has not seen a doctor for over 20 years is found to have a blood pressure of 220/110. Assuming that he has no co-morbidity, which of the following signs would you NOT expect to see on examining his retina? Select one option only.

- [ ] A Cotton-wool spots
- [ ] B Flame haemorrhages
- [ ] C Disc swelling
- [ ] D Drusen
- [ ] E Vitreous haemorrhage

76. A 76-year-old nursing home resident has instructed her solicitor to prepare the paperwork for an Enduring Power of Attorney. You are asked to visit to make an assessment of her. Which one of the following statements about this process is true?

- [ ] A An attorney appointed under an Enduring Power of Attorney can direct where a patient lives
- [ ] B An attorney appointed under an Enduring Power of Attorney can make decisions about medical treatment of a patient
- [ ] C An attorney does not have control over financial assets
- [ ] D A patient must be mentally competent to set up an Enduring Power of Attorney
- [ ] E The fee is set at a standard one of £220 to be paid by all applicants

77. A 76-year-old woman with a previous history of surgery for a ruptured ovarian cyst as a teenager presents with colicky central abdominal pain of 24 hours' duration. She has now started to vomit and on further questioning admits to constipation for the last 12 hours. Which one of the following statements about this patient is true?

☐ A   She should be started on broad-spectrum antibiotics

☐ B   She should be given laxatives and an antiemetic

☐ C   She should be thoroughly examined for a strangulated hernia

☐ D   She should be considered to have appendicitis until proved otherwise

☐ E   The symptoms could be a result of ischaemic bowel

78. Which of the following statements about eyelid conditions is true? Select one option only.

☐ A   Ptosis is always congenital

☐ B   Entropion is usually caused by scarring below the eye, eg as a result of BCC removal

☐ C   Facial nerve palsy causes inability to open the eyes fully

☐ D   Chlamydial infections may cause entropion

☐ E   Bell's palsy always resolves completely

PAPER 4

79. **Which one of the following statements about differences in healthcare between different ethnic groups is true?**

- [ ] A There are no significant differences in primary care management of diabetes for areas of high ethnicity and areas of low ethnicity
- [ ] B Rates of coronary revascularisation are higher in South Asian patients than comparable white patients
- [ ] C Indian children are significantly less likely to consult their GP than other patients
- [ ] D Asians and African–Caribbeans are significantly over-represented among patients with end-stage renal failure
- [ ] E Migrants from the Indian subcontinent tend to have lower average cholesterol levels than people from Anglo-Saxon populations

80. **Which one of the following statements about drug use in the UK is true?**

- [ ] A Over 10 million people in the UK use cannabis
- [ ] B Cannabis cigarettes result in less tar absorption than tobacco cigarettes
- [ ] C Cannabis is classified by the Home Office as a class B drug
- [ ] D Ten per cent of 14-year-old boys have smoked cannabis
- [ ] E Forty-four per cent of injecting drug users are infected with hepatitis C

81. A 5-year-old boy is seen by the practice nurse in her minor injury clinic with a rash. He has had abdominal pain for the last 2 days and his joints are sore. His mother has now noticed a rash on his legs and buttocks. You are asked by the nurse to see him. On examination there are numerous purpuric lesions on the extensor surfaces of his legs and buttocks. Which of the following is a likely diagnosis? Select one option only.

- ☐ A Meningococcal septicaemia
- ☐ B Erythema multiforme
- ☐ C Erythema nodosum
- ☐ D Henoch–Schönlein purpura
- ☐ E Measles

82. Which of the following statements about functional foods is true? Select one option only.

- ☐ A Functional foods are foods that contain medicinal compounds
- ☐ B The USA is the biggest worldwide market for functional foods
- ☐ C Functional foods are controlled by the same regulatory bodies as prescription medicines
- ☐ D Advertisements for functional foods cannot make claims for efficacy without scientific data to back their claims
- ☐ E Functional foods are safe and free from drug interactions

PAPER 4

THEME: DYSPHAGIA

Options

A   Achalasia

B   Barrett's oesophagus

C   Carcinoma of the oesophagus

D   Chronic benign stricture

E   Hiatus hernia

F   Gastro-oesophageal reflux

G   Globus pharyngeus

H   Impacted foreign body

I   Oesophageal perforation

J   Pharyngeal pouch

K   Plummer–Vinson syndrome

For each clinical description below, select the most appropriate diagnosis from the list of options. Each option may be used once, more than once or not at all.

☐   **83.**   A 38-year-old woman complains of slowly progressive dysphagia over several years. She reports belching with regurgitation, and has recurrent episodes of coughing at night.

☐   **84.**   A 48-year-old woman reports that food seems to stick at the back of her throat, which has caused her to choke on occasion. She has no previous history of note other than taking iron tablets for anaemia, which her GP felt was caused by menorrhagia.

85. A 67-year-old man complains that over 4 weeks he has found it progressively more difficult to swallow solids. He mentions that he has lost 12.5 kg (2 stone) over the last 6 months.

86. An 82-year-old man reports that his first mouthful is easily swallowed but he finds it progressively harder to swallow through meals. He often regurgitates undigested food to relieve his symptoms.

87. A 67-year-old woman with longstanding heartburn complains of recent onset of dysphagia, feeling that food sticks just below her sternum. Examination is normal.

88. A 54-year-old woman complains of terrible halitosis and demands something be done to save her social life. Which of the following statements about this problem is true? Select one option only.

A   It may be caused by reduced saliva production
B   It is always the result of local disease
C   It is not related to dental hygiene
D   It is always objective
E   There is seldom an obvious cause on examination

89. A 73-year-old man who has been treated for small cell lung cancer for the last 18 months comes to see you complaining of increasing shortness of breath. On examination you find that he has a red face, stridor, dilated veins over his upper body and face, and swelling in his arms. Which of the following statements about this condition is true? Select one option only.

☐ A He has inferior vena caval obstruction and should be referred urgently

☐ B His stridor will improve with humidified oxygen

☐ C Treatment of his lung primary will improve his symptoms

☐ D Radiotherapy is the only treatment option in this case

☐ E Heliox may be helpful in managing stridor

90. Which one of the following is true regarding the use of exception reporting under the Quality and Outcomes Framework (QOF)?

☐ A Exception reporting removes a patient from the whole of that disease area

☐ B Exception reporting is appropriate where an indicator is inappropriate on economic grounds, eg not doing a cholesterol test on a 90-year-old

☐ C QMAS allows identification of individual patients, allowing verification at practice visits

☐ D APOLLO measures the extent of exception reporting by indicator

☐ E Patients must decline three written invitations before being exception-reported

91. A 45-year-old man presents with ptosis, diplopia and weakness of his arms when lifting them above his head, all of which are worse from late morning onwards. Which of the following is the most likely diagnosis? Select one option only.

☐ A   Myasthenia gravis
☐ B   Polymyalgia rheumatica
☐ C   Multiple sclerosis
☐ D   Rheumatoid arthritis
☐ E   Internuclear ophthalmoplegia

92. Which of the following have been shown in randomised controlled trials to be of benefit in the management of rheumatological disease? Select one option only.

☐ A   Manuka honey
☐ B   Gingko biloba
☐ C   Glucosamine
☐ D   Copper
☐ E   Chondroitin

93. A 51-year-old man presents with flashers in his left eye followed by a curtain descending across his vision. Which of the following statements about retinal detachment is true? Select one option only.

☐ A   It is more common in people with hypermetropia
☐ B   It can usually be treated with medical therapy and bed rest
☐ C   On examination there is a vivid sunset pattern with venous engorgement in the affected eye
☐ D   It may be a sign of malignant melanoma
☐ E   Approximately 50% of patients treated surgically have a good outcome

THEME: STATISTICAL TERMS

Options

A   Confounding factor

B   Evens ratio

C   Exclusions

D   Intention-to-treat analysis

E   Null hypothesis

F   Odds ratio

G   Risk factor

H   Quality-adjusted life-year

I   Sample size

J   Standard deviation

K   Standard error

L   Statistical power

For each situation described below, select the most appropriate description from the list of options. Each option may be used once, more than once or not at all.

94. The risk of having a heart attack in a group of patients taking drug A compared with the control group.

95. An attempt to make subjective outcomes objective.

96. The influence of social class in population studies of the influence of HRT on dementia.

97. An indication of the spread of results around the mean.

98. The inclusion of all patients regardless of event rate.

99. **A 24-year-old man presents with a 3-month history of diarrhoea. He has lost 19 kg (3 stone) over the last 6 months and also reports painful piles. Which one of the following statements about the management of this patient is true?**

- [ ] A He has Crohn's disease
- [ ] B He should be treated with broad-spectrum antibiotics
- [ ] C Left hemicolectomy is the treatment of choice
- [ ] D His piles should respond to topical treatment and a change in diet
- [ ] E Symptoms often recur if patients stop smoking

100. **One of your patients has been diagnosed as having a glioblastoma multiforme. He is due to start radiotherapy next week. He comes to see you with his wife to find out more about the side effects of radiotherapy. Which of the following statements is NOT true? Select one option only.**

- [ ] A Radiotherapy causes minor skin irritation
- [ ] B Radiotherapy may cause cataracts
- [ ] C Radiotherapy causes fatigue
- [ ] D Most patients require one dose of radiotherapy only
- [ ] E Radiotherapy may increase intracranial pressure

101. **Which of the following statements about 5-year survival for different cancers is true? Select one option only.**

- [ ] A The 5-year survival rate for prostate cancer is 80%
- [ ] B The 5-year survival rate for breast cancer is 80%
- [ ] C The 5-year survival rate for colon cancer is 80%
- [ ] D The 5-year survival rate for lung cancer is 40%
- [ ] E The 5-year survival rate for ovarian cancer is 70%

102. A 76-year-old man presents with a lesion on his right hand that has been present for the last 3 weeks and is now 2 cm in diameter. It does not bleed and is non-tender; there is no lymphadenopathy. The lesion is shown in the photograph below.

What is the most likely diagnosis?

- [ ] A   Basal cell carcinoma
- [ ] B   Molluscum contagiosum
- [ ] C   Squamous cell carcinoma
- [ ] D   Keratoacanthoma
- [ ] E   Bowen's disease

THEME: FULL BLOOD COUNT

Options

A   Alcohol consumption

B   Anaemia of chronic disease

C   Aplastic anaemia

D   Chronic renal failure

E   Coeliac disease

F   Iron-deficient anaemia

G   Myeloma

H   Pernicious anaemia

I   Thalassaemia

For each of the situations described below select the most appropriate diagnosis from the list of options. Each option may be used once, more than once or not at all.

□   **103.**   **A 67-year-old woman with longstanding rheumatoid arthritis has an Hb of 9.8 with normal mean corpuscular volume (MCV) and haemoglobin (MCH). Ferritin is normal.**

□   **104.**   **A 77-year-old patient with type 2 diabetes has routine bloods. The haematology report shows a mild anaemia and the film is reported as showing burr cells.**

□   **105.**   **A 79-year-old man with frequent sore throats and bruising has a FBC. This shows a normochromic/macrocytic anaemia, low white cells and thrombocytopenia.**

□   **106.**   **A 59-year-old woman with back pain and fatigue has bloods as part of her investigation. The film shows rouleaux and she has a raised ESR.**

□   **107.**   **A 61-year-old woman with a history of hypothyroidism has routine blood tests as part of a well woman check. These show a raised MCV and blood film oval macrocytes.**

PAPER 4

108. A 34-year-old man presents with itching and burning of his eyelid margins for some weeks; on examination there is redness and scaling on the edges of his eyelids. Which of the following statements about this patient is true? Select one option only.

- [ ] A   He has acute conjunctivitis and should be treated with topical antibiotics
- [ ] B   He has a contact dermatitis
- [ ] C   He should be advised to use dilute baby shampoo to clean the eyelids twice a day and a short course of fucithalmic eye drops
- [ ] D   Most patients with this condition require oral tetracycline
- [ ] E   He should be treated with artificial tears

109. Which one of the following statements about glandular fever is true?

- [ ] A   Subclinical infection is rare
- [ ] B   The presence of stiff neck and headache suggests that meningitis is the diagnosis rather than Epstein–Barr virus infection
- [ ] C   Ninety per cent of symptomatic patients have a severe pharyngitis
- [ ] D   Splenomegaly occurs in 50% of patients
- [ ] E   Corticosteroids shorten the duration of symptoms

110. A 76-year-old man with type 2 diabetes presents with recurrent pain and swelling of his right foot. He has been treated on several occasions for gout but recent blood tests showed normal uric acid levels. He now has a discharging sinus and a fever. Which one of the following statements about this case is true?

- [ ] A   The most likely diagnosis is cellulitis
- [ ] B   The diagnosis of osteomyelitis is a clinical one
- [ ] C   TB is the most common organism responsible in the UK
- [ ] D   Complications include amyloidosis
- [ ] E   Marjolin's ulcer is a chronic infection of the skin seen in patients with osteomyelitis

111. A 42-year-old man reports that he has noticed black tarry stools over the last 2 weeks. He has vomited a small amount of blood. Which one of the following statements about this patient is true?

- [ ] A   Bleeding usually arises from the lower gastrointestinal tract
- [ ] B   If symptoms settle with a proton-pump inhibitor, no further action is required
- [ ] C   The presence of melaena suggests that the primary pathology is localised to the lining of the stomach
- [ ] D   It can result from portal hypertension
- [ ] E   It usually settles with conservative management

PAPER 4

THEME: INFECTIONS IN TRAVELLERS WHO RETURN HOME ILL

Options

A   Amoebic dysentery

B   Dengue

C   Diphtheria

D   Hepatitis A

E   Hepatitis B

F   HIV

G   Influenza

H   Leishmaniasis

I   Malaria

J   Meningitis

K   Rabies

L   Schistosomiasis

M   Tuberculosis

N   Urinary tract infection

PAPER 4

For each of the descriptions below, select the most likely diagnosis from the list of options. Each option may be used once, more than once or not at all.

☐   **112.**   **A previously healthy 43-year-old woman has just got off the plane from The Gambia. She has been on a 2-week package holiday and stayed in a four-star hotel. She had the full course of immunisations recommended but did not take antimalarials because she was staying in a resort. On examination she has a fever, headache, myalgia and vomiting.**

113. A 19-year-old gap year student has just returned from a 6-month placement in South America where he was building a school in a remote community. He has had a slowly enlarging ulcer on his right ankle for 4 months, but is otherwise well.

114. A 53-year-old devout Muslim has returned from the Hajj pilgrimage to Mecca. He has a fever and headache, and is confused.

115. A 24-year-old woman who returned 2 weeks ago from a package holiday to Spain where she indulged her love of seafood. She has developed a profound sense of malaise, vomiting and dark urine with jaundice.

116. A 36-year-old gay man returned from Ibiza 6 weeks ago after a 2-week holiday where he had unprotected sex with a number of men. He has flu-like symptoms, anorexia, nausea and pruritus with pale stools and dark urine.

117. A 37-year-old man, originally from Russia, has recently returned from a trip to his homeland. He reports that he had a sore throat while away and now he feels listless and has dysphagia. On examination he has a temperature of 39°C and a tachycardia of 110. His throat is swollen with a thick membrane over the tonsils.

PAPER 4

118. Two treatments for osteoporosis are compared in a longitudinal trial. The rate of hip fracture for the treatment groups is shown below.

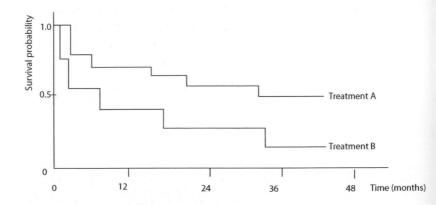

Which of the following statements about this data is true? Select one option only.

- [ ] A   Treatment B reduces the rate of hip fracture more than treatment A
- [ ] B   More than 50% of the patients in treatment group A had experienced a hip fracture by the 12-month point
- [ ] C   Treatment A reduces the rate of hip fracture more than treatment B
- [ ] D   Treatment A reduced the rate of hip fracture significantly more than the placebo
- [ ] E   Treatment B reduced the rate of hip fracture significantly more than the placebo

119. A 76-year-old woman is brought into the surgery by her daughter complaining of swollen legs. These have been present for many years and seem to be slowly getting worse. She has treated diabetes and hypothyroidism but is otherwise well. She has no shortness of breath. Examination reveals lymphoedematous legs to the knee. There are no signs of infection. Which of the following statements about management is true? Select one option only.

☐ A   Four-layer bandaging is often helpful in combination with elevation of the limb

☐ B   Low-dose furosemide is a safe and effective long-term treatment

☐ C   Subclinical infection is often present and a 10-day course of broad-spectrum antibiotics is useful at the start of treatment

☐ D   Patients should be referred for consideration of varicose vein surgery

☐ E   Hypoalbuminaemia is a common cause of lymphoedema and should be treated

120. A 63-year-old man who is a recent immigrant from Tanzania complains about an ulcer on his penis. This is painless and has been present for some months, but is slowly enlarging. On examination he has an ulcer at the base of his glans and an offensive exudate. He also has bilateral inguinal lymphadenopathy. Which of the following is the most likely diagnosis? Select one option only.

☐ A   Balanitis xerotica et obliterans
☐ B   Primary syphilis
☐ C   Cutaneous tuberculosis
☐ D   Penile cancer
☐ E   Malignant melanoma
☐ F   Chancroid

PAPER 4

THEME: NASAL PROBLEMS

Options

A   Acute sinusitis

B   Chronic sinusitis

C   Coryza

D   Deviated nasal septum

E   Foreign body

F   Nasal polyps

G   Nasal vestibulitis

H   Nasopharyngeal carcinoma

I   Perennial rhinitis

J   Septal haematoma

For each patient described below, select the single most likely diagnosis from the list of options. Each option may be used once, more than once, or not at all.

☐   **121.**   **A 46-year-old man with longstanding nasal obstruction. He also has a poor sense of smell.**

☐   **122.**   **It is caused by staphylococci, and frequently affects children.**

☐   **123.**   **A 76-year-old former carpenter presents with unilateral nasal obstruction with epistaxis.**

☐   **124.**   **A 16-year-old girl with persistent itching sneezing and watery rhinorrhoea.**

☐   **125.**   **A 2-year-old boy with unilateral nasal discharge.**

126. You see a 35-year-old man with acute lumbar backache. You conduct a thorough examination to rule out significant pathology. Which of the following is a red flag symptom? Select one option only.

- [ ] A   Unilateral sciatica
- [ ] B   Pain made worse with movement
- [ ] C   Upper motor neurone signs in the legs
- [ ] D   Numbness in buttocks and perineum
- [ ] E   Prolonged incapacity

127. An 88-year-old woman complains that she is unable to read properly and that straight lines appear bent when viewed with her right eye. Her peripheral vision is normal. Fundoscopy reveals yellow spots around the macular area. Which of the following is the most likely diagnosis? Select one option only.

- [ ] A   Macular degeneration
- [ ] B   Cataract
- [ ] C   Glaucoma
- [ ] D   Retinal detachment
- [ ] E   Branch retinal vein occlusion

128. Which one of the following statements about organ donation is true?

- [ ] A   Fifty per cent of the population support organ donation
- [ ] B   Organ donation operates along lines of presumed consent
- [ ] C   Over 2000 people a year die while waiting for a transplant
- [ ] D   Fifty per cent of the population carry a donor card
- [ ] E   Countries where a system of presumed consent operates have three times the rate of organ donation

PAPER 4

129. A 27-year-old man who is known to be an intravenous heroin user presents as an emergency with a persistent fever, blood in his urine and shortness of breath. On further questioning he admits to recent weight loss and night sweats. On examination he has splinter haemorrhages, microscopic haematuria and a systolic heart murmur. Which of the following is the single most likely diagnosis? Select one option only.

- [ ] A Lymphoma
- [ ] B Streptococcal glomerulonephritis
- [ ] C TB
- [ ] D Infectious endocarditis
- [ ] E Legionnaire's disease

130. Which of the following statements about testicular tumours is true? Select one option only.

- [ ] A Testicular tumours are rare in the under-50s
- [ ] B Ninety per cent are benign
- [ ] C They may present with a hydrocele
- [ ] D Testicular tumours are always germ cell in origin
- [ ] E Treatment by lumpectomy is usually possible

THEME: CANCER GENETICS

Options

A   *APC* gene

B   Autosomal dominant inheritance

C   Autosomal recessive inheritance

D   *BRCA*-1 gene

E   Incomplete penetrance

F   *NF1* gene

G   *p53* gene

H   *RB1* gene

I   Sporadic cancer

For each of the statements below, select the most appropriate option from the list of options. Each option may be used once, more than once or not at all.

☐ **131. It is associated with ovarian cancer.**

☐ **132. It is associated with acoustic neuromas.**

☐ **133. It is likely to explain the presence of a specific cancer in most generations of one family.**

☐ **134. This is the causation of most cancers.**

☐ **135. It is associated with bowel cancer.**

136. A 35-year-old woman comes to see you asking if something can be done for the lumps that she has had on her ears since being a teenager. On examination she has the appearance below.

Which of the following statements about this lesion is NOT true? Select one option only?

- [ ] A   They are more common in white people
- [ ] B   They usually recur after excision
- [ ] C   Intralesional triamcinolone may reduce the size of scars
- [ ] D   They are more common in the midline
- [ ] E   May be caused by BCG immunisation

137. A 25-year-old man hobbles into your surgery after twisting his left ankle playing football. Which one of the following statements about the assessment of his injuries is true?

☐ A Lack of malleolar tenderness but inability to weight-bear suggests that a radiograph is not necessary

☐ B Ottawa rules apply only to ankle injuries

☐ C Tenderness at the base of the fifth metatarsal indicates the need for a radiograph of the foot

☐ D The four zones described in the Ottawa rules are the lateral malleolus, medial malleolus, calcaneum and base of the fifth metatarsal

☐ E The malleolar zones extend 2 cm above each malleolus

138. Under which one of the following circumstances is free NHS treatment NOT available in primary care?

☐ A A visitor on a 3-week holiday from Venezuela who has been bitten by a dog

☐ B A visitor from France with a valid European Health Insurance Card (EHIC) requests a repeat prescription of her blood pressure medication

☐ C A Kurdish asylum seeker and his wife request referral for infertility treatment

☐ D A visitor from the USA on a 4-week European tour requests a repeat prescription of her simvastatin

☐ E A 23-year-old Polish barman without a valid EHIC, who has been working in the UK for 9 months, requests a repeat prescription for his asthma inhalers

139. A 45-year-old man presents with a severe headache and neck stiffness. He has been well until a few days ago when he started to develop mild headaches. On examination he is afebrile, has no rash and has some signs of meningism. Which of the following statements about subarachnoid haemorrhage is true? Select one option only.

- [ ] A The mean age is 22 years
- [ ] B Eighty per cent of patients present with collapse
- [ ] C Meningism caused by blood irritating the meninges usually occurs immediately after the onset of the headache
- [ ] D Blood pressure usually falls in the acute phase
- [ ] E A 3rd cranial nerve palsy is common and indicates a posterior communicating artery aneurysm, basilar artery aneurysm or transtentorial herniation

140. A 44-year-old woman complains of epigastric pain radiating to the back, reflux on bending over and general malaise. She has no dysphagia and has gained 5 kg in the last 6 months. Which one of the following statements about this condition is true?

- [ ] A It can be brought on by pregnancy
- [ ] B First-line treatment is a proton-pump inhibitor
- [ ] C It often causes acute severe abdominal pain
- [ ] D Symptoms are usually relieved after meals
- [ ] E It has no long-term complications

141. Under the new GMS Contract you are assigned the role of Caldicott Guardian within the practice. Which one of the following statements about this role is NOT true?

- [ ] A   All uses of identifiable data should be justified
- [ ] B   The minimum identifiable data should be used at all times, eg NHS number rather than full name
- [ ] C   To prevent errors, at least two pieces of identifiable data should be used at every occasion, eg date of birth and NHS number
- [ ] D   Passwords giving access to data should be changed at regular intervals
- [ ] E   Posters should be available for patients to understand how data are used within the practice

142. A 23-year-old man presents with an acutely painful left testicle. The overlying skin is red and he seems to be tender posteriorly. He has a temperature of 38.3°C and feels like he has the flu. The testicle and scrotum are of normal size. During the examination he reports that the testicle feels better when lifted. Which of the following is the most likely diagnosis? Select one option only.

- [ ] A   Acute epididymitis
- [ ] B   Urinary tract infection
- [ ] C   Hydrocele
- [ ] D   Testicular torsion
- [ ] E   Testicular cancer

PAPER 4

THEME: NEURO-OPHTHALMOLOGICAL EXAMINATION

Options

A   Cranial nerve II palsy

B   Cranial nerve III palsy

C   Cranial nerve IV palsy

D   Cranial nerve VI palsy

E   Internuclear ophthalmoplegia

F   Relative afferent papillary defect

G   Romberg's test positive

H   Unterberger's test positive

For each clinical finding described below, select the most appropriate option from the list of options. Each option may be used once, more than once or not at all.

☐   **143.   This would be seen in acute ischaemic optic neuropathy.**

☐   **144.   Ophthalmoplegia on looking laterally.**

☐   **145.   Ophthalmoplegia on looking upwards.**

☐   **146.   It is positive when a patient looking laterally has nystagmus and an apparent lateral rectus palsy.**

☐   **147.   It causes weakness in the superior oblique muscle.**

148. Your practice manager draws to your attention the fact that £250 worth of stamps has disappeared from the office. These have been discovered in the handbag of one of the receptionists. Which of the following actions is appropriate in this situation? Select one option only.

- [ ] A Dismiss the receptionist
- [ ] B Give a verbal warning and record this in her records
- [ ] C Issue a disciplinary fine and dock this from her pay
- [ ] D Report the matter to the police
- [ ] E Make her admit her guilt and apologise to the entire staff for her actions

149. A 58-year-old woman with a previous history of treated hypertension complains of symptoms of bloating over the last few months. She has had no diarrhoea but has lost some weight. On examination there are no abnormalities felt in her abdomen but both legs are oedematous. Which one of the following is the single most appropriate action in managing her problem?

- [ ] A Trial of mebeverine
- [ ] B Pelvic examination
- [ ] C Increase dietary fibre
- [ ] D Try an exclusion diet for 3 months
- [ ] E Refer for Doppler ultrasonography to exclude below-knee deep vein thrombosis

150. Your practice is setting up a smoking cessation clinic and you are asked to write the treatment protocol based on NICE guidance. Which of the following is true with regard to the guidance? Select one option only.

- [ ] A Bupropion may be used in all patients over the age of 18, unless they have a history of epilepsy

- [ ] B Bupropion or nicotine replacement should be started on the chosen stop date

- [ ] C Patients should be reviewed after the first 4 weeks of treatment and their dose reduced at that time if they have been successful

- [ ] D Where patients have previously tried nicotine replacement and failed, combination therapy with bupropion is an effective alternative

- [ ] E Patients should set a stop date and be prescribed enough nicotine replacement products for a period of 2 weeks after this date, at which time their progress should be reviewed

151. A 3-year-old boy is brought in by his mother with crusting weeping lesions around his face. He has had these for 2 days and they seem to be spreading. He has recently started at nursery where another child had a similar rash. Which of the following statements about his management is true? Select one option only.

- [ ] A Topical fusidic acid is highly effective and well tolerated
- [ ] B Where disease is widespread, systemic treatment with amoxicillin is indicated
- [ ] C Topical treatment with mupirocin is usually adequate
- [ ] D If the rash fails to respond to the first-line antibiotic, the diagnosis is likely to be viral
- [ ] E Once on antibiotics, strict hygiene measures are not necessary

THEME: MEDICAL TREATMENT OF PARKINSON'S DISEASE

Options

A   Amantadine

B   Apomorphine

C   Benzhexol

D   Domperidone

E   Entacapone

F   Levodopa

G   Ropinirole

H   Propranolol

I   Sinemet

J   Selegiline

For each of the descriptions below, select the most appropriate from the list of options. Each option may be used once, more than once or not at all.

152. Often combined with a decarboxylase inhibitor to reduce systemic side effects.

153. It may be used to prolong the period before dopamine is needed but studies suggest that it may increase mortality when used in combination with l-dopa.

154. It inhibits l-dopa breakdown and may allow reduction of dopamine dose.

155. It causes rapid-onset benefit of short duration for fluctuating motor responses and on–off symptoms but must be given by injection.

156. It is useful for nausea and vomiting in parkinsonism.

THEME: PREVALENCE OF COMMON CONDITIONS IN PRIMARY CARE IN ENGLAND

Options

A   50

B   1.8

C   4.3

D   7.4

E   75

F   65

G   39.4

For each of the conditions below, select the closest estimate for prevalence (number of cases per 1000 patients) from the list of options. Each option may be used once, more than once or not at all.

- ☐ **157.** Treated hypertension.
- ☐ **158.** Treated asthma.
- ☐ **159.** Treated diabetes (types 1 and 2).
- ☐ **160.** Treated anxiety.
- ☐ **161.** Treated schizophrenia.
- ☐ **162.** Treated depression.
- ☐ **163.** Cancer.

164. **With regard to the NICE guidance on care after a myocardial infarction, which of the following statements about treatment indications is NOT correct? Select one option only.**

- [ ] A   Omega-3 fatty acids are beneficial
- [ ] B   Six months of combination treatment with clopidogrel and aspirin should be given after a non-ST-elevation myocardial infarction (NSTEMI)
- [ ] C   Aldosterone antagonists should be considered if there are signs of heart failure
- [ ] D   ACE inhibitors are indicated
- [ ] E   β Blockers are indicated

165. **A patient with dyspepsia has recently had an endoscopy. The histology report has come back showing *Helicobacter pylori*. Which one of the following statements about this condition is true?**

- [ ] A   Eradication of *H. pylori* will reduce recurrence rates of duodenal ulcer by 90%
- [ ] B   NICE guidelines recommend endoscopy as a cost-effective strategy for patients with dyspepsia but no alarm symptoms
- [ ] C   'Test and treat' refers to a policy of endoscopy followed by proton-pump inhibitor for those who have endoscopy-proved ulcer or reflux
- [ ] D   The MRC-CUBE trial showed test and treat to have significantly lower costs than empirical treatment
- [ ] E   Population screening followed by eradication treatment is effective and feasible in reducing consultations and symptoms

PAPER 4

THEME: SCREENING

A new blood test has been developed to screen for bowel cancer. The results from the pilot trial are shown below:

Disease status	Positive	Negative
Test positive	900	100
Test negative	50	950

Options

A   50/950

B   900/1000

C   100/900

D   900/950

E   100/950

F   50/1000

G   100/1000

H   950/1000

I   950/1050

For each of the statements below, select the most appropriate answer from the list of options. Each option may be used once, more than once or not at all.

☐   **166.**   The sensitivity of the test.

☐   **167.**   The positive predictive value of the test.

☐   **168.**   The specificity of the test.

☐   **169.**   The negative predictive value of the test.

170. Which one of the following statements about stress and burnout is true?

☐ A Burnout is associated with excessive discussions about past mistakes

☐ B Doctors who feel that they see more patients than their peers are more likely to be able to cope with extra workload

☐ C The proportion of health workers reporting stress is 18%

☐ D Doctors are no more likely to commit suicide than the general population

☐ E Female GPs are less likely to experience stress relating to visits than male GPs

171. A 67-year-old man complains of acute onset of left iliac fossa pain associated with diarrhoea and abdominal colic. On examination he has a temperature of 39°C and a tachycardia, with guarding and rebound. Which one of the following statements about his management is true?

☐ A Penicillin is the antibiotic of choice

☐ B Gastroenteritis is usually viral and should settle with fluids and Imodium (loperamide)

☐ C Frequency of attacks can be reduced by removing dietary triggers and using mebeverine after meals

☐ D Increased dietary fibre might help to reduce attacks

☐ E Mesalazine can be used to treat acute attacks

PAPER 4

THEME: SOFT TISSUE CONDITIONS

Options

A Carpal tunnel

B De Quervain's tenosynovitis

C Dupuytren's contracture

D Golfers' elbow

E Plantar fasciitis

F Supraspinatus tendonitis

G Tennis elbow

H Trigger finger

For each scenario described below, select the most appropriate diagnosis from the list of options. Each option may be used once, more than once or not at all.

☐ **172. It is caused by median nerve compression.**

☐ **173. It is characterised by inflammation of the flexor origin at the elbow.**

☐ **174. It causes pain on the radial side of the wrist on abduction of the thumb.**

☐ **175. When recurrent it may require surgical treatment with a lateral release.**

☐ **176. It causes a fixed flexion deformity.**

177. A 19-year-old man has been brought to see you by his mother who is increasingly concerned about his behaviour. He has become withdrawn, is increasingly obsessed with the secret services, and seems to be talking to himself. Which one of the following is the most likely diagnosis?

- ☐ A Hypomania
- ☐ B Alcohol withdrawal
- ☐ C Depression
- ☐ D Schizophrenia
- ☐ E Temporal lobe epilepsy

178. A 54-year-old woman with hypertension presents with a 5-month history of sweating, tachycardia, headache and panic attacks. Her blood pressure has always been difficult to control and she has been labelled as having white coat hypertension. On examination she has a fine tremor and a pulse of 120, and is sweating. Which of the following is the likely diagnosis? Select one option only.

- ☐ A Phaeochromocytoma
- ☐ B Anxiety
- ☐ C Hyperthyroidism
- ☐ D White coat hypertension
- ☐ E Paroxysmal supraventricular tachycardia

PAPER 4

179. An 83-year-old man has been encouraged to attend by his daughter with regard to the appearance of his fingernails. These are yellow and thickened and have been so for a number of years. His daughter thinks that he may have an infection. His previous medical history includes chronic bronchitis and he recently had a pleural effusion drained in hospital. No cause was found. His nails are shown below:

Which of the following is the likely diagnosis?

- [ ] A   Onychogryphosis
- [ ] B   Psoriatic nail involvement
- [ ] C   Tinea unguium
- [ ] D   Yellow nail syndrome
- [ ] E   Trauma

THEME: SEXUALLY TRANSMITTED INFECTIONS

Options

A   Bacterial vaginosis

B   Chlamydia infection

C   Gonorrhoea

D   Herpes simplex

E   Herpes zoster

F   HIV

G   Lymphogranuloma venereum

H   Non-specific urethritis

I   Papillomavirus

J   Syphilis

For each description below, select the most appropriate diagnosis from the list of options. Each option may be used once, more than once or not at all.

☐ **180.** A 28-year-old man presents with a purulent urethral discharge after a one-night stand.

☐ **181.** A 39-year-old man with urethritis, conjunctivitis and arthritis.

☐ **182.** Four weeks after returning from a holiday where she had unprotected sex, a 34-year-old woman presents with painful unilateral inguinal swelling and urethritis. On examination she has a large fluctuant mass in her inguinal region.

☐ **183.** A painless papule develops on the shaft of the penis in a 34-year-old homosexual man. Over the next 3 weeks it breaks down to a superficial ulcer.

☐ **184.** A 29-year-old woman with a new partner complains of fever, malaise with pain, dysuria and itching in the vagina. On examination she has erythematous ulcers on the labia.

PAPER 4

185. With regard to screening trials, which one of the following statements is true?

☐ A Postal screening for *Chlamydia* is popular with high take-up rates

☐ B Magnetic resonance imaging (MRI) is more sensitive than mammography for screening high-risk women for breast cancer

☐ C Screening for undiagnosed abdominal aortic aneurysms reduces deaths with a number needed to screen of 2500

☐ D A trial of nurse-led screening of elderly people for common diseases showed significant reductions in mortality and morbidity

☐ E Screening for type 2 diabetes is cost-effective

186. Which one of the following statements about depression is true?

☐ A A meta-analysis of antidepressants in primary care found a number needed to treat of between 4 and 6

☐ B Fifty per cent of patients treated with antidepressants in primary care achieve remission

☐ C Only 50% of patients in primary care complete a course of antidepressants as prescribed

☐ D Cognitive behavioural therapy (CBT) is significantly more likely to bring about remission than antidepressants

☐ E The use of primary care mental health workers is associated with better outcomes than those achieved in control groups

THEME: ACUTE CEREBROVASCULAR EVENTS

Options

A   Anterior cerebral artery occlusion

B   Cerebellar infarction

C   Diffuse small vessel disease

D   Encephalitis

E   Hypertensive encephalopathy

F   Intracerebral haemorrhage

G   Middle cerebral artery occlusion

H   Multi-infarct dementia

I   Pontine infarction

J   Posterior inferior cerebellar artery occlusion

For each clinical description below, select the most appropriate diagnosis from the list of options. Each option may be used once, more than once or not at all.

187. A unilateral hemiparesis and hemisensory loss affecting the leg more than the arm.

188. A unilateral facial palsy, vomiting and vertigo with dysphagia, ataxia and Horner syndrome.

189. This presents subacutely as progressively increasing dementia.

190. A unilateral hemiparesis affecting the arm and face.

191. It often presents as coma, quadriplegia and multiple cranial nerve signs.

192. Results of a meta-analysis of studies for a new drug are presented below.

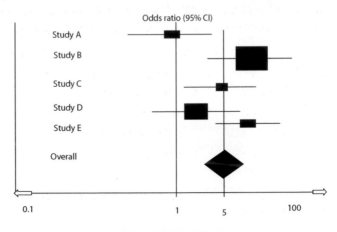

Which one of the following interpretations of this data is correct?

- [ ] A   Study A disproves the null hypothesis
- [ ] B   The meta-analysis suggests an overall odds ratio of 5 but the confidence intervals are wide, suggesting that there may be no effect
- [ ] C   Study D disproves the null hypothesis
- [ ] D   Study D taken on its own proves that the drug is effective
- [ ] E   An odds ratio of 1 suggests no relative risk reduction in the outcome

193. A 76-year-old man with a 4-month history of general malaise has routine blood test that shows a raised serum calcium and raised alkaline phosphatase (ALP). Which of the following statements about possible diagnoses is true? Select one option only.

☐ A Raised calcium and ALP is always caused by malignancy

☐ B Raised parathyroid hormone levels in the presence of a high calcium suggest hyperparathyroidism

☐ C Sarcoidosis causes hypocalcaemia

☐ D Myeloma often presents in this fashion

☐ E It may be a result of excess dietary calcium

194. Which one of the following statements about complementary therapy is true?

☐ A In a trial of acupuncture for tension-type headache, conventional acupuncture was significantly more effective than sham acupuncture

☐ B Over-the-counter use of herbal medications is of no clinical consequence

☐ C St John's wort is less effective than paroxetine

☐ D Studies have shown that herbal treatments are often mixed with conventional medicines

☐ E Homeopathy is not available on the NHS

PAPER 4

THEME: INCONTINENCE

195–200.

Options

A	Anticholinergic	H	Pelvic floor exercises
B	Blood tests	I	Prolapse
C	Desmopressin	J	Reassurance
D	HRT	K	Refer
E	Intermittent self-catheterisation	L	Sibutramine
		M	Ultrasonography
F	Long-term antibiotic	N	Weight loss
G	MSU		

For each stage in the flowchart below, select the most appropriate option from the list. Each option may be used once, more than once or not at all.

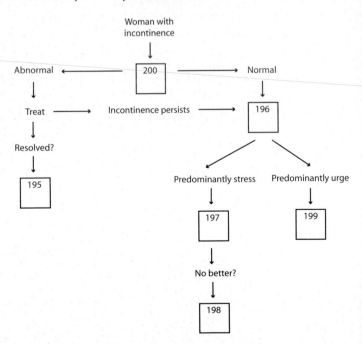

PAPER 4

Paper 4
Answers

1.   E: Condom use may reduce the risk of transmission

Caesarean section is indicated only for gross cervical warts. Carriers are often asymptomatic and perianal warts may, in some cases, be associated with anal intercourse. Warts often worsen during pregnancy and improve afterwards.

2.   C: Warfarin will prevent thrombotic occlusion of stenotic arteries

Aspirin is useful but there is no evidence for use of warfarin. Aggressive management of diabetes, cholesterol and hypertension, as well as smoking cessation, are critical. Cilostazol is a phosphodiesterase inhibitor and may improve walking distance by 50%.

3.   H: Intussusception

Intussusception is the most common cause of intestinal obstruction in infants, usually occurring between 6 and 9 months. A sausage-shaped mass may be felt on palpation and redcurrant jelly stool is often found on rectal examination.

4.   A: Acute appendicitis

Appendicitis is very uncommon below the age of 3. A retrocaecal appendix may have minimal abdominal signs.

5.   F: Infantile colic

Infantile colic usually starts around 2 weeks and lasts up to 3 months. Addition of lactase to feeds may be helpful.

PAPER 4

6.   I: Meckel's diverticulum

Meckel's diverticula are present in 2% of the population. They are usually asymptomatic but may cause symptoms of diverticulitis or rectal bleeding.

7.   L: Pneumonia

Lower lobe pneumonia may present with abdominal pain predominantly rather than respiratory signs.

8.   D: Henoch–Schönlein purpura

Henoch–Schönlein purpura is a vasculitis that typically affects the joints and kidneys and causes a purpuric rash over the buttocks and legs.

9.   C: DKA

DKA should be considered In anyone with symptoms suggestive of diabetes and complaints of abdominal pain should not distract from the symptoms of diabetes.

10.   M: Testicular torsion

A swollen scrotum is tender and red in torsion of the testis, swollen but not red and tender over the upper pole in torsion of the appendage of the testis, whereas an inguinal hernia is tender and inflamed only if strangulated.

11.   A: Her amoxicillin should be changed to ciprofloxacin

This woman is most probably suffering from *Clostridium difficile* infection. Strict hygiene procedures are necessary and alcohol hand washing alone is not sufficient to kill the infection. Confirmation of diagnosis is important to prevent spread.

PAPER 4

12.   B: A partial tear will usually show signs on examination other than tenderness and swelling in the mid-tendon

Achilles tendonitis usually presents with heel pain in young adults. The tendon is intact and treatment involves rest, ice, compression and elevation (RICE) followed by physiotherapy and orthoses. Partial tears often have negative tests for tear but a fusiform swelling. Both methods of treatment are equally efficacious in the first 2–3 days.

13.   E: It may be associated with oesophageal disease

Raynaud's phenomenon often occurs in young women and can be treated with calcium antagonists. It may be part of the CREST syndrome (**c**alcinosis, **R**aynaud's, **oe**sophageal dysmotility, **s**cleroderma and **t**elangiectasia) or cryoglobulinaemia, but this is rare. New onset in middle age should be investigated to exclude connective tissue disease or lymphoproliferative disease.

14.   E: It may be associated with autoimmune disease

Schirmer's test is a test of tear production. Dry eye may be caused by deficiency in the lacrimal glands, not the nasolacrimal duct. Symptoms are usually aggravated by warm air and topical antibiotics help only by their lubricating action, not their antibiotic action. Prolonged use may cause sensitivity.

15.   C: If he is a carrier and she is not they have a 50% risk of offspring being carriers

Cystic fibrosis is a recessive trait. If both parents are carriers the risk of an affected child is 25%, an unaffected child 25% and a child carrying the gene 50%. If she is not a carrier but he is, the risk is 50% of a child being a carrier and 50% not. If he is not a carrier there is still a chance that she will be a carrier because the gene is present in approximately 5% of the population.

PAPER 4

16.   E: Oral dexamethasone

For mild-to-moderate croup a single dose of dexamethasone is often effective in settling symptoms. Supportive measures such as reassurance and treating any associated fever are helpful. Where children have more severe symptoms admission should be considered. For children in extremis, epinephrine nebulisers are effective but close monitoring is necessary because this lasts only 2–3 hours and recurrence is likely.

17.   D: Ischaemic optic neuropathy

18.   A: Pleural effusions are always visible on chest radiograph

Pleural effusions have to be > 300 ml to be seen on a chest radiograph. Exudative effusions may be caused by infection, infarction, tumour or inflammatory processes. Transudative effusions may be the result of hypoproteinaemia, ascites or heart failure.

19.   E: None of the above

Down syndrome is usually caused by a spontaneous mutation during meiosis rather than an inherited trait. Where one parent carries a balanced translocation there is a higher risk of recurrence, but where a mother is under 36 and the baby does not have a translocated chromosome, the recurrence risk is 1/100. Ninety per cent of children survive to only age 5 years, usually because of congenital heart defects.

20.   E: Alcohol consumption is a risk factor only when the weekly consumption exceeds 50 units in men and 42 units in women

Alcohol consumption > 35 units a week doubles risk of stroke. It is estimated that reducing daily salt intake from 10 g to 5 g will reduce systolic BP by 3–5 mmHg.

21.   **E:**   **Manipulation under anaesthetic is best performed 5–7 days after injury**

Treatment in the absence of complications is indicated only where there is cosmetic deformity and is best performed 5–7 days after injury, when swelling has subsided and the bones are more likely to unite. Radiological imaging is seldom helpful other than excluding associated facial fracture. Clear rhinorrhoea may be a sign of CSF leak and prompts further assessment. Septal haematomas should be drained promptly to prevent septal perforation.

22.   **F:**   **Lymphoedema**

Lymphoedema causes chronic painless oedema of the lower legs. Oedema is usually pitting initially but later becomes not pitting. Causes include lymphatic obstruction, eg tumour.

23.   **I:**   **Superficial thrombophlebitis**

Superficial thrombophlebitis usually responds to local heat, elevation and non-steroidal drugs.

24.   **E:**   **Intermittent claudication**

Buerger's test involves elevating the leg until it goes pale, and is a sign of peripheral vascular disease.

25.   **C:**   **Deep vein thrombosis (DVT)**

DVTs may be asymptomatic or may present as a pulmonary embolus (PE).

PAPER 4

26.   H: Ruptured Baker's cyst

Baker's cysts are synovial cysts in the popliteal fossa. They are often seen in rheumatoid arthritis and, if they rupture, may be confused with a DVT.

27.   C: NICE guidelines on social value judgements justify discrimination on the basis of age in some situations

An editorial in the *British Journal of General Practice* in 2007 discussed this area. In older patients, GPs are less likely to seek information on lifestyle, check cholesterol or refer patients with angina. Comparative studies found this to be as likely with GPs, cardiologists and elderly care physicians. Where age is an indicator of benefit or risk, NICE supports discrimination. Elderly people are largely under-represented in trials. QOF exception reporting for stroke is associated with age and female sex.

28.   B: Finasteride is safe and effective

5α-Reductase inhibitors are effective in androgenic baldness. Minoxidil is effective only while being taken. Baldness is a side effect of testosterone therapy, whereas pyrithione zinc is a treatment for dandruff. Cyproterone acetate is used in women with PCOS. Cyproterone acetate is used for severe hypersexuality in men and causes reversible infertility with abnormal sperm. Animal studies have shown an association with hepatic tumours.

29.   E: Intramuscular phenytoin

Absorption of intramuscular phenytoin is slow and erratic. Where used it should be given by slow intravenous injection. Intravenous or buccal lorazepam/intranasal midazolam should be used as a first-line treatment. The maintenance of oxygenation and airway management are essential.

PAPER 4

30.   A: Threadworm infestation

Threadworm is the most common parasitic infection in the UK and typically affects young children causing pruritus ani. The scratching causes re-infection via the faeco-oral route. Occasionally patients or their parents report seeing worms in the toilet. The whole family should be treated, with a second dose 1–2 weeks later. Hookworm is seen in the tropics and tapeworm arises from eating infected meat, and is rare in the UK.

31.   E: Children with dyslexia do not qualify for a 'Statement of Special Educational Needs'

Dyslexia is more common in boys and there is often a positive family history with a dominant inheritance pattern with variable penetrance. Educational support is vital and children often cope better with computers at school, rather than pen and paper. Examination boards are usually able to make concessions.

32.   E: All of the above

Prognosis in petit mal epilepsy is worst in those with generalised seizures, IQ < 90 or frequent seizures. Hyperventilation during an EEG will usually demonstrate the classic 3-second spike.

33.   E: Excision

This is a basal cell carcinoma and should be treated with excision, ideally by a plastic surgeon in this location. Curettage may be appropriate for small lesions on the scalp but recurrence is common. Diclofenac is a treatment for actinic keratosis.

PAPER 4

34.   E: Diabetes increases the risk of developing ischaemic heart disease by 200–300%

Smoking, diabetes and hypertension increase the risk by 200–300% each. The mini-pill is safe, and is the oral contraceptive of choice in smokers over the age of 35. All people with diabetes should be considered for statins.

35.   E: Hyperthyroidism

This is a typical presentation of hyperthyroidism. Bowel transit is often speeded up but diarrhoea is rare. The condition is common, and most cases are caused by Graves' disease or multinodular goitre.

36.   D: Health belief model

Trigger factors may be advice from family or friends, messages from the media or disruption to work.

37.   F: Neighbour's model

Neighbour's model includes connection with the patient, summarising the problem, handing over responsibility for management, safety netting and house keeping.

38.   H: Triaxial RCGP model

Under the triaxial model the problem should be considered under these terms.

39.   G: Pendelton

Pendelton's model was the basis of the video assessment for summative assessment.

40.   E: Helman's folk model

What has happened, why has it happened, why me, why now, what would happen if nothing is done about it and what should I do about it?

41.   C: Acute MI is a risk factor for acute heart failure

Acute heart failure is usually precipitated by acute MI or arrhythmias, although chronic heart failure is usually caused by ischaemic heart disease, hypertension or valve disease. Malignant hypertension may cause acute heart failure.

42.   A: The report on a DS1500 should include the diagnosis, regardless of whether or not the patient knows it

There is space to indicate whether or not the patient is aware of the diagnosis. The form may be given to a patient's representative, and is used when life expectancy is thought to be < 6 months.

43.   B: Avian influenza is spread by contaminated droppings and respiratory secretions

The mortality rate from H5N1 is over 50% but the infectivity for humans is low. Influenza incubation is 1–4 days and infectivity lasts up to 1 week in children. There are reports of resistance to Tamiflu in wild-type influenza virus and this is likely to increase as its use becomes more widespread.

44.   D: Cervical smears have a number needed to screen of 1000 to prevent one death

Liquid-based cytology reduces 'inadequate smear' rates by 75%. The main source of error is subjective interpretation of the smear. The incidence of cancer has fallen by 42% since 1988. Screening occurs at 3-yearly intervals.

PAPER 4

45.   D: Shock, denial, anger/guilt, depression, acceptance

46.   A: This condition should be treated as an emergency and the patient referred to the on-call team

Treatment must be instituted within 48 hours for a good prognosis, and all such patients should be discussed with the on-call ENT team. There are no convincing data to support any particular treatment, but high-dose steroids and aciclovir are widely used. Vertigo is associated with a poor prognosis as is high-frequency loss. Recovery usually takes place over 2–4 weeks.

47.   D: Local steroid injection

Local steroid injection is the most effective treatment for early disease. Splinting and non-steroidals are not effective in the short or medium term. For recurrent disease surgical exploration is indicated.

48.   C: Excessive forward movement of the tibia suggests an anterior cruciate tear

The anterior cruciate ligament (ACL) prevents excessive forward movement of the tibia, whereas the posterior cruciate ligament (PCL) prevents sagging or backward movement. Excessive varus movement of the knee suggests a lateral collateral ligament tear

49.   C: Fluvastatin and erythromycin

Verapamil and β blockers in combination can cause atrioventricular (AV) block. Statins should be stopped while patients are on macrolides.

50.   C: He should be treated with an NSAID and if pain resolves can be discharged

This patient is suffering from acute pericarditis and can be treated with an NSAID and, if well, discharged. If there are signs of pericardial effusion he should have echocardiography.

51.   A: It is caused by excess secretion of ADH by the pituitary

Diabetes insipidus is caused by either insufficient production of ADH (cranial diabetes insipidus) or insensitivity of the kidneys to ADH (nephrogenic diabetes insipidus). Desmopressin is very effective and thiazide diuretics, chlorpropamide and carbamazepine are also used in some cases.

52.   E: It may be iatrogenic

Medications such as thiazide diuretics increase uric acid levels and may precipitate acute attacks of gout. Dietary causes are less common than they once were because of changes in diet; in the past diets rich in purines were often responsible. The photograph demonstrates gouty tophi, which are permanent. This is a clinical diagnosis.

53.   E: Arterial ulcer

This is a typical description of an arterial ulcer, with pain especially at night. Elevating the leg exacerbates pain and three may be a history of ischaemic arterial disease elsewhere.

54.   A: Trigeminal neuralgia

This is a typical history of trigeminal neuralgia. Glossopharyngeal neuralgia affects the distribution of the glossopharyngeal nerve. Ramsay Hunt syndrome causes vertigo, deafness and a rash in the ear. Acoustic neuroma can cause trigeminal nerve signs but they are not paroxysmal.

PAPER 4

55.   J: Risperidone

Risperidone was previously widely used for agitation in elderly confused people. Haloperidol is more appropriate.

56.   H: Haloperidol

Haloperidol is effective for agitation and less likely to cause falls in elderly confused people.

57.   E: Fluoxetine

SSRIs are preferable to tricyclic antidepressants because of the propensity of the latter to cause confusion.

58.   G: Gingko

Gingko seems to be effective but may increase risk of bleeding.

59.   I: Memantine

Memantine has a good side-effect profile and has been shown to halve the risk of deterioration in moderate-to-severe Alzheimer's disease.

60.   E: Methotrexate can be used as a steroid-sparing agent

True power is not affected, but there is frequently significant tenderness. Systemic symptoms are common, with a male:female ratio of 1:3. Most patients require treatment for around 2 years.

61.   C: It may be precipitated by over-zealous use of cotton buds

Otitis externa is an inflammation of the skin of the external auditory meatus and is commonly precipitated by heat, humidity, swimming or trauma. It frequently involves a bacterial component but viral and fungal pathogens may also be seen, particularly after prolonged use of steroid drops. It is often impossible to see the eardrum in the acute phase but use of aminoglycoside drops is safe and effective for short periods. Malignant otitis externa may be seen in immunocompromised individuals, particularly people with diabetes, and may be fatal.

62.   N: Topical clindamycin

Topical metronidazole or clindamycin may produce beneficial results in many patients. In those who do not respond oral antibiotics are indicated.

63.   M: Tacrolimus

Tacrolimus may be used as a steroid-sparing agent or in patients who are resistant to steroids.

64.   F: Emollients

Emollients should be a first-line treatment in all patients with eczema.

65.   A: Benzoyl peroxide

Benzoyl peroxide should be used at a low strength initially and may cause some initial irritation.

66.   C: Calcipotriol

Calcipotriol has few side effects and does not stain clothes. It may be combined with steroids for short periods.

PAPER 4

67.   C: It is an inevitable consequence of noise exposure without ear protection

Noise-induced hearing loss arises from a variety of sources of noise exposure and may be occupational or recreational. Susceptibility depends on the individual and there is some variation according to age and gender. It often affects one ear more than the other, particularly in shooters, and examination findings are usually normal. Audiology typically shows a dip at 4–6 kHz. Treatment is aimed at restoring hearing through aids and managing tinnitus, which often results from hearing loss.

68.   C: Patients with multiple TIAs occurring over a short period of time should refrain from driving until 3 months after attacks have ceased

Isolated TIAs require 1 month off driving and the DVLA needs to be informed only if there is focal neurological deficit, eg visual field loss.

69.   G: UK PDS

The UK Prospective Diabetes Study showed a 56% reduction in heart failure and 44% reduction in stroke with tight blood pressure control.

70.   C: HOPE

The Heart Outcomes Prevention Evaluation Trial study found reductions in myocardial infarction, stroke and cardiovascular deaths in people with diabetes.

71.   B: DREAM

The Diabetes Reduction Assessment with ramipril and rosiglitazone Medication Trial has so far shown that rosiglitazone may reduce the incidence of diabetes.

72.   E: MICRO-HOPE

The Microalbuminuria, Cardiovascular and Renal Outcomes in Heart Outcomes Prevention Evaluation Trial also found that ramipril reduced the incidence of type 2 diabetes if given to those at risk.

73.   D: HPS

The Heart Protection Study gave all participants 40 mg simvastatin and found reduced coronary deaths, strokes and cardiovascular events.

74.   A: Primary nodal osteoarthritis

This is a typical appearance of nodal osteoarthritis. Seropositive arthritis and gout usually cause erythema and pain. Myxoid cysts affect the distal interphalangeal joint but are soft.

75.   D: Drusen

Drusen are a sign of macular degeneration. Malignant hypertension causes cotton-wool spots, flame haemorrhages and disc swelling, whereas vitreous haemorrhage may be a complication of uncontrolled hypertension.

76.   D: A patient must be mentally competent to set up an Enduring Power of Attorney

Where a patient is not competent to set up an Enduring Power of Attorney, an application must be made to the Court of Protection. An attorney has full control over financial assets and can dispose of them as he or she sees fit. The fee can be reduced in cases of hardship or low income. Any fee payable for a medical examination to determine competence is additional, as are solicitors' fees. A Lasting Power of Attorney allows an attorney to make decisions about health and welfare.

PAPER 4

77.   C: She should be thoroughly examined for a strangulated hernia

These symptoms are suggestive of bowel obstruction, probably as a result of adhesions. Strangulated hernias should be excluded, particularly small femoral hernias. Ischaemic bowel is usually seen in patients with pre-existing cardiovascular disease and presents acutely. It usually presents with bloody diarrhoea.

78.   D: Chlamydial infections may cause entropion

Chlamydia trachomatis is a common cause of blindness worldwide and causes entropion, leading to eye trauma. Not all Bell's palsy patients recover and some may need surgery to allow full eyelid closure. Cicatrisation causes an ectropion. Ptosis may develop at any age, eg myasthenia gravis.

79.   D: Asians and African–Caribbeans are significantly over-represented among patients with end-stage renal failure

A survey of 1.8 million patient records (*BMJ* 2004) found significant differences between levels of diabetic care for different groups according to ethnicity and level of deprivation. A study of revascularisation rates in the *BMJ* in 2002 confirmed differences in revascularisation but found no difference in mortality. Indian children are more likely to consult their GP but less likely to use hospital services. The incidence of cardiovascular risk factors, including diabetes, tends to be significantly higher among South Asians.

80.   E: Forty-four per cent of injecting drug users are infected with hepatitis C

Three million people in the UK are estimated to use cannabis. Cannabis cigarettes are associated with four times the levels of tar deposition in the respiratory tract as tobacco cigarettes. Cannabis was reclassified as a class B drug in January 2009. A quarter of 14-year-old boys have tried cannabis. A study in the *BMJ* in 2005 found a prevalence of 44% for hepatitis C and 4% for HIV.

PAPER 4

81.   D: Henoch–Schönlein purpura

HSP is a vasculitis with a typical rash affecting the legs. There may also be urticaria or oedema and nephritis is common. The arthralgia usually lasts a few days only, and usually occurs between the ages of 3 and 8, more frequently in boys. Treatment is supportive.

82.   D: Advertisements for functional foods cannot make claims for efficacy without scientific data to back their claims

The European Union is the biggest worldwide market and is introducing regulation. At present nutritional claims can be made only after assessment and authorisation by the European Food Safety Authority. Many functional foods interact with prescription drugs, eg phytosterols and statins.

83.   A: Achalasia

Achalasia often causes recurrent chest infections resulting from nocturnal aspiration.

84.   K: Plummer–Vinson syndrome

Plummer–Vinson syndrome consists of iron-deficient anaemia and dysphagia as a result of a post-cricoid web.

85.   C: Carcinoma of the oesophagus

Oesophageal carcinoma presents with progressive dysphagia. Regurgitation or blood stained vomiting may also be a feature.

PAPER 4

86.   J: Pharyngeal pouch

Pharyngeal pouches are often associated with recurrent chest infections.

87.   D: Chronic benign stricture

Strictures are usually seen on a background of longstanding reflux.

88.   A: It may be caused by reduced saliva production

Halitosis may be subjective or objective, and usually has an intraoral cause, the most common of which is poor dental hygiene. Reduced saliva production is also a common cause, particularly in patients with salivary gland disease, eg Sjögren syndrome. It may also be a sign of systemic disease such as bronchiectasis or diabetes. Management is aimed at the underlying cause and usually starts with the dentist.

89.   E: Heliox may be helpful in managing stridor

This man has superior vena caval obstruction. Symptoms may be managed in the short term with oral steroids or anticoagulation if thrombus is the cause. Heliox is helpful for stridor because it is of lower density than air. Treatment should be aimed at the site of the obstruction, usually with radiotherapy, not the primary lesion.

90.   D: APOLLO measures the extent of exception reporting by indicator

Exception reporting applies to whole disease areas and indicators. Exception must be clinically justified or by informed dissent, so exclusion on the basis of age alone is not justified.

91.   A: Myasthenia gravis

This is a typical description of myasthenia gravis, with symptoms exacerbated by exertion and preferentially affecting the upper limbs and eyes. Diagnosis may be confirmed by a Tensilon test, injection of a short-acting acetylcholinesterace inhibitor. PMR does not affect eye movements and internuclear ophthalmoplegia and MS would not present in this way.

92.   C: Glucosamine

Randomised controlled trials comparing glucosamine with placebo have shown that at 3 years joint space narrowing in the knee is significantly less in patients taking glucosamine. There is some evidence for chondroitin, but no statistically significant RCT data as yet. Gingko is of proven benefit in memory impairment.

93.   D: It may be a sign of malignant melanoma

Detachment may be a sign of retinoblastoma or melanoma. It is more common in people with myopia and after trauma. All detachments require surgical assessment and most will require surgery. Examination reveals a grey featureless sheet in the affected portion of the retina. Ninety per cent of patients have a good outcome after a single operation.

94.   F: Odds ratio

95.   H: QALY

QALYs quantify both increased longevity and the quality of that extra longevity, eg an increase in life expectancy from 1 year to 5 years, but at a quality of life 50% of the previous, would give 4 × 50% = 2 QALYs.

PAPER 4

96. **A: Confounding factor**

Confounding factors usually relate to pre-existing health or medication usage.

97. **J: Standard deviation**

98. **D: Intention-to-treat analysis**

An example would be a trial of an analgesic whereby all patients are studied according to allocation to control or intervention, regardless of whether they actually took the treatment.

99. **A: He has Crohn's disease**

The mainstay of treatment of Crohn's disease is steroids and sulfasalazine. Surgery should be avoided. The disease can affect any part of the alimentary tract.

100. **D: Most patients require one dose of radiotherapy only**

Palliative radiotherapy is often one dose but, where a cure or longer-term control is the aim, prolonged courses are often necessary. Cerebral oedema is common so many patients are given dexamethasone.

101. **B: The 5-year survival rate for breast cancer is 80%**

Data for 2001 showed 5-year survival rates of 60% for prostate, 50% for colon and 5% for lung cancer. The 10-year survival rate for all cancers is 46% in the UK.

102.   D: Keratoacanthoma

Keratoacanthomas tend to develop on exposed skin such as the hands or face. They grow rapidly and have a central keratin-filled crater. They develop rapidly over 3–4 weeks and spontaneously regress from 6 weeks. The main differential is squamous cell carcinoma.

103.   B: Anaemia of chronic disease

A normochromic/normocytic anaemia with normal iron stores is often seen in chronic disease.

104.   D: Chronic renal failure

Chronic renal failure often causes a normochronic/normocytic anaemia with burr cells on the film. Diabetes is one of the most common causes of chronic renal failure in the UK.

105.   C: Aplastic anaemia

Pancytopenia and macrocytosis are seen in aplastic anaemia.

106.   G: Myeloma

These features are suggestive of myeloma.

107.   H: Pernicious anaemia

Pernicious anaemia can be confirmed with serum testing of antibodies against parietal cells and intrinsic factor. A test dose of vitamin B_{12} followed by a FBC after 1 week will show a rise in reticulocytes.

PAPER 4

108.   C: He should be advised to use dilute baby shampoo to clean the eyelids twice a day and a short course of fucithalmic eye drops

He has blepharitis, a common condition usually caused by staphylococcal infection of the eyelid margin. It may be associated with chronic conjunctivitis and should be treated with meticulous lid cleaning and a short course of topical fucithalmic. Chronic blepharitis may be seen with rosacea and if so should be treated with oral tetracycline.

109.   D: Splenomegaly occurs in 50% of patients

Subclinical infection is very common. After a prodromal phase, lethargy, malaise, headache, stiff neck and dry cough are common symptoms. Fifty per cent of symptomatic patients have a sore throat and pharyngitis. Neither antibiotics nor steroids are effective in shortening the disease. Most symptomatic patients take 4–6 weeks to recover. Ampicillin use is associated with an erythematous rash.

110.   D: Complications include amyloidosis

The most likely diagnosis is osteomyelitis. A radiograph should be performed to confirm the diagnosis. Common organisms include *Staphylococcus aureus*, *Escherichia coli* and *Streptococcus pyogenes*. TB should be considered in those with a history of TB. Marjolin's ulcer is a squamous cell carcinoma that can complicate longstanding osteomyelitis. Clindamycin is a good long-term antibiotic choice because it penetrates bone well. Cephalosporins are an alternative in patients allergic to clindamycin. Surgery is usually necessary once sequestrum has formed.

111.   D: It can result from portal hypertension

Melaena can arise from any point in the upper gastrointestinal tract from swallowed blood caused by epistaxis to duodenal ulcers. NSAIDs and other drugs can cause gastric bleeding. Portal hypertension leads to the development of oesophageal varices. All patients need urgent upper gastrointestinal endoscopy.

112.   I: Malaria

Fever in a returning traveller from an endemic area should be considered to be malaria until proven otherwise, particularly where prophylaxis has not been used.

113.   H: Leishmaniasis

Cutaneous leishmaniasis should be considered in travellers from endemic areas who have non-healing ulcers.

114.   J: Meningitis

Meningitis outbreaks are not uncommon among Hajj pilgrims and where possible participants should be immunised before travel.

115.   D: Hepatitis A

Hepatitis A is usually spread by the faeco-oral route, often through contaminated shellfish. It usually settles with rest.

116.   E: Hepatitis B

Hepatitis B causes no symptoms in 50% of patients. Those who do develop symptoms typically have an incubation period of 30–180 days and develop florid jaundice. Most patients clear the virus successfully and become immune.

117.   C: Diphtheria

Diphtheria is highly contagious and has an incubation period of 2–4 days. It may cause peripheral neuropathy and cardiomyopathy, and can also cause skin ulcers. It is endemic in much of Asia and Russia.

PAPER 4

118. **C:** **Treatment A reduces the rate of hip fracture more than treatment B**

The Kaplan–Meier graph plots the number of a group 'surviving' without an event against time. Thus a treatment that slows the decline in survival is beneficial. This study compares two treatment groups rather than a placebo group.

119. **A:** **Four-layer bandaging is often helpful in combination with elevation of the limb**

Four-layer bandaging is very effective once ischaemia has been excluded and will often reduce swelling to the point where compression hosiery may be used. Low-dose diuretics are of no long-term benefit; nor are antibiotics unless infection is present. Varicose vein surgery is indicated only if there is evidence of venous insufficiency. Hypoalbuminaemia is seldom seen in chronic cases in the community.

120. **D:** **Penile cancer**

Penile cancer is rare in the UK, more commonly seen in patients from Asia and Africa. It is associated with poor hygiene and herpes infections. It is locally destructive and often causes difficulty in retracting the foreskin. The 5-year survival rate with lymph-node involvement is around 50%.

121. **F:** **Nasal polyps**

Nasal polyps tend to cause longstanding nasal obstruction with anosmia and poor taste.

122. **G:** **Nasal vestibulitis**

This may require prolonged courses of anti-staphylococcal antibiotics.

123.   H: Nasopharyngeal carcinoma

Nasopharyngeal carcinoma is more common in patients from Asia and those exposed to wood dusts.

124.   I: Perennial rhinitis

These are classic symptoms of perennial rhinitis.

125.   E: Foreign body

Unilateral nasal discharge in children is almost always caused by a foreign body.

126.   D: Numbness in buttocks and perineum

Urinary incontinence and lower motor neurone signs in the legs with sensory loss suggest cauda equine lesions. Other red flags include night pain, age < 20 or > 55 years, systemic signs and history of malignant disease. Prolonged incapacity is a 'yellow flag' – an indicator of poor prognosis in terms of social functioning. Others include low socioeconomic class.

127.   A: Macular degeneration

This is a typical history of macular degeneration. Cataract causes gradual loss of acuity but not distortion of lines, glaucoma causes loss of peripheral vision while sparing central vision, and retinal detachment causes a segmental loss of visual field as does retinal vein occlusion.

128.   E: Countries where a system of presumed consent operates have three times the rate of organ donation

Around 400 people a year die in the UK waiting for a transplant. Although 90% of the population reportedly support organ donation, only 23% are registered donors. There have been calls to introduce presumed consent, but at present the system operates on a basis of explicit consent. Spain has a policy of presumed consent, but relatives are consulted; it has the highest rate of organ donation in the world.

129.   D: Infectious endocarditis

The classic diagnostic triad of infectious endocarditis is fever, new or changing murmurs and embolic phenomena. Risk factors include intravenous drug abuse, artificial heart valves, congenital defects, eg VSD, and invasive surgical procedures especially dental work.

130.   C: They may present with a hydrocele

Testicular cancer is the most common malignancy in young men. Ninety-two per cent are malignant and are usually seminomas or teratomas. Orchidectomy via an inguinal incision is the treatment of choice. In older patients testicular tumours may be lymphomas.

131.   D: *BRCA*-1 gene

The genes *BRCA*-1 and *BRCA*-2 are associated with familial breast and ovarian cancer. A woman with the *BRCA*-1 mutation has a 40–60% risk of developing ovarian cancer by age 70.

132.   F: *NF1* gene

NF1 is seen in familial neurofibromatosis and these patients have higher incidence of acoustic neuromas.

133.   B: Autosomal dominant inheritance

Autosomal dominant genes are seen in most generations; recessives often skip generations.

134.   I: Sporadic cancer

Oncogenes account directly for the minority of cancers, although they often increase the risk of exposure to other risk factors.

135.   A: *APC* gene

A tumour suppressor gene that is mutated in familial adenomatous polyposis, an autosomal dominant trait with early onset colorectal cancer.

136.   A: They are more common in white people

Keloids are more common in non-white people. They may be seen after minor skin trauma, acne scarring or immunisations. Recurrence after excision may be reduced by topical steroids or intralesional steroid injections.

137.   C: Tenderness at the base of the fifth metatarsal indicates the need for a radiograph of the foot

Application of Ottawa rules results in a sensitivity of almost 100%. The malleolar zones extend 6 cm above each malleolus. The four zones are the malleoli, base of the fifth metatarsal and navicular. Inability to weight-bear requires a radiograph. Ottawa rules have been developed for ankle, knee and foot injuries.

PAPER 4

138. **D:** **A visitor from the USA on a 4-week European tour requests a repeat prescription of her simvastatin**

NHS treatment is available for European Union residents with valid documentation, those in need of immediately necessary treatment, or those who are ordinarily resident in the UK, including asylum seekers and refugees. EHICs apply to immediately necessary and emergency treatment, not planned treatment.

139. **E:** **A 3rd cranial nerve palsy is common and indicates a posterior communicating artery aneurysm, basilar artery aneurysm or transtentorial herniation**

Most patients are over 40 years old. There is often a prodromal period with headache. Fifty per cent present with a seizure or short-lived collapse. Meningism develops 3–12 hours after the bleed. Blood pressure rises acutely. Plantars are usually extensor and fundus examination may show papilloedema.

140. **A:** **It can be brought on by pregnancy**

Hiatus hernia often presents after weight gain or in pregnancy. The initial management should include weight loss, alginates and lifestyle changes. Rolling hiatus hernias can strangulate and also predispose to aspiration and chest infections.

141. **C:** **To prevent errors, at least two pieces of identifiable data should be used at every occasion, eg date of birth and NHS number**

The minimum amount of identifiable data should be used on every occasion, and this includes sharing data within the PCT. Every member of staff with access to information should be trained and audit should be used to monitor compliance.

142. **A:** **Acute epididymitis**

Prehn's sign is indicative of epididymitis. A secondary hydrocele may often develop. Testicular torsion usually causes swelling around the testis rather than the epididymis. Testicular cancer is usually painless.

143. **F:** **RAPD**

RAPD detects afferent lesions affecting one eye. In this case the pupil would not constrict when light is shone into it but would constrict when light is shone into the opposite eye.

144. **D:** **Cranial nerve VI palsy**

The lateral rectus is innervated by cranial nerve VI.

145. **C:** **Cranial nerve IV palsy**

The superior rectus is innervated by cranial nerve IV.

146. **E:** **Internuclear ophthalmoplegia**

This may be a sign of multiple sclerosis.

147.   C: Cranial nerve IV palsy

148.   B: Give a verbal warning and record this in her records

The rules relating to disciplinary procedure are rigid and require two verbal warnings to be given before a written warning, and only then can dismissal take place. Failure to follow this may result in an industrial tribunal. Reporting the matter to the police, punitive fines and ritual humiliation are unlikely to result in rehabilitation of the worker.

149.   B: Pelvic examination

This woman has symptoms consistent with a pelvic mass causing compression of her common iliac veins. Pelvic examination and ultrasonography are mandatory in this situation. Doppler ultrasonography is not reliable in detecting below-knee DVT.

150.   E: Patients should set a stop date and be prescribed enough nicotine replacement products for a period of 2 weeks after this date, at which time their progress should be reviewed

Bupropion should not be used in the under-18s, or pregnant or breast-feeding women. Combination therapy is not recommended. Bupropion should be started 2 weeks before the planned stop date.

151.   C: Topical treatment with mupirocin is usually adequate

Most cases of impetigo are the result of staphylococcal or streptococcal infections. Fusidic acid is associated with high levels of resistance; mupirocin is a better choice for topical treatment. Where there is failure to respond phenoxymethylpenicillin should be added to flucloxacillin, because there is often co-infection with streptococci. Strict hygiene measures (eg not sharing towels) help to prevent spread to siblings.

PAPER 4

152.   F: Levodopa

L-Dopa is usually given with a decarboxylase inhibitor to reduce the dopa dose while maintaining the intracerebral level, reducing nausea and vomiting.

153.   J: Selegiline

Combination of selegiline with L-dopa has been shown to increase mortality in one long-term follow-up study.

154.   E: Entacapone

Entacapone inhibits levodopa breakdown and smoothes out fluctuations, allowing a dose reduction.

155.   B: Apomorphine

Apomorphine may be useful where the patient or a carer is able to give injections.

156.   D: Domperidone

Domperidone is useful adjunctive treatment where iatrogenic nausea occurs.

157–163.

The most recent data from the Office of National Statistics (up to 1998) suggest the following results. The most striking sex differences are seen in anxiety and depression, which are much more common in women.

157.   F: 65

158.   E: 75

159. **D:** 7.4

160. **G:** 39.4

161. **B:** 1.8

162. **A:** 50

163. **C:** 4.3

164. **B:** Six months of combination treatment with clopidogrel and aspirin should be given after an NSTEMI

After an NSTEMI, 4 weeks of aspirin/clopidogrel is indicated, whereas after an acute non-ST-elevation acute coronary syndrome 12 months' treatment is indicated.

165. **E:** Population screening followed by eradication treatment is effective and feasible in reducing consultations and symptoms

NICE guidelines suggest that, for low-risk patients aged under 55, a test-and-treat policy with testing for *H. pylori* is safe and effective. Eradication of *H. pylori* will reduce recurrence rates of duodenal ulcer by 50%. Application of the test-and-treat policy has been shown to reduce referrals for endoscopy by 19%. The CADET-Hp trial demonstrated benefits for test-and-treat compared with acid suppression alone. The MRC-CUBE trial found no improvement in QALYs or costs but symptoms were slightly better. The Bristol Helicobacter Project showed population screening to be effective although the costs of treating asymptomatic people would seem to favour a test-and-treat strategy.

PAPER 4

166.   D: 900/950

Sensitivity = true positives on testing/all positives = 900/(900 + 50)

167.   B: 900/1000

PPV = true positives/test positives = 900/(900 + 100)

168.   I: 950/1050

Specificity = true negatives on testing/all negatives = 950/(100 + 950)

169.   H: 950/1000

NPV = true negatives/test negatives = 950/(50 + 950)

170.   A: Burnout is associated with excessive discussions about past mistakes

There have been numerous studies looking at occupational stress in GPs and this has been shown to average 28%, significantly higher than in the general population, where it averages out at 18%. Female GPs in particular find visits stressful and have been found in some studies to be more likely to self-medicate and to be less likely to seek help than their male counterparts. Availability of occupational health services is less of a problem than lack of use by those in need. GPs who feel they see more patients than their colleagues are more likely to experience burnout.

171.   D: Increased dietary fibre might help to reduce attacks

Acute diverticulitis should be treated with broad-spectrum antibiotics, such as co-amoxiclav or cefradine and metronidazole. Mesalazine is used for colitis and mebeverine for irritable bowel syndrome. Once the acute episode has settled the patient should be referred for a barium enema.

PAPER 4

172.   A: Carpal tunnel

The median nerve is compressed as it passes through the carpal tunnel.

173.   D: Golfers' elbow

Golfers' elbow or medical epicondylitis is characterised by pain in the flexor area of the arm and tenderness over the medial epicondyle.

174.   B: De Quervain's tenosynovitis

De Quervain's tenosynovitis is usually seen in women over the age of 50 and is caused by excessive abduction of the thumb, eg rose pruning.

175.   G: Tennis elbow

Initial therapy for tennis elbow consists of rest, splints and steroid injection; recurrent cases may require surgery.

176.   C: Dupuytren's contracture

Trigger finger causes difficulty in extending the finger but can be overcome. Dupuytren's contracture causes progressive fibrosis that cannot be overcome.

177.   D: Schizophrenia

Schizophrenia is usually associated with thought disorder, persistence, functional deterioration and age at onset < 45 years. The main differential diagnosis is drug-induced psychosis.

178.   A: Phaeochromocytoma

One to two in every 1000 cases of hypertension are caused by phaeochromocytomas. They produce systemic effects and attacks may be paroxysmal. These symptoms, when seen with labile hypertension, should prompt 24-hour urine collection for VMA (vanillylmandelic acid).

179.   D: Yellow nail syndrome

Although this diagnosis is rare, this question demonstrates the changes typical in different nail diseases. Yellow nail syndrome is associated with bronchiectasis, pleural effusion and sinusitis, and causes excessive growth and yellowing of the nails, with all nails affected, and characteristic curvature. Onychogryphosis usually affects toenails only and in particular the great toe. Psoriatic nail changes may be seen in the absence of skin changes but usually produce pitting. Trauma and fungal infections are unlikely to affect all nails.

180.   C: Gonorrhoea

Gonorrhoea usually presents as a purulent cervical or urethral discharge. It may also present with arthritis, rectal discharge and proctalgia or pharyngitis, depending on how it is acquired.

181.   B: Chlamydia infection

Chlamydia is a frequent cause of Reiter syndrome.

182.   G: Lymphogranuloma venereum

LGV is caused by *Chlamydia trachomatis*. There may be a preceding genital lesion in a third of patients.

183.   J: Syphilis

Primary syphilis may be seen on the penis, rectum, cervix or labia. The chancre generally heals in 4–6 weeks.

184.   D: Herpes simplex

Eighty per cent of women with primary herpes infections have cervical or urethral involvement; 50–90% of cases have recurrent lesions within a 12-month period.

185.   B: MRI is more sensitive than mammography for screening high-risk women for breast cancer

A study of postal screening in men and women aged 16–39 years had only a one-third take-up (*BMJ* 2005). The Magnetic Resonance Imaging for Breast Screening (MARIBS) study showed that MRI is more sensitive but less specific than mammography. The Multicentre Aneurysm Screening Study (MASS) found an NNS (number needed to screen) of 352 to prevent one aneurysm-related death but increased operations by up to 400%. Trial of multidimensional assessment of older patients by nurses in the *Lancet* showed no benefits. A combination of risk-factor identification and ultrasonography has been shown to identify 90% of patients with osteoporosis.

186.   A: A meta-analysis of antidepressants in primary care found a number needed to treat of between 4 and 6

Less than 10% of patients in primary care complete a course of antidepressants as prescribed. Meta-analysis of placebo vs SSRI or tricyclic depressant (*Annals of Family Medicine* 2005) showed that, for every person who responds, between three and five did not. A pan-European study of depression in primary care found very low compliance rates, around 10% in some studies. Studies have shown that remission (as opposed to improvement) occurs in only 30% of patients treated with antidepressants. Over a 15-month period, 25% of patients in remission relapsed compared with 76% of patients with residual symptoms. Primary care mental health workers are popular with patients but outcomes are similar.

187.   A: Anterior cerebral artery occlusion

Anterior cerebral artery occlusion causes contralateral hemiparesis and hemisensory loss and often causes dyspraxia. If it affects the dominant hemisphere and expressive dysphasia results.

188.   J: PICA occlusion

The syndrome of PICA may also result from vertebral occlusion.

189.   H: Multi-infarct dementia

Multi-infarct dementia often comes to light during routine investigation of dementia.

190.   G: Middle cerebral artery occlusion

Middle cerebral artery strokes may also cause a contralateral homonymous hemianopia.

191.   I: Pontine infarction

Pontine strokes are usually caused by basilar artery thrombosis and are often fatal.

192.   E: An odds ratio of 1 suggests no relative risk reduction in the outcome

The null hypothesis states that two events are unrelated, ie a drug does not affect the outcome measure. Studies that show a statistically significant difference therefore disprove the null hypothesis. Small studies are prone to either very dramatic or very undramatic results, which often become less so as more data are collected with increased sample size. Confidence intervals that cross the line of no effect are less statistically significant than those that do not.

193.   B: Raised parathyroid hormone levels in the presence of a high calcium suggest hyperparathyroidism

Raised calcium and alkaline phosphatase is usually a result of malignancy but may also be caused by thyrotoxicosis or sarcoidosis. Primary hyperparathyroidism should be suspected where a high calcium level is seen with high parathyroid hormone levels. Excess dietary calcium would not raise ALP, whereas myeloma would usually be seen with a normal ALP and increased protein.

194.   D: Studies have shown that herbal treatments are often mixed with conventional medicines

In a *BMJ* trial in 2005, sham acupuncture showed the same benefit as conventional acupuncture, suggesting a powerful placebo effect. Many patients take over-the-counter herbal medications and several of these can potentially interact with prescription medications, for example gingko and warfarin, St John's wort and the contraceptive pill. A postal survey of patients taking warfarin found 1 in 5 to be taking potentially interacting, over-the-counter drugs (*British Journal of General Practice* 2004). A randomised controlled trial comparing paroxetine and St John's wort in mild to moderate depression found evidence for similar efficacy but fewer side effects in the St John's wort group. A survey of Chinese herbal medicines in the *BMJ* in 2003 found that 13 out of 17 creams for eczema contained steroids. There are four homeopathic hospitals in the UK that treat NHS patients.

195.   J: Reassurance

196.   N: Weight loss

197.   H: Pelvic floor exercises

198.   K: Refer

199.   A: Anticholinergic

200.   G: MSU

Paper 5
Questions

Total time allowed is three hours. Indicate your answers clearly by putting a tick or cross in the box alongside each answer or by writing the appropriate letter alongside the appropriate answer.

1. A 73-year-old man with a history of hypertension and smoking rings the surgery for an emergency visit. On arrival he is pale and sweating and complains of severe abdominal pain radiating to his back. He also reports that he cannot feel his feet. On examination he has a tachycardia and a blood pressure of 80/50 lying. What is the most likely diagnosis? Select one option only.

   ☐ A   Myocardial infarction
   ☐ B   Biliary colic
   ☐ C   Acute pancreatitis
   ☐ D   Ruptured aortic aneurysm
   ☐ E   Perforated duodenal ulcer

2. A 77-year-old man presents with tinnitus. Which of the following statements about tinnitus is true? Select one option only.

   ☐ A   Tinnitus is rare
   ☐ B   Tinnitus is usually caused by drugs
   ☐ C   Tinnitus may be a sign of a brain tumour
   ☐ D   There is no treatment for tinnitus
   ☐ E   Tinnitus is usually constant
   ☐ F   Tinnitus can be diagnosed from history alone
   ☐ G   All patients with tinnitus require ENT referral

PAPER 5

3. **Which one of the following statements about screening for colorectal cancer is true?**

☐ A   Colonoscopy is the only screening method that has been proved to reduce mortality

☐ B   Ninety per cent of patients with colorectal cancer have symptoms of rectal bleeding

☐ C   The national screening for colorectal cancer targets those aged 50–74 years

☐ D   Flexible sigmoidoscopy in women of average risk picks up only 35% of cancers

☐ E   Half of all patients with iron-deficiency anaemia in general practice have been found to have gastrointestinal cancer

4. **A patient with dyspepsia has recently had an upper gastrointestinal endoscopy. His histology comes back positive for *Helicobacter pylori*. Which one of the following statements about the management of this situation is true?**

☐ A   Serological testing is highly sensitive and specific

☐ B   Resistance to metronidazole is common in inner-city areas

☐ C   Eradication therapy involves a combination of amoxicillin and a proton-pump inhibitor

☐ D   Serological testing can be repeated after 4 weeks to confirm eradication

☐ E   Prescriptions for HeliClear (amoxicillin, clarithromycin and lansoprazole) treatment packs are charged one prescription charge where prescriptions are chargeable

5. A 22-year-old amateur rugby player presents with a swollen ear after being punched during a match. Which of the following statements about management of this condition is true? Select one option only.

- [ ] A   Cauliflower ear describes the appearance of acute haematoma in the pinna
- [ ] B   Cauliflower ear is a result of a haematoma becoming infected
- [ ] C   The haematoma should be drained promptly and the ear dressed with a pressure bandage
- [ ] D   Most haematomas will settle spontaneously without active treatment
- [ ] E   Cauliflower ear is easily treated

6. A 44-year-old man with no previous history of note presents with a 2-day history of flu-like symptoms. On examination he has temperature of 39.8°C but normal respiratory rate and his chest is clear. Which of the following statements about the management of influenza is true? Select one option only.

- [ ] A   Influenza immunisation has been shown to increase the number of exacerbations of chronic obstructive airway disease
- [ ] B   There is no effective treatment for influenza
- [ ] C   Oral amantidine is effective for influenza A
- [ ] D   Inhaled oseltamivir is effective against influenza A and B
- [ ] E   In the absence of complications patients should be treated with bed rest, fluids and paracetamol

THEME: CHILD ABUSE

Options

A   Accidental injury

B   Emotional abuse

C   Munchausen syndrome by proxy

D   Neglect

E   Non-accidental poisoning

F   None of them

G   Physical abuse

H   Sexual abuse

For each scenario described below, select the most appropriate description from the list of options. Each option may be used once, more than once or not at all.

☐   **7.   A 3-month-old baby has a bruise on her back. Her mother says that this occurred when she slipped in the bath.**

☐   **8.   An 18-month-old girl from a single parent family attends for her MMR immunisation. The practice nurse notices multiple bruises of different ages on her shins. Her mother denies any knowledge of these.**

☐   **9.   The school nurse advises you that she is concerned about one of your patients who frequently misses school, is often wearing dirty clothes and has been noted to have significant learning difficulties. Reviewing the notes, he has been an infrequent visitor to the practice and he has not completed his immunisation schedule.**

☐   **10.   A 3-year-old girl is brought in by her mother with haematuria, noticed when she went to the toilet. This is the third occasion that this has happened with the child; however, urine cultures have always shown blood only with no signs of infection. She has been investigated by paediatricians and no cause has been found.**

11. A 7-month-old girl who was born at 28 weeks and spent 12 weeks in a special care baby unit attends for a routine child health assessment. On examination you notice a torn frenulum.

12. A 77-year-old woman is seen with recurrent episodes of acute conjunctivitis. Examination reveals the following appearance.

Which of the following is the most appropriate management of this case?

A Topical chloramphenicol for 1 month
B Oxytetracycline for 6 weeks
C Lid cleaning twice daily
D Referral for surgical correction
E Taping of the eyelid

PAPER 5

13. A baby boy is brought in for a routine health check at 18 months. He has dropped from the 75th centile for height and weight at birth to the 9th and his mother reports that he has frequent chest infections. He has been seen on several occasions and been prescribed antibiotics. In between attacks his mother reports that he is well. She is concerned that he might have asthma. Reviewing his notes you notice that he was constipated soon after being born at home but this settled spontaneously. There is no family history of note and he is otherwise well. Which of the following is a possible diagnosis? Select one option only.

- [ ] A   Hypothyroidism
- [ ] B   Coeliac disease
- [ ] C   Cystic fibrosis
- [ ] D α_1-Antitrypsin deficiency
- [ ] E   Asthma

14. A 3-week-old girl is sent to see you by the health visitor after her mother noticed that she was Jaundiced. On examination she is jaundiced with dark urine and pale stools. Examination is otherwise normal. The mother had an uneventful pregnancy and birth and has had vitamin K. Which of the following is a likely diagnosis? Select one option only.

- [ ] A   Biliary atresia
- [ ] B   Vitamin K deficiency
- [ ] C   Rhesus incompatibility
- [ ] D   Physiological jaundice
- [ ] E   Gallstones

THEME: COMPLEMENTARY THERAPISTS

Options

A   Acupuncture

B   Chiropractic

C   Homeopathy

D   Hypnotherapy

E   Kinesiology

F   Magnet therapy

G   Neurolinguistic programming

H   Osteopathy

I   Reflexology

For each description below, select the most appropriate from the list of options. Each option may be used once, more than once or not at all.

☐ **15.** A study in The Lancet in 2005 found evidence that the specific effect of this treatment modality reported in previous trials was a result of placebo effect.

☐ **16.** It has been shown to be effective in treating irritable bowel syndrome.

☐ **17.** It is based on a philosophy that pain and disability are caused by abnormalities in the body's structure and function.

☐ **18.** This treats problems with joints, bones and muscles, and the effects that they have on the nervous system.

☐ **19.** This uses muscle testing to assess functions of the body in the structural, chemical, neurological and biochemical realms.

PAPER 5

20. A 73-year-old mentions at a routine blood pressure check-up that he has to get up four or five times a night to go to the toilet. This is disturbing his wife to the point that he has moved into the spare room. Examination reveals a smooth enlarged prostate and you send blood for PSA (prostate-specific antigen) testing and a urine specimen for culture. This comes back clear and his PSA level is 3.6. Which of the following statements about his management is true? Select one option only.

☐ A   He should be referred for a prostate biopsy

☐ B   Transurethral resection of the prostate is the treatment of choice in this patient

☐ C   Finasteride will provide rapid relief from his symptoms with no risk of postural hypotension

☐ D   Saw palmetto has been shown to have a placebo effect only

☐ E   α Blockers are the first-line treatment in this patient group

21. A 32-year-old woman complains of heavy periods. Which one of the following statements about menorrhagia is true?

☐ A   Menorrhagia is defined as > 90 ml blood loss per month

☐ B   Patients who have completed their families should be offered a hysterectomy if medical therapy fails

☐ C   Norethisterone 15 mg daily from day 5 to day 26 is the first-line medical treatment

☐ D   Tranexamic acid taken from day 5 to day 26 has been proved to reduce blood loss

☐ E   A palpable uterus requires ultrasonography

22. A 43-year-old woman is seen in an emergency appointment complaining that her cold has gone onto her chest, giving her a productive cough and occasional retrosternal chest pain. On examination she has a slight wheeze in her chest but no signs of respiratory distress. She is otherwise fit and well. Which of the following statements about her management is true? Select one option only.

☐ A This condition is usually caused by pneumococci and she should be treated with amoxicillin unless contraindicated

☐ B She should be referred for a radiograph

☐ C A macrolide should be prescribed because this has broader cover than amoxicillin

☐ D She should be advised that she has a viral infection and to take analgesics and antipyretics, with instructions to return if her symptoms worsen

☐ E A cough persisting for more than 5 days suggests secondary bacterial infection

23. Which of the following statements about the management of chickenpox is true? Select one option only.

☐ A All pregnant women who have contact with chickenpox should be treated with aciclovir to avoid congenital chickenpox infection

☐ B Children on long-term steroids should be treated with aciclovir at the onset of the rash

☐ C Normally healthy immunocompetent adults do not need treatment

☐ D Children who are systemically unwell should be given oral aciclovir

☐ E Patients are most infectious in the vesicular stage of the disease

PAPER 5

THEME: CONTRACEPTION

Options

A   Combined oral contraceptive pill

B   Condoms

C   Depo-Provera

D   Diaphragm

E   Femidom

F   Implanon

G   Mirena intrauterine system

H   Progesterone-only pill

I   Sterilisation

J   Triphasic pill

For each of the descriptions below, select the most appropriate form of contraception from the list of options. Each option may be used once, more than once or not at all.

☐ **24.** It should not be removed for at least 6 hours after intercourse.

☐ **25.** It should not be used in women with a history of arterial or venous thrombosis.

☐ **26.** It often causes irregular bleeding and weight gain.

☐ **27.** It has a failure rate of 3% in the over-35 age group.

☐ **28.** It has the lowest failure rate.

☐ **29.** It should not be used in women with a history of osteoporosis.

☐ **30.** It should be changed every 3 years.

31. A 16-year-old girl presents with her mother complaining of late puberty. All of her friends have started their periods a long time ago and she is worried about being teased. She is an infrequent attender and otherwise well. On examination height is on the 25th centile while weight is on the 90th; she has no secondary sexual characteristics and has a webbed neck and broad chest. Which of the following is a likely diagnosis? Select one option only.

- [ ] A Klinefelter syndrome
- [ ] B Hypothyroidism
- [ ] C Down syndrome
- [ ] D Constitutional delay in puberty
- [ ] E Turner syndrome

32. At a 'significant event' meeting one of your colleagues presents the case of a 34-year-old woman who committed suicide after years of domestic abuse, which had gone largely unnoticed by the primary healthcare team. Which one of the following statements about domestic abuse is true?

- [ ] A Women who have been abused visit their GP less often than those who have not
- [ ] B Chronic pain is a common presentation of domestic abuse
- [ ] C Insomnia is the most common presenting complaint in abused women
- [ ] D Only one in four patients with a history of domestic abuse have reported relationship difficulties to their GP
- [ ] E Women who have been abused usually disclose this without prompting rather than on specific questioning

PAPER 5

33. A 6-year-old boy is seen complaining of verrucas. Which of the following statements about treatment of verrucas is correct? Select one option only.

☐ A Where verrucas are resistant to over-the-counter treatments they should be excised

☐ B Cryotherapy results in 90% clear-up rates after one course

☐ C Glutaraldehyde causes a white discoloration of the skin

☐ D Untreated verrucas often resolve spontaneously

☐ E Bleomycin is an effective second-line treatment

34. A 75-year-old man is noted to have the following appearance at a routine appointment.

Which of the statements about this condition is true? Select one option only.

☐ A In Horner syndrome pupils are dilated

☐ B It is always acquired

☐ C The underlying cause does not affect other muscles

☐ D It may be secondary to a cerebrovascular event

☐ E It may be caused by mitochondrial myopathy

THEME: DIET

Options

A ω-3 fatty acids

B Calcium consumption

C Fibre

D Fish consumption

E Five servings of fruit and vegetables a day

F Olive oil consumption

G Probiotics

H Red meat consumption

I Sorbitol

For each description of a piece of research relating to diet below, select the most appropriate food from the list of options. Each option may be used once, more than once or not at all.

☐ **35.** In a study of 25 000 people over 9 years, consumption of this foodstuff was associated with a doubling of the incidence of rheumatoid arthritis.

☐ **36.** A meta-analysis in The Lancet in 2006 looking at 250 000 people found a reduction of 26% in the risk of stroke with consumption of this foodstuff.

☐ **37.** The EPIC prospective cohort study found that consumption of this foodstuff would give a 60-year-old an extra year's life expectancy.

☐ **38.** The 12-year follow-up of 5000 elderly people found a 31% reduction in atrial fibrillation in patients consuming this foodstuff at least once a week.

☐ **39.** It was shown in the EPIC study to increase the risk of bowel cancer by 35%.

40. An 82-year-old man comes to see you having been diagnosed with cataract by a local optician. Which of the following statements about cataract is NOT true? Select one option only.

- ☐ A Cataracts may result from infection
- ☐ B They may cause similar symptoms to macular degeneration
- ☐ C They may cause diplopia in one eye only
- ☐ D They are seen only in elderly people
- ☐ E Recurrence of symptoms after surgery is not uncommon

41. A 67-year-old man presents with painful ulcers in his mouth. Examination reveals the lesions below.

What is the likely diagnosis?

- ☐ A Aphthous ulcers
- ☐ B Herpes virus
- ☐ C Contact dermatitis
- ☐ D Lichen planus
- ☐ E Candida infection

42. A 56-year-old man presents with unprovoked, painless, macroscopic haematuria. Dipstick testing confirms the presence of blood but no leukocytes or nitrites. Which of the following may be a cause of these symptoms? Select the single most appropriate answer from the list below.

☐ A Renal colic
☐ B Beetroot consumption
☐ C Urinary tract infection
☐ D Bladder tumour
☐ E Renal trauma
☐ F All of the above

43. Which of the following patients is NOT suitable for referral under the 2-week rule for suspected brain tumours? Select one patient only.

☐ A A 23-year-old woman who has been previously fit and well complaining of severe headache, worse in certain postures
☐ B A 62-year-old man with new-onset epilepsy
☐ C A 72-year-old woman who has noticed that overnight she can no longer do the *Times* crossword
☐ D A 46-year-old man with unilateral cranial nerve III and IV palsies of new onset
☐ E A 17-year-old girl complaining of flashing lights in one eye, nausea and headache

PAPER 5

THEME: EAR DISEASE

Options

A   Cerumen

B   Cholesteatoma

C   Chronic suppurative otitis media

D   Exostoses

E   Glomus tumour

F   Glue ear

G   Granuloma

H   Keratosis obturans

I   Otitis externa

J   Otitis media

For each statement described below, select the single most likely diagnosis. Each option may be used once, more than once, or not at all.

☐ **44.** The tympanic membrane has a crust of wax on the drum.

☐ **45.** There is a large perforation revealing most of the middle ear.

☐ **46.** Removal of debris in the canal with a probe is very painful.

☐ **47.** The commonest cause of this condition is streptococcal infection.

☐ **48.** It is a painless condition often seen in surfers.

49. Which of the following statements about the management of eye injuries is NOT true? Select one option only.

- [ ] A Exposure of the cornea to acid is less severe than to alkali
- [ ] B Orbital injury followed by diplopia to up- or down-gaze may be a sign of orbital fracture
- [ ] C Reduced visual acuity after trauma may be a sign of retinal damage
- [ ] D Corneal abrasion can be confidently diagnosed from history alone
- [ ] E Penetrating injuries can be excluded only by a radiograph

50. One of your patients is due to have his hip replaced but is very concerned about the risk of deep venous thrombosis. He comes to see you for advice on the prevention of DVT. Which one of the following statements is correct?

- [ ] A Fluid balance is not an important risk factor
- [ ] B Travel of more than 3 hours' duration in the 4 weeks before and after surgery should be avoided
- [ ] C Female patients should stop using the combined oral contraceptive pill 2 weeks pre-operatively
- [ ] D Patients with risk factors for DVT should use low-molecular-weight heparin following hip replacement until discharge
- [ ] E Anticoagulants should be stopped 2 weeks before elective surgery as a matter of course

51. As part of their annual review for hypertension, your patients have urea and electrolytes measured. Significant numbers are now coming back with evidence of chronic renal impairment. Which one of the following statements about this condition is true?

- [ ] A   Most laboratories now provide a measurement of the patient's true glomerular filtration rate (GFR), which is a definitive guide to renal function

- [ ] B   Patients with an eGFR > 60 ml/minute per 1.73 m^2 do not have renal impairment

- [ ] C   A blood pressure treatment goal of < 125/75 mmHg is indicated for patients with proteinuria

- [ ] D   A high-protein diet is required in patients with proteinuria to replace urinary losses

- [ ] E   ACE inhibitors are contraindicated in patients with only one kidney

52. A 29-year-old woman presents to her GP with an acute onset of lateral rectus palsy. On reviewing her notes you find a reference to an episode of paraesthesia in her left leg 2 years ago, which settled spontaneously over 2 weeks. What is the most likely diagnosis? Select one option only.

- [ ] A   Multiple sclerosis
- [ ] B   Sarcoidosis
- [ ] C   Radiculopathy
- [ ] D   Transient ischaemic attack
- [ ] E   Hydrocephalus

53. You are called out to visit a 21-year-old student complaining of lethargy, fever, neck pain and a rash. On examination he is photophobic and has a non-blanching rash on his abdomen. Which of the following statements about management of this case is true? Select one option only.

- [ ] A Antibiotics should not be given until blood cultures and a lumbar puncture have been performed
- [ ] B In patients with proven anaphylaxis with penicillin, cefotaxime may be used
- [ ] C Benzylpenicillin is the first-line drug of choice in community-acquired infections
- [ ] D Rifampicin should be given to all close contacts
- [ ] E Childhood contacts may be given ciprofloxacin as an alternative to rifampicin

54. A 3-year-old girl is brought in by her parents with a 3-week history of violent paroxysms of coughing that end in an inspiratory whoop. She often vomits with the coughing attacks. She and her parents are exhausted. Which of the following statements about whooping cough is true? Select one option only.

- [ ] A Compliance with the normal immunisation schedule provides 100% protection against whooping cough
- [ ] B Coughing may last up to 8 weeks
- [ ] C It should be treated with amoxicillin
- [ ] D Treatment with antibiotics will significantly shorten the duration of the illness
- [ ] E Parents should be reassured that, although dramatic, the disease is almost always benign

THEME: LEGISLATION AFFECTING GENERAL PRACTICE

Options

A   Access to Health Records Act

B   Civil Contingencies Act

C   Data Protection Act

D   Disability Discrimination Act

E   Equality Act 2006

F   Freedom of Information Act

G   Health and Safety at Work Act

H   Human Rights Act

I   None of the above

For each of the descriptions relating to practice management below, select the most appropriate piece of legislation from the list of options. Each option may be used once, more than once or not at all.

☐ **55.   It requires practices to have a major incident plan.**

☐ **56.   It requires practices to audit accessibility of services.**

☐ **57.   It can be used for a patient to access practice prescribing data.**

☐ **58.   It contains provisions to prevent gender discrimination.**

☐ **59.   Charges for the request cannot be made to the patient.**

60. Which of the following statements about common eye conditions is NOT true? Select one option only.

- [ ] A Subconjunctival haemorrhages are never a sign of significant pathology

- [ ] B Acute bacterial rather than viral conjunctivitis will often resolve without antibiotics

- [ ] C A pterygium is a benign wedge-shaped growth that may extend from the margin of the cornea to impede the visual axis

- [ ] D A pinguecula is a benign growth that does not impede on the visual axis

- [ ] E Episcleritis can be managed in primary care with topical NSAID drops

61. A 23-year-old woman complains of feeling tired all the time, finding it impossible to go to work. On further questioning she admits to tearfulness, apathy and poor sleep. She feels guilty that she cannot pull herself together and is convinced that her partner will leave her. Which one of the following statements about her management is correct?

- [ ] A She should have appropriate investigations to rule out an organic cause for her symptoms, eg hypothyroidism

- [ ] B Counselling should always be used before drug treatment

- [ ] C She has bipolar disorder

- [ ] D Grading as mild, moderate or severe is a subjective process, according to the impact on her life

- [ ] E She has a poor long-term prognosis

62. A 63-year-old man started simvastatin 2 months ago for hypercholesterolaemia. When seen for review, he complains that the pills do not suit him. Which of the following statements about statins is true? Select one option only.

- [ ] A   They have no major drug interactions
- [ ] B   They cause myalgia in 10% of patients
- [ ] C   They may interfere with sleep
- [ ] D   They can be used safely with fibrates
- [ ] E   A CK level of twice normal should prompt cessation of treatment

63. A 2-year-old girl is brought in by her mother with a unilateral nasal discharge. Which of the following statements is most likely to be true in this situation? Select one option only.

- [ ] A   A tumour of the postnasal space is a probable cause for her discharge
- [ ] B   Inorganic foreign bodies such as beads are more dangerous than organic ones
- [ ] C   Foreign bodies usually present soon after insertion
- [ ] D   Foreign bodies can be safely removed in general practice with a wax hook
- [ ] E   Unilateral blood-stained discharge is unlikely to be caused by a foreign body
- [ ] F   Attempted removal may result in aspiration of foreign bodies

64. Which of the following symptoms is NOT a symptom of fibromyalgia? Select one option only.

- [ ] A   Hyperalgesia, particularly over bony parts of the body
- [ ] B   Pain localised to one limb
- [ ] C   Tenderness on rolling the skin
- [ ] D   Abdominal pain
- [ ] E   Headache

65. A 76-year-old woman with a long history of smoking has had an ulcer on her lower lip for 6 months. The lesion is shown below.

What is the likely diagnosis?

- [ ] A   Squamous cell carcinoma
- [ ] B   Aphthous ulcer
- [ ] C   Basal cell carcinoma
- [ ] D   Keratoacanthoma
- [ ] E   Herpes simplex

PAPER 5

THEME: TESTICULAR SWELLINGS

Options

A   Epididymal cyst

B   Epididymo-orchitis

C   Femoral hernia

D   Hydrocele

E   Inguinal hernia

F   Lymphoma

G   Patent processus vaginalis

H   Seminoma

I   Teratoma

J   Testicular torsion

K   Torsion of the hydatid of Morgagni

L   Varicocele

For each of the clinical histories below, select the most appropriate diagnosis from the list of options. Each option may be used once, more than once or not at all.

☐ **66.** A 17-year-old boy with a sudden onset of severe scrotal pain, nausea and vomiting. On examination the testis is hard, swollen and very tender.

☐ **67.** A 77-year-old man with a history of prostatism complains of a tender swollen testicle, dysuria, rigors and frequency. On examination the testicle is swollen and tender.

☐ **68.** A 12-month-old baby boy is brought in by his mother with a painless swelling of the testis. On examination there is a smooth swelling that extends into the groin.

☐ **69.** An 82-year-old man with a painless smooth swelling on his right testicle that has only been present for 4 weeks.

70. A 23-year-old man complains of a dull ache in his scrotum at the end of the day, particularly after exercise. There is a swelling on examination that is present on standing and disappears when supine.

71. A 76-year-old man complains of a painful lump in his groin. On examination there is a very tender swelling lateral to the pubic tubercle.

72. Which one of the following is NOT one of the subject areas that is covered specifically by the GMC's *Good Medical Practice*?

A   Good clinical care
B   Maintaining good medical practice
C   Teaching and training, appraising and assessing
D   Rational prescribing
E   Relationships with patients

73. A 45-year-old man presents in a state of some anxiety, having noticed blood in his semen on ejaculating. Which of the following statements about this condition is true? Select one answer only.

A   A third of cases are idiopathic
B   The most common cause is prostate cancer
C   Infection is rare in the under-40 years age group
D   May be part of a systemic disorder
E   Patients under the age of 65 can be reassured if a midstream urine is clear

PAPER 5

477

74. Your practice is invited to submit a plan for practice-based commissioning (PBC). Which one of the following statements about this scheme is true?

- [ ] A Savings can be spent only on improving patient care
- [ ] B Participation in PBC is covered by a local enhanced service
- [ ] C Administration costs of running a PBC scheme are funded out of savings from the scheme
- [ ] D Practices that participate will receive an uplift to their global sum to incorporate their PBC budget
- [ ] E Commissioning decisions are made only by GPs

75. According to NICE guidance on suspected lung cancer, which of the following persistent symptoms (for more than 3 weeks) is NOT an indication for an urgent chest radiograph? Select one option only.

- [ ] A Clubbing
- [ ] B Cough
- [ ] C Dyspnoea
- [ ] D Splinter haemorrhages
- [ ] E Supraclavicular lymphadenopathy

76. A meta-analysis of studies for a new drug to prevent complications of diabetes has looked at the following individual outcomes:

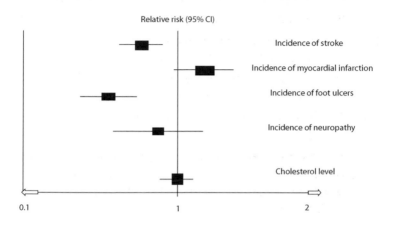

Which one of the following statements about this drug is true?

☐ A The drug brings about a statistically significant reduction in the incidence of neuropathy

☐ B The drug reduces the risk of foot ulcers

☐ C The drug increases the risk of stroke

☐ D The drug reduces the risk of macrovascular complications

☐ E The data suggest a net benefit from the drug

THEME: MEDICAL STATISTICS

Options

A   Case–control study

B   Confidence intervals

C   Cross-sectional study

D   Kaplan–Meier method

E   Longitudinal study

F   Negative predictive value

G   Randomised controlled study

H   Odds ratio

I   Positive predictive value

J   Prevalence

K   Sensitivity

L   Specificity

M   Standard deviation

For each description below, select the most appropriate from the list of options. Each option may be used once, more than once or not at all.

☐ **77.** **The probability that an event occurs divided by the probability it does not.**

☐ **78.** **The proportion of true negatives correctly identified by a test.**

☐ **79.** **The Framingham study.**

☐ **80.** **It is useful for studying diseases with low prevalence.**

☐ **81.** **It demonstrates the proportion of a population surviving at a given time.**

THEME: CARDIOVASCULAR TRIALS

Options

A   4S trial

B   AFFIRM trial

C   ELITE study

D   EPHESUS study

E   GREACE trial

F   Heart Protection Study

G   HOPE trial

H   HOT study

I   Physicians' Health Study

J   WOSCOPS trial

For each statement about the findings of landmark studies in cardiovascular medicine, select the name of the study from the list of options. Each option may be used once, more than once or not at all.

☐   **82.**   Confirmed the benefits of statins as secondary prevention in patients with hypercholesterolaemia.

☐   **83.**   It showed that long-term secondary prevention treatment with statins to achieve an LDL-cholesterol < 2.6 mmol/l significantly reduced morbidity and mortality.

☐   **84.**   It indicates that in patients over 65 years of age with AF, a policy of anticoagulation and rate control is superior to attempting to maintain sinus rhythm in reducing thromboembolic events.

☐   **85.**   It randomised patients to receive either 40 mg simvastatin or placebo regardless of cholesterol levels.

☐   **86.**   It demonstrated the benefits of ramipril in reducing morbidity and mortality in high-risk patients.

PAPER 5

87. A 47-year-old man complains of gradually increasing pain, swelling and stiffness in his right knee, particularly towards the end of the day. He is overweight but takes no regular medication. He had meniscal surgery in his 20s but has no other history of note. Which of the following statements about his condition is NOT true? Select one option only.

☐   A   The history is typical of osteoarthritis

☐   B   Exercise and weight loss will improve function and symptoms

☐   C   Simple analgesia such as paracetamol may be effective

☐   D   He should be referred for joint replacement

☐   E   Steroid joint injection may give temporary relief

88. Which one of the following statements about new developments in the management of back pain is true?

☐   A   In a study of first presentation of back pain in primary care, 90% of patients were found to have made a full recovery within 6 weeks

☐   B   Addressing psychological factors at initial presentation has been shown to improve functional outcome

☐   C   Rigid application of backache management guidelines has been shown to be cost-effective in terms of reduced secondary-care referrals

☐   D   A Cochrane review has shown no difference in short- and long-term outcomes for spinal manipulation, usual care and 'back school' (physiotherapy-led classes aimed at back problems)

☐   E   A randomised controlled trial of physiotherapy compared with simple advice has shown significant objective benefits for the physiotherapy group

89. A 37-year-old man who has had asthma since childhood is seen in the asthma clinic. His asthma has been poorly controlled over the last 3 years and he has seen a number of different practitioners. In an attempt to gain control over his asthma his inhaled steroids have been increased on several occasions and he has had several prolonged courses of oral steroids. He comments that he has put on a lot of weight over the last 5 years and bruises easily. He finds that he is tired all the time and finds it difficult to get out of a chair. On examination he has purple striae over his abdomen and urinalysis is positive to glucose. What is the likely diagnosis? Select one option only.

- ☐ A   Addison's disease
- ☐ B   Diabetes mellitus
- ☐ C   Hypothyroidism
- ☐ D   Cushing syndrome
- ☐ E   Conn syndrome

90. Your local PCT is setting up a local enhanced service to try to reduce the level of chlamydial infection in girls under the age of 18 in the area. Which one of the following statements about this problem is true?

- ☐ A   Encouraging condom use is the only realistic goal of intervention
- ☐ B   Modifiable risk factors include low educational attainment and age less than 18
- ☐ C   The number of diagnoses in genitourinary medicine (GUM) clinics has increased by 300% since 1995
- ☐ D   Risky sexual behaviour is almost exclusively the result of alcohol use
- ☐ E   Teenage pregnancy rates are at their highest level since 1986

PAPER 5

91. A 57-year-old man with controlled hypertension has come in to ask for some antibiotics for his toenails, which the chiropodist told him he could get. On examination he has thickened yellow great toenails with normal surrounding tissue. The other nails are normal. Which of the following statements about the management of this condition is true? Select one option only.

☐ A Fungal nail infection is a clinical diagnosis

☐ B With appropriate topical antifungal therapy 90% of cases will resolve in a 12-month period

☐ C Where extensive disease is present oral fluconazole is indicated

☐ D Antifungal choice should be guided by microscopy, culture and sensitivity results

☐ E Tea tree oil is ineffective for fungal nail infection

92. A 32-year-old woman complains of persistent dandruff that is worse in winter but never truly clears. She has tried all the over-the-counter remedies and wants to try prescription treatment. She has not been seen for dermatological problems before but reports eczema on her elbows and knees. On examination she has silvery scale on her scalp, elbows and knees. This can be removed but causes pinpoint bleeding. Which of the following statements about her condition is true? Select one option only.

☐ A She should use Nizoral shampoo

☐ B She should use a tar-based shampoo

☐ C She should be reassured and continue her normal routine

☐ D She should use systemic steroids to get control of her eczema and scalp condition

☐ E She should be referred for PUVA

THEME: RHEUMATOLOGICAL CONDITIONS

Options

A   Colchicine

B   Intra-articular steroid injection

C   Intramuscular steroid injection

D   Methotrexate

E   Oral steroids

F   Physiotherapy

G   Probenecid

H   Referral for surgery

I   Rest

J   Splinting

For each of the scenarios described below, select the most appropriate treatment from the list of options. Each option may be used once, more than once or not at all.

☐ 93.   De Quervain's tenosynovitis not responding to rest and a wrist support.

☐ 94.   Early morning stiffness and pain in shoulders with raised ESR.

☐ 95.   Acutely swollen erythematous first MTP (metatarsophalangeal) joint.

☐ 96.   Acute onset of lumbar backache when lifting with right-sided sciatica.

☐ 97.   A patient with fibromyalgia complains of multiple tender points in her shoulders; examination reveals normal range of movement but numerous trigger points within the muscles.

98. Your local PCT wishes to increase the role of pharmacists in primary care. Which one of the following statements about the evidence for their role is true?

- ☐ A Pharmacist follow-up of patients after discharge from hospital reduced morbidity and mortality
- ☐ B Pharmacist follow-up after admission has been shown to be popular with patients
- ☐ C Telephone follow-up of non-compliant patients by pharmacists reduces costs and mortality
- ☐ D Pharmacists are unable to prescribe
- ☐ E Pharmacist medication reviews are more cost-effective than usual care

99. An obese 54-year-old lorry driver comes to see you about his snoring, saying that his wife thinks that, at times, he is not breathing at night. Which of the following statements is true regarding this situation? Select one answer only.

- ☐ A Sleep apnoea is more common in women than in men
- ☐ B Sleep apnoea is seen only in adults
- ☐ C Sleep studies are an effective screening tool
- ☐ D Surgery is an option for severe sleep apnoea
- ☐ E Continuous positive airway pressure is an effective treatment for sleep apnoea
- ☐ F Daytime symptoms of snoring are daytime somnolence, headaches and poor concentration

100. A 45-year-old woman presents with intense itching around her perineum, particularly at night. On examination you see excoriation only. Which one of the following statements about this condition is true?

- ☐ A This condition is frequently caused by the presence of a foreign body
- ☐ B Where atrophic changes are seen over the perineum the probable diagnosis is chronic eczema
- ☐ C Multiple areas of hypertrophic change suggest that vulval intraepithelial neoplasia may be the cause
- ☐ D It always results from local rather than systemic pathology
- ☐ E It should be treated initially with Elocon and antihistamines

101. Which of the following statements about osteoporosis is true? Select one option only.

- ☐ A Osteoporosis can be diagnosed on radiographs of the lumbar spine
- ☐ B A *T* score of less than −2.0 is diagnostic of osteoporosis
- ☐ C HRT is an effective treatment for prevention of osteoporosis in postmenopausal women
- ☐ D Bisphosphonates are the only treatment for established osteoporosis
- ☐ E Depo-Provera may cause osteoporosis

PAPER 5

102. A 92-year-old man presents with 3-week history of painless swelling on the side of his neck. He does not have any systemic symptoms and has a history of diet-controlled diabetes. On examination there is a hard rubbery mass in the side of his neck.

What is the likely diagnosis?

- ☐ A   Lymphoma
- ☐ B   Parotid adenoma
- ☐ C   Tuberculosis
- ☐ D   Metastatic deposits
- ☐ E   Sarcoma

103. With regard to the assessment of heart failure in general practice, which of the following statements is NOT true? Select one option only.

☐   A   Resting heart rate > diastolic pressure suggests left ventricular dysfunction

☐   B   Natriuretic peptide levels are a useful screening test to determine which patients should be referred for echocardiography

☐   C   A normal ECG suggests that significant systolic dysfunction is very unlikely

☐   D   A displaced apex beat is suggestive of left ventricular enlargement

☐   E   Raised serum urea is a useful screening test with high specificity in heart failure

104. A 49-year-old man who smokes has routine blood tests done as part of a 'well man' check. His full blood count comes back with a haematocrit of 57% and a haemoglobin of 17.8 g/dl. Which one of the following statements about his condition is correct?

☐   A   He has leukaemia and should be referred urgently to a haematology department

☐   B   He is at risk of stroke

☐   C   First-line treatment is radiotherapy

☐   D   The condition is always the result of clonal proliferation of red cells

☐   E   Splenomegaly is uncommon

PAPER 5

THEME: CONNECTIVE TISSUE DISEASES AND VASCULITIS

Options

A   Churg–Strauss syndrome

B   Dermatomyositis

C   Fitz–Hugh–Curtis syndrome

D   Polyarteritis nodosa

E   Relapsing polychondritis

F   Rheumatoid arthritis

G   Sjögren syndrome

H   Systemic lupus erythematosus

I   Systemic sclerosis

J   Wegener's granulomatosis

For each clinical scenario below, select the most likely diagnosis from the list of options. Each option may be used once, more than once or not at all.

☐ **105.** A 35-year-old woman with 3 months of malaise, weight loss and arthralgia. She has also noticed a rash on either side of her nose.

☐ **106.** A 46-year-old woman complains of dry mouth, dry eyes and dyspareunia. She has been treated in the past for a seropositive arthritis but this has been in remission recently.

☐ **107.** A 32-year-old woman complains of recurrent pain and tenderness of her nose, ears and windpipe.

☐ **108.** A 55-year-old man with a previous history of idiopathic perforation of the nasal septum presents with dyspnoea and haemoptysis.

109. A 56-year-old man with asthma and rhinitis has been the finding over the last few months that his asthma has been increasingly difficult to manage. He had routine blood tests recently which showed an eosinophilia only. He now presents with a purpuric rash and nodules below the skin.

110. A 42-year-old man with long-standing nasal obstruction presents to you in surgery. Examining him you find what you think are nasal polyps. Which of the following statements about nasal polyps is true? Select one answer only.

☐ A   Polyps are very sensitive

☐ B   Polyps are relatively common in children

☐ C   Surgical polypectomy is curative

☐ D   Polyps may be associated with cystic fibrosis

☐ E   Polyps are a frequent cause of recurrent epistaxis

☐ F   Polyps often resolve without treatment

111. With regard to the Quality and Outcomes Framework (QOF) of the General Medical Services Contract (GMSC), which one of the following statements is correct?

☐ A   The QOF is compulsory

☐ B   The Minimum Practice Income Guarantee protects practices against poor performance in the QOF

☐ C   One in 20 practices is likely to receive a random anti-fraud QOF visit each year

☐ D   The maximum points score is 1050

☐ E   QOF is designed to reward practices for good clinical performance

THEME: PERIPHERAL NEUROPATHY

Options

A   Autonomic neuropathy

B   Charcot–Marie–Tooth syndrome

C   Drug-induced neuropathy

D   Guillain–Barré syndrome

E   Leprosy

F   Motor neurone disease

G   Painful diabetic neuropathy

H   Porphyria

I   Vitamin B$_{12}$ deficiency

For each scenario described below, select the most appropriate diagnosis from the list of options. Each option may be used once, more than once or not at all.

☐ **112.** A 67-year-old man with long-standing epilepsy treated with phenytoin complains of numbness in his feet.

☐ **113.** A 56-year-old schoolteacher who was seen with a viral URTI (upper respiratory tract infection) 6 weeks ago complains of numbness and weakness in his feet, which is gradually extending up his legs. On examination he has no tendon reflexes but normal plantar reflexes.

☐ **114.** A 45-year-old woman with long-standing type 1 diabetes complains of burning pains, pins and needles, and increased sensitivity to touch in her feet.

☐ **115.** An 81-year-old man with gradual onset of weakness and tremor in his right hand. On examination he has weakness, wasting and fasciculation of his thenar eminence.

☐ **116.** A 45-year-old woman who has recently arrived in the UK from the Sudan is applying for asylum. She has been living in a refugee camp in Chad for 2 years and is malnourished. She has paraesthesiae and numbness affecting her legs and routine bloods show a macrocytosis.

117. A 34-year-old woman presents with red eye, photophobia and blurred vision. Which of the following statements about iritis is true? Select one option only.

☐ A   Pupils always react normally to light but this may be painful

☐ B   It is usually triggered by acute infection

☐ C   It is associated with autoimmune disease

☐ D   It can be managed in primary care

☐ E   It does not result in long-term complications

118. With regard to confidentiality and patient records, which one of the following statements about patient records is true?

☐ A   Records may include abbreviations where these are in common usage

☐ B   They may contain statements of personal opinion about patients as long as the author is identifiable

☐ C   Electronic records may use coding systems developed in house as long as a cipher is available to decode them

☐ D   They may be written in any colour of ink as long as they are legible and the author is identifiable

☐ E   Records should be written in a style that would be comprehensible to another doctor

PAPER 5

119. A 73-year-old man with treated hypertension presents with 'chilblains' that are not getting better. On examination his pulse is irregular and his foot has the following appearance.

What is the likely diagnosis?

- ☐ A   Cellulitis
- ☐ B   Thromboembolism
- ☐ C   Venous ulcer
- ☐ D   Chilblains
- ☐ E   Raynaud's phenomenon

120. A 67-year-old man who has treated hypertension is seen accompanied by his wife. They have just returned from a family reunion where they saw his brother for the first time in 25 years, who commented on how his appearance has changed. On examination you note large hands, a large tongue, frontal bossing of the skull and malocclusion of the jaw. Which of the following is a likely diagnosis? Select one option only.

- [ ] A Pituitary apoplexy
- [ ] B Growth hormone deficiency
- [ ] C Hypopituitarism
- [ ] D Acromegaly
- [ ] E Gigantism

121. Which of the following are NOT features of thyroid eye disease? Select one option only.

- [ ] A Proptosis
- [ ] B Ophthalmoplegia
- [ ] C Periorbital oedema
- [ ] D Reduced visual acuity
- [ ] E Pretibial myxoedema

PAPER 5

THEME: CHILDHOOD INFECTIONS

Options

A   Chickenpox

B   Coxsackievirus

C   Cytomegalovirus

D   Epstein–Barr virus

E   Hand, foot and mouth disease

F   Measles

G   Mumps

H   Parvovirus B19

I   Rubella

J   Scarlet fever

For each description below, select the most appropriate diagnosis from the list of options. Each option may be used once, more than once or not at all.

☐   122.   A low-grade fever followed by a lacy reticular rash on the legs and a slapped cheek appearance.

☐   123.   After a 4-day prodromal phase with malaise, conjunctivitis and fever, photophobia cough and nasal congestion develops. Small red lesions with blue centres appear on mucous membranes followed by a rash spreading down from the forehead.

☐   124.   After a 4- to 8-week incubation period a prodromal phase of malaise and anorexia precedes severe pharyngitis with splenomegaly and lymphadenopathy.

☐   125.   If acquired in pregnancy it may cause heart malformations, blindness, deafness and learning disability.

☐   126.   It may cause a severe pneumonia.

127. With regard to the management of constipation in palliative care, which of the following statements is true? Select one option only.

☐ A Co-danthramer is safe to use in patients with incontinence

☐ B Laxatives should not be prescribed routinely, because most patients will manage with increased dietary fibre and exercise

☐ C Movicol should be used no more than three times a day

☐ D Spinal cord compression or bowel obstruction should be excluded in all patients with constipation in a palliative care setting

☐ E Co-danthramer may colour urine black

128. Which one of the following statements about renal stones is true?

☐ A Larger stones are more likely to cause symptoms than smaller stones

☐ B Renal stones are always the result of metabolic conditions

☐ C Recurrent *Proteus* urinary tract infection suggests that renal stones might be present

☐ D Renal stones that pass into the bladder tend to persist as bladder stones

☐ E Renal colic should be managed with opioids as first-line treatment

PAPER 5

THEME: WEIGHT LOSS

Options

A   Atkin's diet

B   Bariatric surgery

C   Orlistat

D   Rimonabant

E   Sibutramine

For each of the statements below, select the most appropriate treatment from the list of options. Each option may be used once, more than once or not at all.

☐   **129.   A cannabinoid receptor antagonist that acts centrally.**

☐   **130.   It is taken three times a day.**

☐   **131.   It is suitable for otherwise healthy patients with a body mass index of 27.**

☐   **132.   The most common side effects are depression and anxiety.**

☐   **133.   It may cause a significant increase in blood pressure.**

134. Which one of the following statements about access to GP services is true?

☐ A Compliance with access targets is measured by a telephone audit of free appointments

☐ B An annual survey of patients is part of the payment process, and includes questions on patients' satisfaction with current opening hours

☐ C To qualify for payment, patients must be able to see a GP within 24 hours

☐ D The results of the patient survey must be discussed with a patient group to qualify for the full payment

☐ E Access targets only applies to surgery consultations

135. A 32-year-old man requests an HIV test. He has previously been an intravenous drug abuser and has in the past worked as a rent boy to fund his drug addiction. As part of his pre-test counselling you have a detailed discussion about the disease. Which of the following statements about HIV is NOT true? Select one option only.

☐ A HIV testing may give false positive results in the first 3 months after exposure

☐ B It is estimated that 27% of HIV-positive people in the UK are unaware of their status

☐ C The risk of acquiring HIV through a percutaneous needle-stick injury is 0.3%

☐ D The risk of acquiring HIV through mucocutaneous exposure is 0.1%

☐ E The median time to developing AIDS is at least 10 years

136. A 57-year-old man with myeloma is suffering increasing breakthrough pain on his current medication but is keen to maintain his mobility. You decide to prescribe fentanyl patches. Which of the following statements about fentanyl patches is true? Select one option only.

- [ ] A They are changed every 48 hours
- [ ] B They must not be cut in half
- [ ] C They come in 25 mcg/h, 50 mcg/h and 100 mcg/h strengths
- [ ] D Peak plasma concentrations are reached in 12 hours
- [ ] E They must not be used on the same site as heat pads

137. Which of the following statements about ischaemic heart disease is NOT true? Select one option only.

- [ ] A It is the leading cause of death in industrialised nations
- [ ] B It may be caused by vasculitis
- [ ] C It affects men and women equally
- [ ] D It may present with heart failure
- [ ] E Smoking increases the risk of ischaemic heart disease by two to three times

THEME: SKIN CONDITIONS

Options

A   Atopic dermatitis

B   Erysipelas

C   Erythrasma

D   Hand, foot and mouth disease

E   Impetigo

F   Lichen planus

G   Pityriasis versicolor

H   Pompholyx

I   Psoriasis

J   Urticaria

For each description below, select the most appropriate diagnosis from the list of options. Each option may be used once, more than once or not at all.

☐ **138.** Shiny papules arranged in a lacy pattern on flexor surfaces of the body.

☐ **139.** An itchy erythematous rash in the groin that does not respond to topical antifungals.

☐ **140.** Attacks may be precipitated by salicylates, certain foods and preservatives.

☐ **141.** Isolated lesions may be treated with topical antibiotics.

☐ **142.** A spreading superficial infection caused by *Streptococcus pyogenes*.

THEME: SICK NOTES

Options

A   Med 3

B   Med 4

C   Med 5

D   Med 6

E   Private sick note

F   Self-certification

For each scenario described below, select the most appropriate certificate from the list of options. Each option may be used once, more than once or not at all.

☐ **143.** A 35-year-old man who has just been discharged from hospital after an emergency appendectomy requests a backdated sick note to cover the time from his admission.

☐ **144.** A 13-year-old boy who is prone to school absence and has been told by the school that he must obtain a doctor's note for each absence. He is seen, having missed school the previous day apparently as a result of diarrhoea.

☐ **145.** A 23-year-old man who works in a carpet factory has been off work for 3 days with flu-like symptoms. He is now fit to work but requests a sick note.

☐ **146.** The man in the previous question telephones the surgery to say that his employer is refusing to accept self-certification and insists on a doctor's note.

☐ **147.** A 47-year-old man with long-term depression who is waiting for an incapacity benefit medical has been told that he needs a sick note to cover him until this takes place.

☐ **148.** It does not record any clinical information about the patient.

149. A 46-year-old man complains of a painless swelling on the back of his wrist, present for many months. It is slowly enlarging and he is bothered by its appearance. He has no previous medical history of note. On examination the lump is fluctuant and you note the following appearance.

What is the likely primary diagnosis?

- [ ] A   Acute rheumatoid arthritis
- [ ] B   Baker's cyst
- [ ] C   Ganglion
- [ ] D   Lipoma
- [ ] E   Sebaceous cyst

150. According to NICE guidance, which of the following statements about statins is true? Select one option only.

- [ ] A   In primary prevention trials there were no statistically significant reductions in incidence of stroke
- [ ] B   Statins should be used for all patients with a 10-year cardiac risk > 15%, unless contraindicated
- [ ] C   In primary prevention trials the number needed to treat (NNT) to prevent one myocardial infarction after 5 years of treatment was 37
- [ ] D   The choice of statin used should reflect the patient's cholesterol level
- [ ] E   Statin treatment for secondary prevention should be initiated when the 10-year cardiac risk score is > 10%

151. A 7-year-old girl who was treated in A&E 2 weeks ago for a 'strep throat' is brought in by her mother complaining of aches and pains in her joints, a temperature and general lethargy. On examination she has a sinus tachycardia, a pink rash in the shape of rings on her trunk and a systolic murmur. Which of the following statements about her management is true? Select one option only.

- [ ] A   She has Lyme disease and should have blood taken for serology and start appropriate antibiotics
- [ ] B   She has scarlet fever and should start a prolonged course of phenoxymethylpenicillin
- [ ] C   She has juvenile-onset rheumatoid arthritis and should be referred to a paediatric rheumatologist
- [ ] D   She has rheumatic fever and should be admitted for appropriate treatment
- [ ] E   She has Henoch–Schönlein purpura and can be reassured

THEME: BIAS

Options

A Inclusion bias

B Recording bias

C Observer bias

D Lack of blinding

E Placebo effect

F Publication bias

G None of the above

Published research is often assumed to be of good quality if it has been accepted by a peer-reviewed journal. There are many examples, however, of poor quality research that biases results. This may also apply to everyday situations in clinical practice. For each situation or piece of research below, select the most appropriate description for the form of bias.

152. At your practice's annual QOF visit the assessor points out that according to the Apollo software the most frequently recorded blood pressure (the statistical mode) is 140/90.

153. A meta-analysis of studies of efficacy of ibuprofen against osteoarthritis, which includes randomised controlled trials published in English language journals.

154. A study of 17 patients with chronic functional pain who were given six sessions of acupuncture. At 6-month follow-up 10 of them reported that they were significantly better.

155. A renal physician is studying the effects of a new ACE inhibitor on progression to end-stage renal failure. He recruits patients from his clinic by inviting suitable patients to join the trial.

156. A trial comparing monthly bisphosphonate injections with oral therapy for osteoporosis shows a lower incidence of nausea and headache in the oral group.

157. A drug representative comes to see you after surgery to discuss some new research that he is sure you will find very interesting. His company manufactures a novel anti-Alzheimer's drug given monthly by depot injection. New trial data have just been released from a randomised controlled trial, which he breathlessly presents to you. The data for performance in three areas over the 3-year period are shown below.

Cognitive area assessed	Drug A	Usual care	Difference (95% CI)	p value
	Change from baseline	Change from baseline		
Mini-mental test score	1	−2	3 (−0.04 to 3.04)	0.07
Verbal fluency	0.05	−0.03	0.08 (−0.01 to 0.11)	0.004
Carer-rated quality of life	5.3	−1	6.3 (2.3 to 6.3)	0.002

Which one of the following conclusions may be correctly drawn from these data?

- [ ] A Improvement in quality-of-life scores might be a result of a placebo effect
- [ ] B There is a statistically significant benefit from drug A in mini mental test scores
- [ ] C Verbal fluency improvement is minimal and does not reach statistical significance
- [ ] D There is objective improvement in quality of life
- [ ] E These data support an economic argument for prescribing the drug

THEME: RASHES

Options

A   Erythema ab igne

B   Erythema chronicum migrans

C   Erythema infectiosum

D   Erythema multiforme

E   Erythema neonatorum

F   Erythema nodosum

For each description below, select the most appropriate from the list of options. Each option may be used once, more than once or not at all.

☐ **158.** **A 19-year-old student with tender nodules on her shins.**

☐ **159.** **A 5-day-old baby with red papules on her face arms and legs. She is otherwise well.**

☐ **160.** **A 56-year-old woman with Crohn's disease complains of bruises on her lower legs.**

☐ **161.** **A 32-year-old who has been feeling lethargic and has aches in his joints for several months since a summer camping trip to the New Forest. He has been told by his girlfriend that he has a red line across his shoulders and base of his back.**

☐ **162.** **A 79-year-old man with chronic abdominal pain is noted to have a reticulated erythematous area on his abdomen. He is otherwise well.**

THEME: BREAST LUMPS

Options

A   Breast abscess

B   Breast carcinoma

C   Ductal carcinoma *in situ*

D   Fat necrosis

E   Fibroadenoma

F   Gynaecomastia

G   Mammary duct ectasia

H   Mastitis

I   Referred pain

For each clinical scenario below, select the most appropriate diagnosis from the list of options. Each option may be used once, more than once or not at all.

163. A 33-year-old woman who is 6 weeks post partum presents with gradual onset of pain in the lateral aspect of her left breast. On examination there is a hot tender swelling in this position.

164. A 67-year-old man has found a lump below his right nipple. On examination he has a nodular non-tender lesion beneath the areola.

165. A 27-year-old woman has noticed a painless lump in her breast. On examination there is a small, hard and mobile lump in the breast.

166. A 56-year-old woman has noticed a hard lump in her right breast. She recalls bruising the area a few weeks ago, but has no other history of note. On examination there is a hard lump with puckered skin over it.

167. A 53-year-old perimenopausal woman complains of persistent discharge from the nipple. There is a tender lump adjacent to the nipple.

168. A 61-year-old man with hypertension and diabetes has felt short of breath since suffering an upper respiratory tract infection 1 week ago. On examination he has bilateral basal crepitations and swollen ankles. His ECG is shown below (heart rate 113/minute, QT interval 290 ms).

Heart Rate: 113 bpm
QT Interval: 290 ms

Which one of the following statements about this case is true?

☐ A He should be started on warfarin

☐ B He should be given amiodarone to try to restore sinus rhythm

☐ C He should be referred to an outpatients department for consideration of permanent pacemaker insertion

☐ D He should be given 300 mg aspirin and oxygen, and admitted via blue-light ambulance

☐ E Flecainide can be safely given in this situation

PAPER 5

THEME: ANALGESIA IN PALLIATIVE CARE

169–173.

Options

A   Cyclizine

B   Dexamethasone

C   Diclofenac

D   Dihydrocodeine

E   Hyoscine hydrobromide

F   Midazolam

G   Morphine

H   Paracetamol

I   Pregabalin

For each stage in the analgesic ladder shown opposite, select the most appropriate from the list of options. Each option may be used once, more than once or not at all.

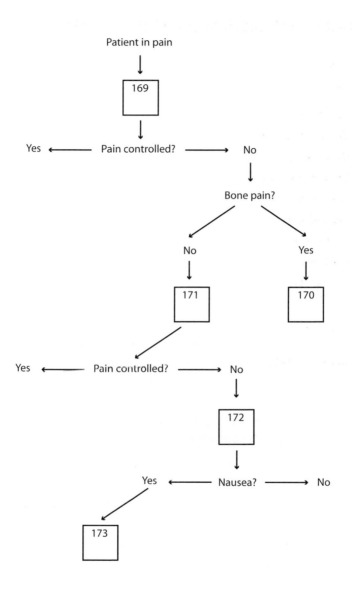

THEME: ECZEMA

Options

A Asteatotic eczema

B Eczema herpeticum

C Guttate psoriasis

D Lichenified eczema

E Nummular eczema

F Paget's disease

G Pompholyx

H Seborrhoeic eczema

I Varicose eczema

For each clinical description below, select the most appropriate diagnosis from the list of options. Each option may be used once, more than once or not at all.

174. Small itchy blisters appearing on the palms of the hands and soles of the feet, which may rupture and become infected.

175. It is seen in patients with long-standing eczema that has been poorly controlled.

176. It is seen on the legs of patients with long-standing venous insufficiency.

177. It is often seen in middle-aged men; coin-shaped lesions are seen usually on the legs.

178. Dry cracked skin on the legs of elderly women, with a crazy paving pattern.

179. A meta-analysis looks at the available data on a new drug for the treatment of pain in osteoarthritis. The data are presented below.

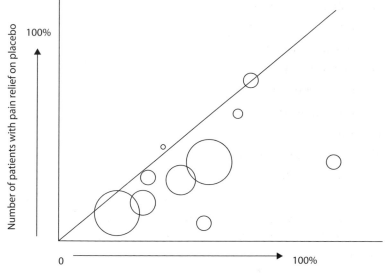

Number of patients with pain relief on drug A

Which of the following statements is true about these data? Select one option only.

☐ A   All of the studies included demonstrate a positive benefit from drug A compared with placebo

☐ B   The studies all have similar outcomes

☐ C   The trials all have similar numbers of patients

☐ D   The data suggest that overall there is a positive benefit for drug A

☐ E   The data suggest that there is no statistically significant difference between drug A and placebo

THEME: MANAGEMENT OF ACUTE ASTHMA IN CHILDREN

180–190.

Options

A   < 33% predicted

B   > 50% predicted

C   < 50% predicted

D   Admit to hospital

E   Cyanosis

F   Epinephrine (adrenaline)

G   Intravenous hydrocortisone

H   Nebulised salbutamol

I   Oral salbutamol

J   Oral steroids

K   Oxygen

L   Respiratory rate normal

M   Salbutamol via spacer

N   Tachypnoea

O   Theophylline

For each stage in the flowchart opposite, select the most appropriate action from the list of options. Each option may be used once, more than once or not at all.

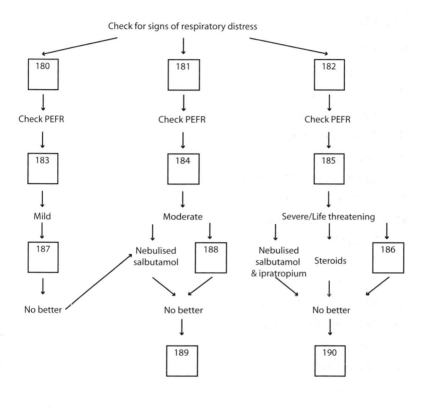

Check for signs of respiratory distress

| 180 | 181 | 182 |

Check PEFR · Check PEFR · Check PEFR

| 183 | 184 | 185 |

Mild · Moderate · Severe/Life threatening

| 187 | Nebulised salbutamol | 188 | Nebulised salbutamol & ipratropium | Steroids | 186 |

No better · No better · No better

| 189 | 190 |

THEME: MANAGEMENT OF NEWLY DIAGNOSED AF

191–197.

Options

A   24-hour ECG

B   β Blocker

C   Digoxin

D   Echocardiogram

E   FBC/U&Es/TFTs

F   Flecainide

G   Reduce alcohol/caffeine

H   Refer for ablation

I   Refer for cardioversion

Select the option from the list that is most appropriate for each stage in the flowchart opposite. Each option may be used once, more than once or not at all.

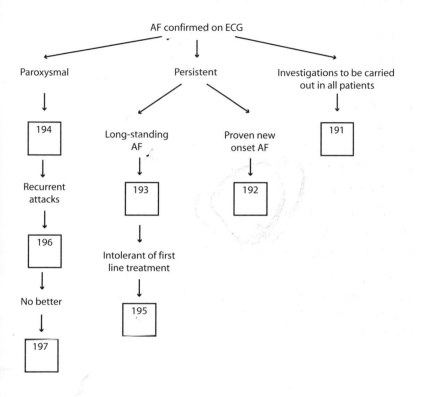

198. A 46-year-old woman complains of difficulty hearing and years of ear pain and dizziness. Her audiogram is shown below.

What is the most likely diagnosis? Select one option only.

☐ A Menière's disease

☐ B Presyacusis

☐ C Glue ear

☐ D Noise-induced hearing loss

☐ E Otosclerosis

199. You attend a meeting sponsored by a drug company at which one of the local consultants presents data from a trial of a new inhaler. Patients in the control group received usual care whereas those taking the new treatment as monotherapy had a weekly visit from a trained asthma nurse who measured their peak flow and assessed them for side effects. The data are shown below.

Which one of the following statements about these findings is true?

- A The intensive follow-up from the asthma nurse may have resulted in greater compliance in the intervention group
- B The data show a statistically significant benefit for the conventional treatment
- C The data show a statistically significant benefit for the new treatment
- D The intervention and control groups are identically matched
- E The data suggest that the drop-out rate as a result of side effects was lower in the new treatment group

200. A 76-year-old man recently started on goserelin (Zoladex) for prostate cancer is seen complaining that the treatment just does not seem to suit him. Which of the following statements about goserelin is true? Select one option only.

- [ ] A   It may cause acute spinal cord compression in patients with prostate cancer
- [ ] B   It may cause gynaecomastia
- [ ] C   It may cause hair loss
- [ ] D   It may cause hypercalcaemia
- [ ] E   All of the above

Paper 5
Answers

1.   D: Ruptured aortic aneurysm

This presentation is typical of a ruptured aneurysm. Neurological symptoms suggest involvement of the spinal arteries. The diagnosis is usually confirmed by the finding of a pulsatile mass in the abdomen.

2.   C: Tinnitus may be a sign of a brain tumour

Tinnitus is the sensation of sound not brought about by simultaneous, externally applied, mechanoacoustic signals. It is very common, with up to a third of the population experiencing it at some time in their lives. Less than 1% seek treatment, however. Unilateral tinnitus may be the only sign of an acoustic neuroma and these patients should he referred. All patients require examination because almost every ear disease may cause tinnitus from ear wax to cholesteatoma. Symptoms usually come and go, being worse particularly at night. Hearing loss is a particularly frequent cause and treatment of this usually helps, as do white noise generators or pillow loud speakers.

3.   D: Flexible sigmoidoscopy in women of average risk picks up only 35% of cancers

Of patients with iron-deficiency anaemia in general practice, 11% were found to have gastrointestinal cancer. The presence of a latent phase with pre-cancerous lesions makes colorectal cancer ideal for screening. Faecal occult blood (FOB) testing is the only screening method proved to cut death rates. The proposed screening programme will start in 2010 and screen the age group 60–69 years. The CONCeRN study (Colorectal Neoplasia Screening with Colonoscopy in Average-Risk Women at Regional Naval Medical Centers) showed low sensitivity for colonoscopy in women of average risk. Rectal bleeding occurs in fewer than 50% of colorectal cancers.

PAPER 5

4.   B: Resistance to metronidazole is common in inner-city areas

Breath-testing, CLO testing and stool antigen tests are sensitive and specific. Eradication therapy involves high-dose amoxicillin, clarithromycin and lansoprazole. Prescriptions for combination helicobacter eradication treatments (eg amoxicillin, clarithromycin and lansoprazole) are charged one prescription charge where prescriptions are chargeable. Serological testing takes 6–12 months to return to normal.

5.   C: The haematoma should be drained promptly and the ear dressed with a pressure bandage

Trauma to the ear resulting in subchondral haematoma requires prompt treatment to prevent avascular necrosis of the ear cartilage. Failure to do so results in the permanent cosmetic appearance of cauliflower ear, which is very difficult to remedy.

6.   E: In the absence of complications patients should be treated with bed rest, fluids and paracetamol

Oral oseltamivir is effective against influenza A and B, as is inhaled zanamivir. Influenza immunisation reduces the number of exacerbations in patients with COPD. Oral amantidine is of no benefit in influenza A.

7.   G: Physical abuse

Bruises are common in mobile toddlers but very rare in babies. Bruises on the face, back and buttock are often a sign of non-accidental injury. The presence of an apparent bruise from birth on the buttocks or base of spine is usually a Mongolian Blue Spot, not uncommon in patients of Asian or Mediterranean descent, and is not associated with trauma.

8.   A: Accidental injury

Bruises on the shins are common in toddlers as they learn to walk.

9. D: Neglect

Neglect may present as failure to thrive, poor hygiene, and emotional and developmental delay.

10. C: Munchausen syndrome by proxy

Munchausen syndrome by proxy is very difficult to diagnose but should be considered in patients with unusual symptoms.

11. G: Physical abuse

A torn frenulum is often a sign of abuse. Premature babies and spending time on an SCBU are associated with abuse.

12. D: Referral for surgical correction

This woman has an entropion and the lashes are irritating the cornea and causing recurrent infections.

13. C: Cystic fibrosis

The combination of failure to thrive and respiratory symptoms should prompt exclusion of cystic fibrosis. Ten per cent of patients with CF have neonatal constipation caused by meconium ileus. α_1-Antitrypsin deficiency presents with COPD later in life. Asthma would normally present with wheeze or recurrent nocturnal cough, with normal growth.

14. A: Biliary atresia

Obstructive jaundice in a newborn child should be considered to be biliary atresia until proven otherwise. Physiological jaundice appears after 2–3 days and begins to disappear from 7 days. Haemolytic jaundice appears within the first 24 hours. Vitamin K deficiency should not occur in a child who has had vitamin K and usually presents with bleeding.

PAPER 5

15.   C: Homeopathy

This study compared 110 double-blind conventional medicine trials with 110 matched homeopathy trials for the same condition. The evidence for a homeopathy benefit was weak but pointed to a placebo effect.

16.   D: Hypnotherapy

The *Drugs and Therapeutics Bulletin* in 2005 recommended, on the basis of trial data, that hypnotherapy was useful for functional gastrointestinal disorders.

17.   H: Osteopathy

For more about osteopathy, see www.osteopathy.org.uk

18.   B: Chiropractic

For a detailed description of chiropractic, see www.chiropractic-uk.co.uk

19.   E: Kinesiology

For more information about kinesiology, see www.kinesiology.co.uk

20.   E: α Blockers are the first-line treatment in this patient group

Surgery should be reserved for patients with bladder outflow obstruction or in those in whom medical therapy fails. Finasteride is effective but takes some weeks to work. Its mode of action is to shrink the prostate. Saw palmetto has been shown to be an effective treatment for prostatism.

21.   E: A palpable uterus requires ultrasonography

NICE guidance suggests that medical treatment should be hormonal, with Mirena for long-term use, and the combined oral contraceptive pill (COCP) or tranexamic acid during bleeding for short-term use. Norethisterone is effective but has to be taken three times daily for 21 days each cycle. Menorrhagia is subjective. A palpable uterus requires ultrasonography to exclude fibroids or tumour. Transcervical hysteroscopic endometrial resection (TCRE) is often effective in those without fibroids.

22.   D: She should be advised that she has a viral infection and to take analgesics and antipyretics, with instructions to return if her symptoms worsen

Acute bronchitis is commonly viral, but in a previously healthy individual with mild symptoms bacterial infections are usually self-limiting. Options include deferred prescriptions with advice sheets or simple reassurance.

23.   B: Children on long-term steroids should be treated with aciclovir at the onset of the rash

Healthy children do not need treatment unless systemically unwell. This is usually a sign of bacterial infection and they should be treated for this, usually with hospital admission. Children and adults who are immunocompromised should be treated at the first signs of disease. Adults should be treated with oral aciclovir within 24 hours of the rash. Pregnant women are only at risk of passing the disease to their children if they are not immune.

24.   D: Diaphragm

The efficiency of a diaphragm is increased by using it together with spermicide.

PAPER 5

25.   A: COCP

The POP is, however, safe.

26.   C: Depo-Provera

This usually settles down in time.

27.   B: Condoms

Condoms have a higher failure rate of 6% in the under-35s because of their intrinsically higher fertility.

28.   G: Mirena intrauterine system

Mirena has been shown to have a lower failure rate than sterilisation, which has a failure rate of about 1:1000.

29.   C: Depo-Provera

Depo-Provera may cause reduction in bone density and is not suitable for long-term use.

30.   F: Implanon

Implanon is a subdermal progesterone-only contraceptive that needs to be removed after 3 years.

31.   E: Turner syndrome

Turner syndrome results from the karyotype 45 XO and is associated with streak ovaries and absence of sexual characteristics. Short stature is common and IQ is often low. Klinefelter syndrome affects boys and has the karyotype 47 XXY.

32.   B: Chronic pain is a common presentation of domestic abuse

Abused women use all aspects of health care more often. High consultation frequency, chronic pain and high number of prescriptions for analgesics are all suggestive of abuse. Women found to be abused in one primary-care survey were almost twice as likely to disclose this on questioning than of their own accord (*British Journal of General Practice* 2007) and two-thirds of patients with a history of domestic abuse have reported relationship difficulties to their GP.

33.   D: Untreated verrucas often resolve spontaneously

For verrucas that warrant treatment, first-line treatment should be over-the-counter salicylic acid, although this turns the affected area white. Glutaraldehyde is effective but may turn skin brown and cause sensitisation. Second-line treatment is cryotherapy, although up to four cycles may be needed. Surgery or bleomycin should be reserved for those lesions that resist cryotherapy.

34.   E: It may be caused by mitochondrial myopathy

Ptosis may be unilateral, bilateral, congenital or acquired. Where the pupil is constricted, the diagnosis is usually Horner syndrome. Ptosis with a dilated pupil suggests oculomotor palsy. Other causes include mitochondrial myopathy, myotonic dystrophy and myasthenia.

35.   H: Red meat consumption

36.   E: Five servings of fruit and vegetables a day

Consumption of three servings a day was associated with an 11% reduction.

PAPER 5

37.   F: Olive oil consumption

The EPIC study also adjusted the traditional Mediterranean diet to make it more acceptable to northern European palates without reducing its effectiveness.

38.   D: Fish consumption

A separate trial found a 31% decrease in stroke incidence in those who eat fish at least four times a week.

39.   H: Red meat consumption

This finding was consistent through all of the populations studied.

40.   D: They are seen only in elderly people

Congenital cataracts may be caused by metabolic defects or congenital infection. Unilateral cataract in early stages may cause refractive errors, resulting in monocular diplopia. Painless loss of vision may be a symptom of cataract and macular degeneration. Posterior capsular opacification may be treated with YAG laser after surgery.

41.   D: Lichen planus

This is the typical appearance of oral lichen planus with the appearance of grains of salt on a background of erythema. There is a small risk of malignant transformation and these patients should be followed up in the maxillofacial surgery department.

42.   D: Bladder tumour

Painless macroscopic haematuria should be considered to be the result of renal tract cancer until proven otherwise. A UTI would be associated with dysuria and leukocytes and nitrites. Beetroot may discolour the urine but would not affect dipstick results. Trauma and colic are associated with pain, although haematuria may be a sign of a coagulopathy.

43.   E: A 17-year-old girl complaining of flashing lights in one eye, nausea and headache

This patient has migraine. Referral criteria under the 2-week rule include new-onset focal neurological signs, symptoms attributable to raised intracranial pressure or new-onset epilepsy, or new symptoms of intellectual impairment.

44.   B: Cholesteatoma

Attic crust, a patch of wax adherent to the drum, may be a sign of underlying cholesteatoma.

45.   C: Chronic suppurative otitis media (CSOM)

CSOM is associated with perforations in the central part of the eardrum and are often referred to as safe perforations. Attic perforations are more often associated with cholesteatoma and require active management.

46.   H: Keratosis obturans

Keratosis obturans, unlike wax, is very painful to remove and needs specialist treatment.

47.   J: Otitis media

Acute suppurative otitis media is caused by streptococci in 30% of cases.

48.   D: Exostoses

Exostoses are often seen in water sports enthusiasts. It seldom causes problems but if the ear is completely occluded surgery can be successful.

49.   D: Corneal abrasion can be confidently diagnosed from history alone

Corneal abrasion causes identical symptoms to a foreign body and this should be excluded by clinical examination. Commotio retinae describes oedema to the retina after trauma; this usually resolves spontaneously but trauma may cause retinal detachment. A suspicious history of penetrating foreign body should always prompt a search for an intraocular foreign body.

50.   B: Travel of more than 3 hours' duration in the 4 weeks before and after surgery should be avoided

NICE guidelines suggest the following: mobility, avoiding dehydration, and mechanical and pharmacological prophylaxis. The COCP should be stopped 4 weeks before elective surgery. Patients with risk factors for DVT should use LMW heparin for 4 weeks after hip surgery.

51. **C: A blood pressure treatment goal of < 125/75 mmHg is indicated for patients with proteinuria**

The result measured by laboratories is an estimated GFR (or eGFR), which assumes standard body surface area and race. Patients who have, for instance, had an amputation could receive erroneous results. An eGFR between 60 and 89 ml/minute correlates with mild renal impairment. Stage 5 chronic kidney disease is defined as an eGFR < 15 ml/minute. A low-protein diet has been shown to reduce the death rate in chronic renal disease. Patients with only one kidney are prone to renal impairment and should all be considered for ACE inhibitors. Patients with moderate to severe chronic renal impairment should follow a diet restricted in potassium.

52. **A: Multiple sclerosis**

Multiple sclerosis is characterised by the presence of multiple focal neurological deficits separated in place and time. They may affect any neurological system. Sarcoidosis does cause isolated cranial nerve lesions but would not normally cause sensory deficits as well. Hydrocephalus causes impaired consciousness.

53. **C: Benzylpenicillin is the first-line drug of choice in community-acquired infections**

Antibiotic therapy should not be delayed. Chloramphenicol should be used in cases of anaphylaxis to penicillin. Cefotaxime may be used for patients who are intolerant of but not allergic to penicillin. Ciprofloxacin, although unlicensed for this, is the prophylaxis of choice for adults, and rifampicin for children.

PAPER 5

54. **B:** **Coughing may last up to 8 weeks**

Treatment with antibiotics will reduce infectivity but not shorten disease. Immunisation provides 95% protection only and relies on a degree of herd immunity. Where treated a macrolide should be used. Infants less than 6 months old and any unwell child should be admitted to hospital. Bronchiectasis and pneumonia are complications.

55. **B:** **Civil Contingencies Act**

PCOs have primary responsibility to plan for disasters but they rely on individual practices to have plans in place for disasters.

56. **D:** **Disability Discrimination Act**

The DDA places a statutory requirement on practices to monitor access for the disabled and consider making reasonable adjustments where necessary.

57. **F:** **Freedom of Information Act**

58. **E:** **Equality Act 2006**

59. **F:** **Freedom of Information Act**

Reasonable charges may be made to cover costs of photocopying but not for the actual request.

60. **A:** **Subconjunctival haemorrhages are never a sign of significant pathology**

Subconjunctival haemorrhages are usually a result of simple local trauma, eg coughing or sneezing, but may be a signs of skull fracture or blood dyscrasias. Episcleritis that does not settle should be referred. Differentiation should be made from scleritis, which is very painful and often affects vision.

61. **A:** **She should have appropriate investigations to rule out an organic cause for her symptoms, eg hypothyroidism**

Diagnosis of depression involves the exclusion of organic disease, lack of obvious environmental factors and persistence. Bipolar disorder comprises alternating hypomania or mania and depression. Grading is objective and uses validated tools such as the Beck depression scores. Prognosis for patients with a single episode is generally good. NICE guidelines recommend antidepressants as first-line treatment. Counselling can be appropriate in some cases but patient choice and availability are important factors in choosing treatment modality.

62. **C:** **They may interfere with sleep**

One of the common side effects of statins is insomnia. Traditionally they have been given in the evening because plasma cholesterol levels are thought to be highest after evening meals. Five per cent of patients report myalgia but myositis or rhabdomyolysis is much rarer. Statins interact with fibrates and macrolides in particular. The *BNF* advises that statins should be stopped if the creatine kinase is five times normal.

63. **F:** **Attempted removal may result in aspiration of foreign bodies**

The peak age for insertion of foreign bodies is 2–3 years. Organic foreign bodies are more irritant and the discharge frequently becomes bloody with time. Unilateral nasal discharge is almost always caused by a foreign body. Removal with a wax hook should not be attempted in general practice because of the risk of pushing the foreign body posteriorly, resulting in aspiration. Always check the other nostril and the ears. These children are often serial offenders.

64. B: Pain localised to one limb

Patients with fibromyalgia have pain in all quadrants of the body, but no objective cause. Diagnostic criteria exist such as the American College of Rheumatology classification, which can be used in doubtful cases.

65. A: Squamous cell carcinoma

This lesion is an SCC. Treatment is by wedge excision.

66. J: Testicular torsion

The testis is usually found to be riding higher than the contralateral side.

67. B: Epididymo-orchitis

Bacterial epididymo-orchitis is more common in elderly men, usually as a result of reflux of infected urine or prostatic fluid. Younger patients are more likely to have chlamydial or gonococcal infections.

68. G: Patent processus vaginalis

PPV is usually seen in infants and should be treated in the same way as an inguinal hernia.

69. F: Lymphoma

Lymphomas comprise 7% of testicular tumours and are usually seen in elderly people. They are usually non-Hodgkin's lymphomas and the prognosis is poor.

70. L: Varicocele

Varicoceles are usually obvious because they have a 'bag of worms' feel to them. They are sometimes found during the course of infertility investigations.

71.   C: Femoral hernia

Although more common in women femoral hernias can be seen in either sex at any age. They are much more likely to strangulate than inguinal hernias.

72.   D: Rational prescribing

Although not one of the seven areas covered explicitly, these might fall under the other headings, eg rational prescribing could be considered under maintaining good medical practice.

73.   A: A third of cases are idiopathic

The most common cause of haematospermia in the under-40s is infection, usually prostatitis or urethritis. Trauma is also a common cause. Coagulopathies may present in this way, as may prostate cancer, although this is a rare presentation.

74.   A: Savings can be spent only on improving patient care

PBC is covered by a direct enhanced service. Administration costs do not come out of savings. Practices that do not participate are not disadvantaged. Commissioning decisions can be made by any member of the primary healthcare team. PCTs will continue to deal with contracting and payments.

75.   D: Splinter haemorrhages

Splinter haemorrhages are a sign of endocarditis. Other signs of suspected lung cancer include weight loss, signs of superior venal caval (SVC) obstruction, lymphadenopthay or chest/shoulder pain.

PAPER 5

76.   B: The drug reduces the risk of foot ulcers

In this meta-analysis the outcome measures are adverse events, so data appearing to the right of the line of no effect (1) suggest an increase in that event with the drug, whereas data on the left (relative risk < 1) suggest that outcome measure is less likely to occur, ie a beneficial effect. The increase in MI could cause an overall increase in death rate, negating the benefits in reduced stroke.

77.   H: Odds ratio

The odds ratio is particularly useful in binary outcomes (i.e. yes or no), eg in case–control studies.

78.   L: Specificity

79.   E: Longitudinal study

A longitudinal study follows subjects over time, continuously monitoring risk factors or outcomes, or both. It is, however, prone to bias.

80.   A: Case–control study

Longitudinal studies have to be extremely large to have sufficient power to study rare diseases. Case–control studies collect cases and identify age- and sex-matched controls.

81.   D: Kaplan–Meier method

Kaplan–Meier method demonstrates results with proportion surviving on the *y* axis and time on the *x* axis.

82.   A: 4S trial

83.   E: GREACE trial

84.   B: AFFIRM trial

85.   F: Heart Protection Study

86.   G: HOPE trial

87.   D: He should be referred for joint replacement

Joint replacement at this age should be considered only if conservative measures fail. He should be treated with weight loss, physiotherapy and simple analgesia initially. Joint injection is effective for acute flare-ups, but repeated injections produce side effects.

88.   D: A Cochrane review has shown no difference in short-and long-term outcomes for spinal manipulation, usual care and 'back school' (physiotherapy-led classes aimed at back problems)

A study of Norwegians presenting with a first episode of backache (*Spine* 2005) found that only 76% had resolved at 12 weeks and 6% were still absent from work at 12 weeks. Poor prognosis was associated with high levels of psychological distress. A paper in the *BMJ* in 2005 described an attempt to provide psychological therapy at presentation but there was no impact on recovery rates or absenteeism. A paper in the *British Journal of General Practice* in 2006 confirmed the importance of positive coping skills. Rigid application of RCGP guidelines with provision of fast-track physiotherapy and triage services did not reduce drug costs, sick notes or referrals. The *BMJ* 2004 randomised controlled trial comparing simple advice and physiotherapy found significant subjective benefits (such as improved mental health) but no benefit in terms of objective measurements of mobility. The study in the *BMJ* in 2003 comparing manual therapy (spinal mobilisation with gentle passive exercise) and physiotherapy with usual GP care found faster recovery and lower costs for manual therapy.

89.   D: Cushing syndrome

This patient has iatrogenic Cushing syndrome caused by excessive steroid use. Addison's disease is caused by adrenal failure whereas Conn syndrome is characterised by electrolyte abnormalities. Cushing syndrome may be seen in people with asthma taking inhaled steroids only.

90.   C: The number of diagnoses in GUM clinics has increased by 300% since 1995

Risky behaviour is multifactorial and relates to alcohol consumption, inability to say 'no', low self-esteem and deprivation, including living in care. Encouraging condom use is helpful but empowering people to take positive steps to improve their health is also important. At-risk people seldom visit their GP. Teenage pregnancy rates are at their lowest level since 1986.

91.   D: Antifungal choice should be guided by microscopy, culture and sensitivity results

Dystrophic nails may result from numerous causes of which fungal infection is only one. Accurate microbiological diagnosis should guide treatment. Topical treatments have a 40% success rate; oral treatment will clear up 85% of cases. Terbinafine, griseofulvin or itraconazole are the systemic antifungals of choice. There is some evidence for the use of tea tree oil.

92.   B: She should use a tar-based shampoo

This patient has scalp psoriasis. Use tar-based shampoo followed, if necessary, by either Betnovate scalp application or salicyclic-containing shampoo to soften the scale.

93.   B: Intra-articular steroid injection

Where De Quervain's tenosynovitis is not responding to rest and splinting an injection in the tendon sheath is appropriate. In refractory cases surgery may be necessary.

94.   E: Oral steroids

This is a typical description of polymyalgia rheumatica.

95.   A: Colchicine

This history is suggestive of gout. Colchicine or non-steroidals are an appropriate first-line treatment. Where intolerant, steroids by mouth or probenecid may be helpful.

96.   F: Physiotherapy

Rest makes backache worse. Maintaining activity, adequate analgesia and physiotherapy are all helpful.

97.   C: Intramuscular steroid injection

Where trigger points are present, local injection of steroid often mixed with local anaesthetic may provide benefit.

98.   C: Telephone follow-up of non-compliant patients by pharmacists reduces costs and mortality

Studies in the *BMJ* showed no benefit from pharmacist intervention and furthermore found that this intervention was not popular with patients. Telephone follow-up has proved effective in a 2-year trial in Hong Kong (*BMJ* 2006) but this might not be generalisable to the UK. Pharmacists have had prescribing rights since 2006. The efficiency of pharmacist medication reviews has been limited by the inability to access medical records, which should change with the advent of electronic patient records. Community pharmacists are paid to carry out medication usage reviews.

PAPER 5

99. E: CPAP is an effective treatment for sleep apnoea

Surgery is an effective treatment for snoring but much less so for moderate-to-severe sleep apnoea. The only effective treatments here are CPAP and sometimes mandibular advancement devices where the mandible is pulled forward. Daytime symptoms are caused by sleep apnoea, rather than simple snoring. Children may get sleep apnoea as a result of lymphoid hyperplasia, with a peak age of 5 years, and this may be cured by adenotonsillectomy.

100. C: Multiple areas of hypertrophic change suggest that vulval intraepithelial neoplasia (VIN) may be the cause

Lichen sclerosis et atrophicus causes atrophic change, whereas VIN causes hypertrophic change. Biopsy is often required to confirm these diagnoses. Patients should be tested for diabetes and consideration should be given to a psychosexual cause. Where no cause is found, hydrocortisone is the first-line treatment. Lichen sclerosis may require short courses of Betnovate.

101. E: Depo-Provera may cause osteoporosis

Osteoporosis may be suggested by plain radiograph, but DEXA (dual energy X-ray absorptiometry) scanning is needed to confirm diagnosis. A T score < -2.5 is diagnostic. HRT may reduce fractures but the NNT is 40 and risks are considered to outweigh benefits when used for this alone. Depo-Provera causes osteoporosis but this is thought to reverse on cessation of treatment.

102. A: Lymphoma

This is a classic description of a lymphoma, which usually feels rubbery hard and is painless.

103. **E:** **Raised serum urea is a useful screening test with high specificity in heart failure**

A study in the *BMJ* (2000) concluded that a combination of clinical assessment, resting ECG and bloods for natriuretic peptide was the best way to detect patients likely to have heart failure.

104. **B:** **He is at risk of stroke**

This patient has polycythaemia rubra vera. First-line treatment is venesection and stopping smoking. Splenomegaly is common. This picture can also be seen in people who have been living at altitude. There is a 20% risk of progressing to myelofibrosis.

105. **H:** **Systemic lupus erythematosus**

SLE may affect virtually any part of the body. Flare-ups may be precipitated by pregnancy or menstruation. A characteristic butterfly rash is diagnostic but seen in only 50% of cases.

106. **G:** **Sjögren syndrome**

Sjögren syndrome (keratoconjunctivitis sicca) is seen in 50% of people with rheumatoid arthritis and is caused by damage to secretory glands all over the body.

107. **E:** **Relapsing polychondritis**

Relapsing polychondritis affects cartilage in the ear, nose, larynx and trachea. It may be associated with arthritis. Treatment is with steroids.

108. **J:** **Wegener's granulomatosis**

Wegener's granulomatosis is a necrotising vasculitis that affects the lungs and may affect the nasal septum. Radiographs show pulmonary infiltrates.

PAPER 5

109.   A: Churg–Strauss syndrome

Churg–Strauss syndrome has an initial asthmatic phase followed by a vasculitic phase, which may be fatal. A post-vasculitic phase follows with allergic symptoms.

110.   D: Polyps may be associated with cystic fibrosis

Nasal polyps are insensitive areas of swelling in the sinus and nasal mucosa, caused by persistent inflammation. They are a sign of underlying inflammation, rather than a disease in themselves, and failure to treat the underlying cause will result in recurrence rates of 50% after nasal polypectomy. They are rare in children, and where seen may be a sign of underlying cystic fibrosis. Bleeding suggests that polyps are neoplastic.

111.   C: One in 20 practices is likely to receive a random anti-fraud QOF visit each year

QOF rewards practices for good clinical and organisational care. The maximum QOF score was 1050 in years 1 and 2 but is now 1000.

112.   C: Drug-induced neuropathy

Phenytoin is a common cause of drug-induced peripheral neuropathy.

113.   D: Guillain–Barré syndrome

Guillain–Barré syndrome usually follows a prodromal illness and causes an ascending peripheral neuropathy. Demyelination may extend to the respiratory and bulbar centres and may also cause Bell's palsy.

114.   G: Painful diabetic neuropathy

Painful diabetic neuropathy is a common complication of diabetes and is seen increasingly with duration of diabetes. There is some evidence that tight diabetic control will reduce the risk of developing this complication (DCCT – Diabetes Control and Complications Trial).

115. F: Motor neurone disease

Motor neurone disease causes a motor neuropathy often initially affecting hands or feet.

116. I: Vitamin B$_{12}$ deficiency

Vitamin B$_{12}$ deficiency is usually seen in developed countries as a consequence of pernicious anaemia but it may also be seen as a consequence of malnutrition.

117. C: It is associated with autoimmune disease

A red eye with pain, photophobia and lacrimation is typical of iritis; examination may reveal a flare in the anterior chamber (like dust in a beam of sunlight) and in recurrent cases a fixed pupil with adhesions. Most cases are idiopathic but may be associated with autoimmune disease, particularly Reiter syndrome. It should be managed by ophthalmology because of the need for definitive diagnosis and long-term complications such as glaucoma, cataract and retinal detachment.

118. A: Records may include abbreviations where these are in common usage

Medical records should be: factual, consistent and accurate; relevant and useful; include medical observations, relevant disclosures and treatment plans. They do not include unnecessary jargon, irrelevant speculation or personal opinions about patients. Paper records should be photocopiable. Medical records are specifically exempt from the Disability Discrimination Act.

119. B: Thromboembolism

This appearance is the result of an embolic event causing an ischaemic ulcer. He has an irregular heartbeat and an echocardiogram showed dilated cardiomyopathy. Other causes include aneurysms and peripheral vascular disease.

120. D: Acromegaly

These are typical features of acromegaly, resulting from high levels of growth hormone occurring after skeletal maturity. Where this occurs before maturity gigantism occurs. Pituitary apoplexy results in hypopituitarism. Hypopituitarism may result in a range of conditions including hypothyroidism, diabetes insipidus, amenorrhoea and failure to lactate, according to the hormones affected.

121. E: Pretibial myxoedema

Pretibial myxoedema is often found in Graves' disease, but is not a feature of thyroid eye disease because it affects the legs. The condition is caused by an autoimmune process and tends to relapse and remit, usually occurring within 12 months of the onset of hyperthyroidism. Treatment usually involves steroids but surgery may be necessary.

122. H: Parvovirus B19

Parvovirus B19 is usually mild in children but can cause arthralgias and arthritis in adults. It may cause fetal hydrops in pregnancy or aplastic crises in patients with chronic haemolytic disease.

123. F: Measles

Koplik's spots on mucous membranes, particularly opposite the second molars, are pathognomonic of measles.

124. D: Epstein–Barr virus

The pharyngitis usually resolves after 5–7 days but contact sports should be avoided for 6–8 weeks because of splenomegaly.

125.   I: Rubella

Congenital rubella is acquired in the first trimester, but has been largely eliminated in the developed world as a result of immunisation.

126.   F: Measles

Measles may cause croup, bronchiolitis and pneumonia.

127.   D: Spinal cord compression or bowel obstruction should be excluded in all patients with constipation in a palliative care setting

Movicol may be used up to eight times a day. Co-danthramer may be irritant in patients with incontinence and colours urine red. Consideration to laxative prescribing should be part of the process of prescribing opioids.

128.   C: Recurrent *Proteus* UTI suggests that renal stones might be present

Larger stones are often immobile and therefore less likely to pass into the ureter. Renal stones can be caused by bilharzia, which is caused by a tropical parasite. Stones that reach the bladder usually continue into the outside world. Most bladder stones form *in situ*. NSAIDs are the first-line management option.

129.   D: Rimonabant

Rimonabant has been shown to be effective in dieting and also complements behaviour modification in smoking cessation. Rimonabant has recently been temporarily withdrawn due to concerns over suicide rates.

130.   C: Orlistat

Orlistat is a lipase inhibitor and prevents absorption of fat.

PAPER 5

131. A: Atkin's diet

Pharmacological therapy is not licensed at BMIs < 30 without co-morbidity.

132. D: Rimonabant

One in 12 patients taking rimonabant reports depression and anxiety. Insomnia and nausea are also common.

133. E: Sibutramine

Up to 10% of patients have a significant increase in blood pressure on sibutramine.

134. B: An annual survey of patients is part of the payment process, and includes questions on patients' satisfaction with current opening hours

Access is a direct enhanced service and is therefore optional. The access targets are to be seen by a healthcare professional within 24 hours and a GP within 48 hours. Access now includes provision for extended hours. A plan for extended hours needs to be agreed with the PCT to provide 30 minutes of pre-bookable appointments per 1000 registered patients, to be provided outside the core hours of 0800–1830. Patient satisfaction survey results need to be considered as part of the planning and PCTs may use questionnaire responses to confirm compliance. Since the revisions of 2006/7 the 'two working days' target refers to 'consult a GP', rather than 'see a GP', and can now include telephone or email consultations.

135. A: HIV testing may give false positive results in the first 3 months after exposure

HIV testing is 99.9% sensitive and specific once the 3-month window has passed. In the first 3 months after infection however ELISA testing may give false negative results and a repeat at 3 months is recommended.

136.   E: They must not be used on the same site as heat pads

Heat pads increase absorption and may cause overdose. The Durogesic D-Trans brand may be cut in half. They are changed every 72 hours and peak concentration is reached after 24 hours, so patients should continue using other analgesia during the changeover. Similarly, side effects may persist for some hours on stopping.

137.   C: It affects men and women equally

Men are affected approximately 50% more frequently by ischaemic heart disease. Other risk factors include smoking, hypertension, hypercholesterolaemia and diabetes. Vasculitis, eg polyarteritis nodosa, may cause ischaemia.

138.   F: Lichen planus

Lichen planus may follow contact sensitivity to chemicals and drugs. White lesions are often seen on the buccal mucosa.

139.   C: Erythrasma

Erythrasma results from corynebacterial infections. It fluoresces with Wood's light and usually responds to 2 weeks of erythromycin.

140.   J: Urticaria

Identification of triggers in urticaria is important in managing symptoms.

141.   E: Impetigo

All children with impetigo should be excluded from school until lesions have crusted over. Widespread lesions may need systemic antibiotics.

PAPER 5

142.   B: Erysipelas

Elderly people and those with diabetes are particularly sensitive to erysipelas, which spreads via the lymphatics.

143.   C: Med 5

A Med 5 allows a doctor to sign a sick note based on information from another doctor.

144.   E: Private sick note

This is a request for a non-DSS sick note and should be treated as a request for a private sick note.

145.   F: Self-certification

Absence up to 7 days should be certified via the self-certification system. Where employers refuse to accept this a private sick note should be issued.

146.   E: Private sick note

147.   B: Med 4

A Med 4 should include details on the disabling effects of the condition, treatment and progress.

148.   D: Med 6

A Med 6 can be used where clinical information may be harmful to the patient, and should prompt the issue of a request for a formal medical report.

149.   C: Ganglion

This is a ganglion, typically seen over the dorsum of the wrist. Treatment may be by aspiration but it frequently recurs. Definitive treatment involves surgery. It may be seen in chronic rheumatoid arthritis or as a new symptom.

150.   A: In primary prevention trials there were no statistically significant reductions in incidence of stroke

Statins should be initiated with a 10-year risk of 20%; 10-year risk scores are valid only for primary prevention. In trials of statins in primary prevention the NNT was 95.   Patients should start on the most cost-effective statin, usually generic simvastatin.

151.   D: She has rheumatic fever and should be admitted for appropriate treatment

The diagnosis of rheumatic fever requires the presence of recent streptococcal infection and the fulfilment of Jones' criteria. These are two major criteria or one major and two minor criteria. Major criteria are carditis, migratory polyarthritis, Sydenham's chorea, erythema marginatum and subcutaneous nodules. Minor criteria are fever, raised ESR or CRP, and ECG changes. Treatment involves penicillin, bed rest, aspirin and steroids for carditis.

152.   B: Recording bias

The most likely explanation is recording bias, where the nurse or doctor subconsciously rounds the blood pressure up or down at the target for the QOF. Another possibility of course is fraud.

PAPER 5

153. A: Inclusion bias

Inclusion bias, in this case only English language, removes published data from the meta-analysis and may be culturally significant.

154. E: Placebo effect

Placebo effect is most likely in this study where there is no control group and no blinding.

155. A: Inclusion bias

This is another example of inclusion bias where the inclusion of patients is not systematic and will not be representative of the patient population, because patients with co-morbidity or other poor prognostic features are often not invited to join the trial.

156. D: Lack of blinding

In a trial comparing two different treatment delivery systems, it is very difficult to conceal allocation and hence lack of blinding is a potent source of bias. This can be got around by giving each group a dummy pill and live injection or vice versa.

157. A: Improvement in quality of life scores might be a result of a placebo effect

The p values for verbal fluency and carer-rated quality of life are < 0.05, suggesting a small but definite statistical effect. Carer-rated quality of life is subjective and based on the opinions of carers who are not blinded and hence may be wishfully thinking; it might be a placebo effect because the control group is receiving usual care whereas the intervention group receives a monthly injection. No analysis is done on costs or admission rates, so it is not possible to make an economic evaluation.

158. F: Erythema nodosum

Erythema nodosum may be caused by mycoplasma infections, strepto-coccal infections and sarcoidosis as well as inflammatory bowel disease.

159. E: Erythema neonatorum

This condition usually presents shortly after birth and naturally resolves in time.

160. F: Erythema nodosum

Erythema nodosum lesions are initially red but over 2–4 weeks take on the appearance of bruises.

161. B: Erythema chronicum migrans

Lyme disease causes a rash that spreads out from the original tick bite to form a circular rash. As it expands it may take on the appearance of a linear rash unless viewed in its entirety.

162. A: Erythema ab igne

Chronic use of hot water bottles or heat pads can cause the development of an erythematous reticular rash on the affected site. It has even been reported in heavy users of laptop computers.

163. A: Breast abscess

Initially the brawny area is hard but later may become fluctuant.

164. B: Breast carcinoma

Around 1% of breast cancers are found in men, more commonly in Klinefelter syndrome. The prognosis is worse in men.

PAPER 5

165.   E: Fibroadenoma

Fibroadenomas are often described as a breast mouse. Prognosis is excellent.

166.   D: Fat necrosis

Fat necrosis arises at the site of a haematoma and clinically resembles carcinoma.

167.   G: Mammary duct ectasia

This condition arises around the time of the menopause. The main differential is breast cancer.

168.   A: He should be started on warfarin

Patients with atrial fibrillation (AF) of more than 48 hours' duration should be anticoagulated for 6 weeks before attempted cardioversion because of the risk of atrial thrombus giving rise to stroke. Flecainide should be used only in a structurally normal heart and where there is no ischaemic heart disease.

169.   H: Paracetamol

Paracetamol is the first choice for mild pain.

170.   C: Diclofenac

Diclofenac should be used for bone pain with consideration of referral for palliative surgery or radiotherapy.

171.   D: Dihydrocodeine

A moderate strength opioid should be added in at stage 2.

172.   G: Morphine

A strong opiate should be added in at stage 3, either orally as MST or oxycodone, transdermally as fentanyl or via syringe driver.

173.   A: Cyclizine

An antiemetic should be added for nausea.

174.   G: Pompholyx

175.   D: Lichenified eczema

Lichenification refers to thickening of the skin to form a leather-like appearance.

176.   I: Varicose eczema

Varicose eczema typically shows brown pigmentation as a result of haemosiderin deposition. It is associated with venous ulceration.

177.   E: Nummular eczema

This tends to be worse in the winter and better in the summer.

178.   A: Asteatotic eczema

This results from dehydration of the epidermis.

179.   D: The data suggest that overall there is a positive benefit for drug A

This is a L'Abbe plot. Each circle plotted represents a separate data-set. Data that cross the line indicate a small effect; data a long way from the line indicate a strong effect.

180. **L:** Respiratory rate normal

181. **N:** Tachypnoea

182. **E:** Cyanosis

183. **B:** > 50% predicted

184. **C:** < 50% predicted

185. **A:** < 33% predicted

186. **K:** Oxygen

187. **M:** Salbutamol via spacer

188. **J:** Oral steroids

189. **D:** Admit to hospital

190. **D:** Admit to hospital

191. **E:** FBC/U&Es/TFTs

192. **I:** Refer for cardioversion

193. **B:** β Blocker

194. **G:** Reduce alcohol/caffeine

195. **C:** Digoxin

196. **B:** β Blocker

197. **I:** Refer for cardioversion

198. **A:** Menière's disease

Menière's disease initially causes no permanent hearing loss but in time a low-frequency sensorineural loss often develops.

199. **A:** The intensive follow-up from the asthma nurse may have resulted in greater compliance in the intervention group

There is no information on sample size, drop-out rates or markers of statistical significance such as p values, so conclusions cannot be drawn on size of effect. The protocol with nurse follow-up opens the door to observer bias and the Hawthorne effect, where a population being intensively observed has better than expected results. The normal treatment group could contain patients on low-dose steroids, high-dose steroids, long-acting β agonists or even oral steroids. Direct comparisons cannot therefore be made without knowing the characteristics of the groups.

200. **E:** All of the above

Initial treatment with goserelin may increase testosterone levels and cause a tumour flare. Cover with an antiandrogen for the first 2 weeks is necessary to prevent cord compression in patients with metastatic disease.

PAPER 5

INDEX

Locators in **bold** refer to the answers sections.